Problem-Based Pain Managemen

D0864325

Problem-Based Pain Management

Eric S. Hsu

Clinical Professor, Department of Anesthesiology, David Geffen School of Medicine at University of California Los Angeles, Santa Monica, CA, USA

Charles Argoff

Professor of Neurology, Albany Medical College, and Director, Comprehensive Pain Center, Albany Medical Center, Albany, NY, USA

Katherine E. Galluzzi

Professor and Chair, Department of Geriatrics, Philadelphia College of Osteopathic Medicine, Philadelphia, PA, USA

Raphael J. Leo

Associate Professor, Department of Psychiatry, State University of New York at Buffalo, School of Medicine and Biomedical Sciences, Erie County Medical Center, Buffalo, NY, USA

Andrew Dubin

Program Director and Associate Professor, Physical Medicine and Rehabilitation, Albany Medical College, Albany, NY, USA

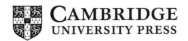

CAMBRIDGE
UNIVERSITY PRESS

CAMBRIDGE
UNIVERSITY PRESS

University Printing House, Cambridge CB2 8BS, United Kingdom

Published in the United States of America by Cambridge University Press, New York

Cambridge University Press is part of the University of Cambridge.

It furthers the University's mission by disseminating knowledge in the pursuit of
education, learning and research at the highest international levels of excellence.

www.cambridge.org
Information on this title: www.cambridge.org/9781107606104

First published 2013

Printed and bound in the United Kingdom by CPI Group Ltd, Croydon CR0 4YY

A catalog record for this publication is available from the British Library

Library of Congress Cataloging in Publication data
Problem-based pain management / Eric S. Hsu ... [et al.].
      p. ;   cm.
Includes bibliographical references and index.
ISBN 978-1-107-60610-4 (Paperback)
I. Hsu, Eric S.
[DNLM: 1. Pain Management.   2. Diagnosis, Differential.   3. Pain–diagnosis. WL 704.6]
RC71.5
616.07′5–dc23   2013014285

ISBN 978-1-107-60610-4 Paperback

Contents

List of contributing authors   *page* ix
Preface   xi

Section 1 Headache

1	Migraine headache	1
2	Cluster headache	8
3	Tension-type headache	13
4	Chronic daily headache	18
5	Post-lumbar-puncture headache	23

Section 2 Head pain

6	Trigeminal neuralgia	27
7	Temporomandibular joint syndrome and orofacial pain	32
8	Occipital neuralgia	37

Section 3 Neck and shoulder

9	Neck strain/sprain	41
10	Cervical radiculopathy	46
11	Cervical facet syndrome	51
12	Cervicobrachial pain syndrome, cervical dystonia, and spasmodic torticollis	55
13	Brachial plexopathy	59
14	Thoracic outlet syndrome	63

15   Shoulder arthritis   67

16   Shoulder bursitis and tendinitis   72

17   Rotator cuff tear   77

Section 4 Upper limb

18   Elbow degenerative joint disease and elbow bursitis   83

19   Tennis and golfer's elbow: lateral and medial epicondylitis   88

20   Nerve entrapments at the elbow   92

21   Hand and wrist arthritis   97

22   Carpal tunnel syndrome   102

Section 5 Thorax

23   Costosternal, costochondral, and costovertebral syndromes   107

24   Intercostal neuralgia   114

25   Post-thoracotomy, post-cardiac surgery, and post-mastectomy
      pain syndromes   120

26   Thoracic spinal pain   125

Section 6 Abdomen and pelvis

27   Acute and chronic pancreatitis   131

28   Functional abdominal pain   137

29   Groin pain, ilioinguinal, iliohypogastric, and genitofemoral
      neuralgia   146

30   Coccydynia   152

31   Interstitial cystitis   156

32   Pelvic pain and endometriosis   161

Section 7 Spine

33   Acute and chronic back pain, back strain and sprain   167

34 Compression fracture 180

35 Lumbosacral radicular pain and lumbar radiculopathy 185
With contributions from Jeffrey Loh

36 Sciatica and piriformis syndrome 192

37 Lumbar spinal stenosis 196

38 Lumbar facet syndrome 200

39 Sacroiliac joint pain 204

40 Lumbar post-laminectomy syndrome 211
With contributions from Christine Lee and Talin Evazyan

Section 8 Hip and lower limb

41 Hip arthritis and bursitis pain 217

42 Meralgia paresthetica 222

43 Knee arthritis and bursitis pain 227

44 Knee sprains and tendinitis 232

45 Degenerative joint disease pain of the ankle, foot, and toe 238

Section 9 Pain syndromes and special topics

46 Myofascial pain syndrome 243

47 Fibromyalgia pain syndrome 249

48 Pain in rheumatism 258

49 Herpes zoster and post-herpetic neuralgia 268

50 Complex regional pain syndrome I (RSD) and II (causalgia) 275

51 Painful polyneuropathy 281

52 Pain in human immunodeficiency virus-related neuropathy 288

53 Central pain and neurologic disorders 297

54 Phantom limb pain 303

55 Burn pain 307

56 Acute postoperative pain management   314

57 Pain during pregnancy, childbirth, and lactation   319

58 Sickle cell disease   325

59 Pain in critical care   331

60 Pediatric pain   337

61 Geriatric pain   347

62 Cancer pain, palliative and end-of-life care   353

63 Opioid tolerance, physical dependence, and addiction   360

Index   368

Contributing authors

Talin Evazyan, MD
Department of Anesthesiology, David Geffen School of Medicine at University of California Los Angeles, Santa Monica, CA, USA

Christine Lee, MD
Department of Anesthesiology, David Geffen School of Medicine at University of California Los Angeles, Santa Monica, CA, USA

Jeffrey Loh, MD
Department of Anesthesiology, David Geffen School of Medicine at University of California Los Angeles, Santa Monica, CA, USA

Preface

Pain management is an essential part of clinical practice for all healthcare providers. However, there is no suitable choice for a quick, concise, and pertinent reference book covering the diagnosis and management of common pain syndromes. There are a few comprehensive and cumbersome books with more detailed information, but these are suitable for use only as academic textbooks or as resources in research. On the other hand, thinner books are usually geared toward review and preparation for the subspecialty board exams in pain medicine, and illustrated atlases on interventional pain procedures serve only as instruction manuals for various options in the diagnosis and treatment of pain.

In preparing this book I am very privileged to have collaborated with four outstanding co-authors in neurology, psychiatry, physical medicine and rehabilitation, and internal medicine/gerontology. This is a new book that consists of problem-based chapters geared toward real-world pain management. All the chapters follow a standard, easy-to-read, and quick-access format covering (1) clinical presentation, (2) signs and symptoms, (3) laboratory tests, (4) imaging studies, (5) differential diagnosis, (6) pharmacotherapy, (7) non-pharmacologic approaches, (8) interventional procedures, (9) follow-up, and (10) prognosis.

This is a pocket-size book and an e-book. Although this first edition is in black and white, illustrations and colorful icons could be used in future editions to catch the eye at a glance and facilitate reading and comprehension. The book is planned to be regularly updated, with a new edition every four or five years.

In addition to this practical reference book on pain management, readers may also find it useful to refer to a number of other books published by Cambridge University Press for further information, including *Stahl's Essential Psychopharmacology*, *Essential Neuropharmacology*, and *Essential Pain Pharmacology*.

We anticipate that the market for this book will be very wide, encompassing primary care, anesthesiology, physical medicine and rehabilitation, neurology, psychiatry, and any specialty with an interest in pain management. This book is intended for medical students, for residents, fellows, and trainees in medicine, for mid-level providers such as nurse practitioners and physician assistants, and it may also prove useful as a quick update for the practicing attending physician and consultant. The book may also have a potential use in the pharmaceutical industry, as an aid to facilitate marketing and promotion.

Our aim is to provide the tools for an education in the proper diagnosis and treatment of a wide range of acute and chronic pain conditions. We hope that our book may also inspire various research and development teams to take an interest in the clinical study of pain. We hope that the book will enhance the understanding of painful conditions, eliminate the barriers to adequate treatment, and improve the quality of life of pain patients and their loved ones.

The team at Cambridge University Press offers tireless effort to guide authors throughout the journey to publication. I would like to thank Deborah Russell, editorial director of medicine; Jane Seakins, assistant editor/publishing assistant; and Hugh Brazier, copy-editor.

The book is dedicated to my wife and children, who have encouraged me throughout, and have provided the motivation to accomplish this project.

Eric S. Hsu

Headache

Migraine headache

Clinical presentation

It is important to recognize just how significant a problem migraine headache is. It has been estimated that migraine affects 11% of the United States population, with an estimated cost of lost work productivity due to migraine of over 10 billion dollars annually. Since migraine is highly prevalent, quite costly to our overall healthcare and general economy, and potentially disabling, it is one of the most important chronic pain problems that practitioners evaluate and treat.

The migraine attack may be divided into four phases; however, it is important to recognize that not all affected individuals will experience each phase, and for some individuals the migraine attack is not uniform. Thus a migraineur may actually experience a spectrum of migraine headaches. With this in mind, the four migraine phases to consider when evaluating a person with suspected migraine are (1) the premonitory phase, (2) the aura phase, (3) the headache phase, and (4) the resolution phase.

During the premonitory phase, migraineurs may note depression, irritability, restlessness, fatigue, and changes in bowel function, appetite, or fluid balance, among other symptoms. The aura phase may precede or occur during the migraine episode. Aura is uncommon, and 70–80% of migraineurs do not experience this; however, keep in mind that many of the patients who experience migraine with aura will also experience episodes of migraine without aura.

The most frequently experienced aura is visual with scintillations and/or fortification spectra. Some patients will experience loss of vision during the aura. Other aural symptoms may include alterations in sensation (numbness or tingling) or motor function (hemiparesis). Because these tend to occur on one side of the body, and because visual abnormalities have multiple causes other than migraine, clinicians must consider other non-migraine-related etiologies of these symptoms such as stroke and epilepsy, especially in a newly diagnosed person, but sometimes even after the diagnosis of migraine has been made.

It is essential to recognize that the headache phase is characterized by a combination of pain and associated non-painful symptoms, and this recognition is in many instances vital to establishing the diagnosis. For example, four characteristic features of this phase are: moderate to severe pain intensity, pain worsened by activity or head movement, throbbing pain, and unilateral pain. However, many patients will experience bilateral pain that is not throbbing, yet experience the other characteristics of the headache phase of migraine. Why is this important to consider? Because recognition of it is vital to making the correct headache diagnosis, which in turn is more likely to lead to effective treatment (compared to making an incorrect diagnosis). Nausea is experienced more commonly than emesis during a migraine. Other symptoms may include osmophobia, photophobia, and phonophobia.

During the resolution phase, some patients may experience a sense of euphoria, but others feel totally "wasted" and "washed-out."

Signs and symptoms

Table 1.1 shows the diagnostic criteria established by the International Headache Society to be used when considering a diagnosis of migraine without aura or migraine with aura.

Laboratory tests and diagnostic investigations

The purpose of diagnostic testing when evaluating a patient with suspected migraine is to rule out other causes, e.g., secondary causes of migraine such as (migrainous) headaches. Even if there are no obvious concerns of such after taking the history, the physical and neurologic examination findings may raise suspicion of a secondary headache.

It should be kept in mind that although most published guidelines do not recommend blood tests and/or neuroimaging for all patients with migraine, published guidelines are most effective when considered in association with one's clinical judgment. Thus, the managing clinician must decide for each individual patient whether or not formal diagnostic testing is appropriate. For example, also take into account if the patient has a change in headache character or severity, increased frequency, a lack of family history, a later age of onset – there are many other clinical situations in which the clinician's judgment may lead to consideration of laboratory testing and neuroimaging.

Imaging studies

With respect to neuroimaging, when ordering this on an elective basis the clinician should be fully aware that an MRI scan of the brain will provide more

Table 1.1 International Headache Society diagnostic criteria for migraine without aura and migraine with aura

---

Migraine without aura
A At least five attacks fulfilling B–D
B Headache attacks lasting 4–72 hours (untreated or unsuccessfully treated)
C Headache has at least two of the following characteristics:
   (1) Unilateral location
   (2) Pulsating quality
   (3) Moderate or severe intensity (inhibits or prohibits activities)
   (4) Aggravation by walking, climbing stairs, or similar routine physical activity
D During headache at least one of the following:
   (1) Nausea and/or vomiting
   (2) Photophobia and phonophobia
E At least one of the following:
   (1) History, physical, and neurologic examination do not suggest secondary headache
   (2) History and/or physical and/or neurologic examinations do suggest
       such a disorder (secondary headache) but it is ruled out by appropriate
       investigations
   (3) Such a disorder is present, but migraine attacks do not occur for the first time in
       close temporal relation to the disorder

Migraine with aura
A At least two attacks fulfilling B
B At least three of the following four characteristics:
   (1) One or more fully reversible aura symptoms indicating focal cerebral cortical and/or
       brainstem dysfunction
   (2) At least one aura symptom develops gradually over more than 4 minutes, or two
       or more symptoms occur in succession
   (3) No aura symptom lasts more than 60 minutes. If more than one aura symptom is
       present, accepted duration is proportionately increased
   (4) Headache follows aura with a headache-free interval of less than 60 minutes
       (it may also begin before or simultaneously with the aura)
C At least one of the following:
   (1) History, physical, and neurologic examination do not suggest secondary
       headache
   (2) History and/or physical and/or neurologic examinations do suggest
       such a disorder (secondary headache) but it is ruled out by appropriate
       investigations
   (3) Such a disorder is present, but migraine attacks do not occur for the first time in
       close temporal relation to the disorder

---

detail than a CT scan of the brain; in practice, many patients who are referred for a headache consultation have had a CT scan completed but not an MRI. This often requires the patient having to undergo two procedures instead of potentially one (MRI).

Differential diagnosis

It is important to differentiate migraine from other primary headaches, e.g., tension type or cluster, since treatment approaches may be different. One should also keep in mind that migraine is a familial disorder, and thus taking a careful family history is an essential part of the evaluation.

Migraine must also be differentiated from "migrainous" headaches, which may be associated with a secondary headache disorder or coexist with such. Each of the following headache characteristics should prompt one to consider a secondary headache disorder, and further investigation:

- The first or worst headache of the patient's life, especially if rapid in onset and severe in intensity
- New-onset headache associated with fever and/or meningeal signs
- A change in frequency, severity, or clinical features of the attack from what the patient usually experiences
- New progressive headache that persists for days
- Precipitation of headache with Valsalva maneuvers (i.e., coughing, sneezing, bearing down)
- The presence of focal neurological signs or symptoms (e.g., diplopia, loss of sensation, weakness, ataxia)
- New onset of headaches after the age of 55 years
- Post-traumatic headache
- Unusual headache character that does not fulfill the criteria for migraine or any other clear headache disorder
- Remember that certain patients with intracranial aneurysms, other cerebrovascular abnormalities including stroke, intracranial hemorrhage, vasculitis/arteritis, venous thrombosis, and arterial dissections, as well as patients with a CNS infection or idiopathic intracranial hypertension, may experience migrainous headaches before or after the event.

Thus, when evaluating a person with suspected migraine, it is important to consider the most common as well as the less common as part of the evaluation.

Pharmacotherapy

It is important for patients to keep a headache diary, not only to document the number of headache days per month but also to annotate the functional impact that the headache may have on that person. Pharmacotherapy is usually divided into acute/abortive/symptomatic therapies and prophylactic/preventive therapies. While almost all patients with migraine will need some form of acute therapy, prophylactic therapies are generally reserved for: (1) those whose headaches impair their ability to function at least 4 days per month, (2) those for whom the use of acute therapies is either contraindicated or not helpful, (3) those whose headaches are generally disabling, and (4) those who are consistently using acute therapies more than twice weekly.

Fortunately, there are many acute therapies currently available. For mild to moderate headaches, the use of aspirin or other non-steroidal anti-inflammatory drugs (NSAIDs), or acetaminophen, may be sufficient and acceptable, especially if they are not used too frequently.

Certain non-prescription analgesics combine caffeine with acetaminophen or aspirin, for example, based upon the potential for caffeine to enhance the benefit of these agents. Prescription agents may combine butalbital with acetaminophen and caffeine. However, although widely prescribed, analgesics are also widely overused by many migraineurs, with resulting daily or near daily use of multiple tablets. This frequently leads to medication-overuse headache, also known as analgesic-rebound headache. In this setting, the patient is likely to believe that only if he/she continues to take the medication will there be relief, when in fact the opposite may be best. Patients with medication-overuse headache need to be counseled to taper the offending medication(s), and when this is successfully completed, many patients are dramatically improved with far fewer headaches overall.

More specifically targeted acute therapies for migraine include the triptans, dihydroergotamine, and ergotamine. These targeted therapies are each believed to bind to serotonin-1 (5-HT$_1$) receptors, presynaptically, in various locations including portions of the trigeminal nerve, certain blood vessels, and the brain. Triptans do this in a more selective fashion than ergotamine and dihydroergotamine.

The currently available triptans include sumatriptan, eletriptan, almotriptan, naratriptan, frovatriptan, zolmitriptan, and rizatriptan. Several of these are available in more than one form, a factor that may be important for individual patients. For example, sumatriptan is available as a tablet, a nasal spray, or a subcutaneous injection as well as in combination with naproxen; rizatriptan is available as a tablet or as a rapidly dissolvable oral tablet; and zolmitriptan is available as a tablet, a rapidly dissolvable oral tablet, or a nasal spray. Naratriptan and frovatriptan each have a longer serum half-life than the other triptans, and this might be considered when choosing a triptan for a person whose headaches last more than one day at a time or for whom the use of another triptan resulted in headache relief but recurrence after several hours.

Choosing the best acute treatment for a patient should be based on the severity of the headache, its functional impact, and its frequency, as well as on consideration of the patient's overall medical condition. The contraindications for the triptans, as for any treatment, must be reviewed and followed. Triptans as well as ergot-type agents are contraindicated in individuals who have a history of ischemic heart disease, myocardial infarction, certain forms of migraine with aura, and other vascular conditions.

Opioids are commonly prescribed for various acute pain conditions; their use in migraine management should be as limited as possible in most settings, because of concerns for analgesic rebound as well as general concerns regarding abuse and misuse of these agents.

Migraineurs should be considered for prophylactic treatment when their headaches occur frequently enough (2–4 times a month) and are disabling enough (lasting several days without normal function per episode); if acute treatments are ineffective or contraindicated; if acute treatment is being utilized/required more than twice weekly on a consistent basis; or when headaches are so frequently debilitating that there is significant life disruption associated with them.

There are many available agents to consider for migraine prevention, including those specifically approved by the US Food and Drug Administration (FDA) for migraine prevention, such as beta-blockers (propranolol and timolol) and certain anticonvulsants (depakote and topiramate), as well as others that may be used in an off-label manner. These would include various antidepressants (especially tricyclics), verapamil, and gabapentin, for example.

It may take a month or more for a patient to achieve a therapeutic response to prophylactic therapy. A 50% reduction in headache frequency and severity is considered a good response to prophylactic therapy. A subtype of migraine, chronic migraine, should be diagnosed when the patient experiences 15 or more headaches a month for at least three consecutive months, each lasting 4 hours or more per day, and at least eight of which are clearly migraine. Recognizing this may be important for treatment, as the FDA recently approved the use of botulinum toxin A (Botox) for the treatment of chronic migraine. This medication is used via provider-administered injections.

Non-pharmacologic approaches

Various herbal remedies have been considered for migraine, including feverfew, butterbur, magnesium, co-enzyme Q10, riboflavin, and others. Acupuncture is sometimes recommended, especially when there has not been an adequate response to medical therapies or if these are poorly tolerated or contraindicated. Regular aerobic exercise has also proved to be of value to many who suffer from migraine. Cognitive behavioral approaches may be helpful as well, especially for pediatric patients.

Interventional procedures

These are not commonly used for most patients with migraine. However, for the small subset of patients who are particularly resistant to other treatments, interventions including various types of nerve blocks, radiofrequency lesioning, and occipital nerve stimulation have been offered. None of these has been studied to the extent that many of the other migraine therapies have.

Follow-up

Regular follow-up is advised to monitor the patient's response to treatment and to make appropriate changes in therapy.

Prognosis

For many people, although not all, migraines eventually go into remission and sometimes disappear completely, particularly as they get older. Estrogen decline after menopause may be responsible for remission in some women.

REFERENCES AND FURTHER READING

Bigal ME, Lipton RB. Overuse of acute migraine medications and migraine chronification. *Curr Pain Headache Rep* 2009; **13**: 301–7.

Buse DC, Rupnow MF, Lipton RB. Assessing and managing all aspects of migraine: migraine attacks, migraine-related functional impairment, common comorbidities, and quality of life. *Mayo Clin Proc* 2009; **84**: 422–35.

Holland S, Silberstein SD, Freitag F, *et al.* Evidence-based guideline update: NSAIDs and other complementary treatments for episodic migraine prevention in adults: report of the Quality Standards Subcommittee of the American Academy of Neurology and the American Headache Society. *Neurology* 2012; **78**: 1346–53.

International Headache Society (IHS). *The International Classification of Headache Disorders*, 2nd edn, 1st revision. Oxford: IHS, 2005. ihs-classification.org/_downloads/mixed/ICHD-IIR1final.pdf (accessed May 17, 2013).

Manack A, Turkel C, Silberstein S. The evolution of chronic migraine: classification and nomenclature. *Headache* 2009; **49**: 1206–13.

Silberstein SD, Holland S, Freitag F, *et al.* Evidence-based guideline update: pharmacologic treatment for episodic migraine prevention in adults: Report of the Quality Standards Subcommittee of the American Academy of Neurology and the American Headache Society. *Neurology* 2012; **78**: 1337–45.

2

Cluster headache

Clinical presentation

Cluster headache is a primary, not secondary, headache disorder considered to be a form of neurovascular headache. The headache attacks are characterized as unilateral, severe, lasting a few minutes to several hours.

The two main types of cluster headache are episodic cluster headache, in which the affected individual has experienced at least two headache periods (see below for signs and symptoms) lasting 1 week to 1 year with a headache-free interval of at least 1 month, and chronic cluster headache, in which the headache attacks occur for more than 1 year and either the headache-free interval is less than 1 month or there is no period of remission.

Although the mechanism of cluster headache is not completely understood, proposed mechanisms include serotonergic, hemodynamic, autonomic, circadian rhythm, histaminergic, mast cell, and trigeminal. Positron emission tomography (PET) scan studies have demonstrated abnormal activation of the hypothalamus during cluster headaches, and some have hypothesized that hypothalamic dysfunction may explain why the headaches often come in clusters.

Cluster headache prevalence in males is estimated to be 0.4–1%. Age of onset is mid-adult, with men affected at a younger age (30) than women. This is one of the few primary headache disorders that is more common in males than females.

Signs and symptoms

Attacks are associated with severe, horrible, unilateral boring and lancinating head pain. The patient may feel as if the eye is being moved or pushed. The pain is felt within the first divisions of the trigeminal nerve as well as along the carotid artery and neck. Attacks are often nocturnal and may recur from once every other day up to eight times daily.

Autonomic features, including ptosis, miosis, conjunctival injection, eyelid swelling, sweating over the forehead and face, lacrimation, and rhinorrhea, all on the side of the pain, are often present. Patients often describe feeling agitated during an attack.

A typical cluster period occurs 1–2 times each year and lasts as long as several months at a time. Between 10% and 15% of sufferers report side-change in different episodes. Rarely, patients with typical cluster headache describe experiencing an aura such as that described in migraine before an attack.

The majority of patients with cluster headache describe periodicity: cluster attacks recurring at approximately the same time each day throughout the cluster cycle. It is estimated that 75% of attacks occur between 9:00 p.m. and 10:00 a.m., and approximately 50% of patients experience nocturnal attacks that disrupt their sleep, usually within 2 hours after falling asleep.

The physical examination during an attack may demonstrate ipsilateral lacrimation and conjunctival injection or ptosis. A mild Horner's syndrome, bradycardia, facial and/or scalp tenderness, carotid tenderness, and facial pallor may also be present ipsilateral to the pain. During an attack, the patient may appear in severe distress, screaming in pain and pressing on the painful area in an attempt to get relief.

Table 2.1 shows the International Headache Society diagnostic criteria for cluster headache.

Laboratory tests and diagnostic investigations

The diagnosis of cluster headache is generally based on the integration of information gained from performing a detailed history and physical. Key findings include the typical attack description and the periodic nature of the attacks.

Imaging studies

Clinicians may consider ordering an imaging study (preferably an MRI of the brain) to exclude other etiologies in certain patients.

Differential diagnosis

The differential diagnosis includes acute herpes zoster or post-herpetic neuralgia, carotid artery dissection, trigeminal neuralgia, pain due to a subarachnoid hemorrhage, temporal (giant cell) arteritis, cluster-like headache associated with a brain tumor, and sinusitis.

Table 2.1 International Headache Society diagnostic criteria for cluster headache

A At least five attacks fulfilling B–D
B Severe or very unilateral orbital, supraorbital, and/or temporal pain lasting 15–180 minutes if untreated [note 1]
C Headache is accompanied by at least one of the following signs, which have to be present on the pain side:
(1) ipsilateral conjunctival injection and/or lacrimation
(2) ipsilateral nasal congestion and/or rhinorrhea
(3) ipsilateral eyelid edema
(4) ipsilateral forehead and facial sweating
(5) ipsilateral miosis and/or ptosis
(6) a sense of restlessness or agitation
D Attacks have a frequency from one every other day to 8 per day [note 2]
E Not attributed to another disorder [note 3]

Notes:
(1) During part (but less than half) of the time-course of cluster headache, attacks may be less severe and/or of shorter or longer duration.
(2) During part (but less than half) of the time-course of cluster headache, attacks may be less frequent.
(3) History and physical and neurologic examinations do not suggest any of the disorders listed in groups 5–12 (head and/or neck trauma; cranial or cervical vascular disorder; nonvascular intracranial disorder; a substance or its withdrawal; infection; disorder of homoeostasis; disorder of cranium, neck, eyes, ears, nose, sinuses, teeth, mouth or other facial or cranial structures; psychiatric disorder), or history and/or physical and/or neurologic examinations do suggest such disorder, but it is ruled out by appropriate investigations, or such disorder is present, but attacks do not occur for the first time in close temporal relation to the disorder.

Pharmacotherapy

The goal of pharmacotherapy is to prevent the attack or adequately control its symptoms if it is already under way.

The acute, rapid, and severe acuity of a typical cluster attack limits the benefits of symptomatic treatment. Thus, almost all patients with cluster headache should be treated with preventive treatment.

Consider the use of prednisone to help a patient achieve remission. Prednisone should be used at a dose of 60–80 mg daily for 1 week and then tapered by 10 mg per day. Verapamil is a generally well-tolerated calcium channel blocker that can be an effective prophylactic agent for cluster headache. Doses as high as 480 mg per day may be required to maximize benefit. The clinician should keep in mind that verapamil may take several weeks to be effective and the dose may need to be increased gradually, so abortive therapy with prednisone is often required concurrent with the institution of a prophylactic agent such as verapamil. Consider lithium carbonate or valproic acid if verapamil is not effective enough. Other calcium channel blockers that might be considered include nimodipine and diltiazem.

Patients should be treated with preventive medication for a somewhat longer period than their typical cluster headache cycles. If the typical cluster lasts 1 month, maintain the patient for at least 6 weeks before considering a taper of the prophylactic regimen. Tapering may not be appropriate for patients with the chronic form of cluster headache.

Acute treatments for cluster headache attacks include sumatriptan. Subcutaneous sumatriptan 6 mg may quickly abort an attack within 5–10 minutes in many patients; however, this drug should not be given more than twice daily, leaving patients with more than two attacks in a day in need of another treatment.

Non-steroidal anti-inflammatory drugs (NSAIDs) including ibuprofen, naproxen, ketoprofen, and ketorolac may be used in a non-specific manner. Ketorolac if effective may be especially useful, since it is currently available in parenteral, intranasal, and oral preparations, giving the patient a great deal of flexibility. However, keep in mind that this can only be used safely on a limited basis, because of concerns for gastrointestinal and renal side effects.

Dihydroergotamine (DHE) administered intramuscularly or subcutaneously is also effective. Ergot suppositories at bedtime may be considered for individuals whose attacks are often nocturnal. Contraindications of ergots include peripheral and/or cardiovascular disease, and the prescriber should be aware of these. Patients who are not responsive to medical or non-pharmacologic therapy may benefit from being hospitalized and treated with parenteral DHE and metoclopramide every 8 hours, sometimes for several days to break the cycle. See *Interventional procedures*, below, for other considerations for medically refractory patients.

Non-pharmacologic approaches

Oxygen is often an effective acute treatment for cluster headache. Oxygen can be delivered via face mask or nasal cannula for 10–15 minutes. This can be done in an urgent care setting, or under certain circumstances it may be appropriate for home use.

Interventional procedures

Ipsilateral occipital nerve blocks may help certain patients. Percutaneous glycerol injections into the trigeminal cistern, percutaneous radiofrequency trigeminal rhizotomy, and decompression of the nervus intermedius have been reported but are not uniformly effective.

Deep brain stimulation of the hypothalamus has been recently reported to be of some benefit in a series of cluster headache patients. Limited success has been reported with the use of botulinum toxin for the prevention of cluster headache.

Follow-up

Patients will need to be followed at regular intervals to ensure adequate treatment response, as well as to monitor for adverse effects of treatment.

Prognosis

In fewer than 15% of patients with episodic cluster headache, spontaneous remission may occur. Thus, for most patients, after the onset, cluster headache remains a problem for the entire life.

Episodic cluster headache may transform into chronic cluster headache in 4–13% of patients. It is uncommon for chronic cluster to transform into episodic cluster headache. Male patients who develop cluster headache later in life tend to have a more difficult course.

REFERENCES AND FURTHER READING

Bahra A, May A, Goadsby PJ. Cluster headache: a prospective clinical study with diagnostic implications. *Neurology* 2002; **58**: 354–61.

International Headache Society (IHS). *The International Classification of Headache Disorders*, 2nd edn, 1st revision. Oxford: IHS, 2005. ihs-classification.org/_downloads/mixed/ICHD-IIR1final.pdf (accessed May 17, 2013).

Leone M, Franzini A, Broggi G, Bussone G. Hypothalamic deep brain stimulation for intractable cluster headache: a 3 year follow-up. *Neurol Sci* 2003; **24** (Suppl 2): S143–5.

Nesbitt AD, Goadsby PJ. Cluster headache. *BMJ* 2012; **344**: e2407. doi: 10.1136/bmj.e2407.

Newman LC, Goadsby P, Lipton RB. Cluster and related headaches. *Med Clin North Am* 2001; **85**: 997–1016.

3

Tension-type headache

Clinical presentation

Tension-type headache (TTH) is the most common form of primary headache. Approximately 40% of people experience a headache at least once annually. The mechanism of TTH is not known.

As its name suggests, the etiology of the pain associated with tension-type headache for many years was thought to result from the muscular contraction of pain-sensitive structures of the cranium. However, more recently the International Headache Society (IHS) has concluded, based on currently available research findings, that it is not appropriate to use the terms *muscular contraction headache* or *tension headache*, because no research supports muscular contraction or muscle tension as the sole pain etiology.

The term *tension headache* was also used by some to imply that "stress" and "psychological" factors were the essential causes of the disorder. We now know that more muscle contraction occurs during a migraine headache than in TTH and that many individuals experience TTH in the absence of any clear or obvious stress.

Of interest is that certain patients may experience both TTH and migraine headache – and, as will be summarized below, this is important when considering treatment options. TTH has a lifetime prevalence of 88% in females and 69% in males and is more commonly experienced in middle life compared with other ages.

The two main groups of TTH are episodic and chronic TTH. Episodic TTH occurs on less than 15 days per month and chronic TTH, affecting approximately 3% of the population, occurs 15 days per month for at least 6 months.

The best available evidence suggests that episodic TTH is not a familial disorder, but there is some evidence that chronic TTH may be associated with familial aggregation.

Signs and symptoms

To diagnose TTH, the following signs and symptoms should be present.

First, according to IHS criteria, 10 episodes of a headache that fit the criteria for TTH must be experienced by a person before TTH can be diagnosed.

Symptoms include bilateral pain, pain quality that is a steady ache or perceived as steady tightening pressure, pain that is mild or moderate in its intensity, and pain that is not made worse by physical activity. The location of the pain is characteristically frontal-occipital and the pain is typically *not* throbbing. The pain is more constant in quality, and less severe, than that experienced during a migraine headache. It is often described as a band-like or vise-like sensation around the head.

Nausea and vomiting do not typically occur, but either photophobia or phonophobia can occur. The headache most commonly lasts several hours, but shorter and longer durations do occur. It does not suddenly awaken a person from sleep.

The physical examination needs to be completed to help exclude other causes of headache, and the neurological examination should be normal in a person with TTH.

Laboratory tests and diagnostic investigations

Specific laboratory tests should be ordered only if, during the evaluation of a patient with suspected TTH, another diagnostic possibility other than TTH is suspected. The laboratory findings should be unremarkable in patients with TTH.

Imaging studies

A neuroimaging study, preferably an MRI of the brain, should be strongly considered, and completed when a patient's headache pattern has changed suddenly, affecting the patient adversely. If the relevant neurological examination is abnormal, and/or if the headache presentation, including age of onset, is not consistent with one of the common primary headache disorders, one should suspect a secondary headache disorder

Differential diagnosis

Many medical conditions are associated with headache, and the quality of such a headache may be somewhat reminiscent of TTH. A non-exhaustive list of such conditions includes depression, glaucoma, brain abscess, sinusitis, temporal arteritis, temporomandibular joint syndrome, stroke, various infections, and subdural hematoma.

While headaches associated with intracranial mass lesions may initially be difficult to clearly distinguish from TTH, these tend to progress in severity and frequency and may become associated with focal or other formal neurological findings and complaints – findings not seen with TTH.

It is important to distinguish between migraine headache and TTH, although some patients may experience both headache types:

- Migraine pain is typically unilateral; TTH pain is bilateral.
- Migraine pain is often throbbing; the pain of TTH is more of a steady ache or a pressure/squeezing sensation.
- Migraine pain is moderate to severe in intensity; TTH pain is mild to moderate in intensity.
- Migraine headache is worsened by physical activity; TTH is not affected by physical activity.

If the location of the headache is primarily frontal, TTH and sinus headache may be confused. In contrast to TTH, "true" sinus headaches are characterized by fever, purulent nasal discharge, and sinus tenderness.

Pharmacotherapy

Choice of treatment certainly depends upon the clinical situation and goal of therapy. Episodic TTH may require only acute, symptomatic therapy, whereas chronic TTH may be best managed with a prophylactic approach as well as the use of acute symptomatic therapies.

TTH is often treated symptomatically with over-the-counter (OTC) medications including aspirin, ibuprofen, naproxen sodium, ketoprofen, and acetaminophen. Patients often choose an OTC combination product containing one or more OTC analgesics with, for example, caffeine (e.g., Excedrin).

Prescription-strength non-steroidal anti-inflammatory drugs (NSAIDs) have been used when OTC agents fail to help the patient. An older combination preparation containing acetaminophen and isometheptene, among other ingredients, may be helpful. Widely prescribed and possibly effective in the short term are the butalbital/caffeine/acetaminophen or aspirin-containing combination products (e.g., Fioricet/Fiorinal/Esgic). These are also available combined with codeine.

There is a significant risk of overuse of these agents, and quite insidiously a patient may wind up using these daily to treat a headache which by that time may have transformed from TTH to rebound headache. The prescriber must absolutely be aware of and monitor for the overuse of these agents to avoid rebound headache, as rebound headache is *not* TTH and the result will be a headache syndrome that is much more difficult to treat. This can occur with the use of intranasal opioids (e.g., butorphanol) as well.

Patients should restrict their use of such symptomatic medications to no more than 3 days weekly, and preferably no more than 2 days weekly, to try to minimize this occurrence. This may pose a challenge to the primary care and other providers, since it appears that these agents are commonly prescribed by emergency room providers. Nearly any medication can be overused – *any*! Therefore match the use of acute versus prophylactic treatment of TTH to the individual patient. For chronic TTH, for example, the sheer number of headaches experienced each month essentially precludes the regular use of symptomatic treatment, to prevent and avoid rebound headache.

Another important point when using these agents is that the provider must be as clear as possible with the patient about the presence of acetaminophen and/or an NSAID in the medication, and about the need to avoid inadvertently using too much acetaminophen or a dangerously high NSAID total dose daily, since so many OTC and prescription analgesics contain these agents.

Prophylactic medications are not commonly used in TTH but may be appropriate for certain patients depending upon the headache frequency and severity. Specifically, consider this approach when the patient is experiencing significant headache-related functional impairment 3 or more days monthly.

As is the case with migraine headache, since overuse of symptomatic treatments can lead to adverse consequences, including rebound headache, the frequency of TTH experienced by a patient may dictate prophylactic therapies for each individual.

Antidepressant medications are the most commonly used prophylactic agents for TTH. Tricyclic antidepressants including nortriptyline, amitriptyline, doxepin, and others can be effective for patients with TTH. Low starting doses – e.g., 10 mg at bedtime – may need to be titrated to effect. Anticholinergic and other side effects need to be monitored for and addressed if present. The selective serotonin reuptake inhibitors (SSRIs) such as fluoxetine may play a role as well, although they have not been evaluated in large studies.

Other prophylactic medications that have been used to treat TTH include various calcium channel blockers, divalproex sodium, and occasional daily use of a long-acting NSAID. Evidence suggests that beta-blockers are not particularly effective prophylactic agents for TTH.

Of interest is that triptan medications do not appear to be helpful from a symptomatic/abortive point of view for patients who experience TTH only. However, patients who experience both TTH and migraine headache appear to respond to triptan therapy for what would appear to be a TTH.

Non-pharmacologic approaches

As would be the case for any pain syndrome, non-pharmacologic treatments are used either alone or in combination with pharmacotherapy. Non-pharmacologic treatments may be considered for all patients with TTH but should be especially considered for those patients with TTH with significant headache-related disability, coexisting mood or anxiety disorders, difficulty managing stress or other documented non-medical triggers, and medication overuse.

It should also be kept in mind that certain patients prefer non-pharmacologic therapies. Relaxation, biofeedback, and cognitive behavioral therapy are considered first-line preventive options. Acupuncture may be helpful for some. Butterbur extract and vitamin B_2 have shown efficacy in more than one randomized trial and are thus potentially useful interventions. Patient education regarding TTH may be generally helpful for patients.

Interventional procedures

There is no robust consistent evidence to support the use of specific interventional procedures for the management of TTH.

Follow-up

Patients require regular follow-up to assist in the safe and appropriate use of their OTC and prescribed treatments, as well as to monitor for the development of new complaints or findings.

Prognosis

Most patients with episodic TTH will not develop chronic TTH, and with available therapies, used properly, they can continue to live productive lives.

REFERENCES AND FURTHER READING

Bendtsen L, Evers S, Linde M, *et al.* EFNS guideline on the treatment of tension-type headache: report of an EFNS task force. *Eur J Neurol* 2010; **17**: 1318–25.

Crystal SC, Robbins MS. Tension-type headache mimics. *Curr Pain Headache Rep* 2011; **15**: 459–66.

Sacco S, Ricci S, Carole A. Tension-type headaches and systemic medical disorders. *Curr Pain Headache Rep* 2011; **15**: 438–43.

4

Chronic daily headache

Clinical presentation

Chronic daily headache (CDH) may result in significant pain and suffering, loss of productivity, reductions in quality of life, and enormous overall economic costs to society. CDH should be viewed as a term that does not describe one distinct entity but in fact applies to several specific headache types associated with frequent headaches.

The prevalence of CDH in adults is approximately 4%, with the majority of patients experiencing chronic tension-type headache, chronic migraine, or medication-overuse headache. Women are affected 2–3 times more often than men.

The next section will review these headache types based upon the typical duration of headache, first those whose duration is typically more than 4 hours (chronic migraine, chronic tension-type headache, medication-overuse headache, new daily persistent headache, and hemicrania continua) and then those whose duration is typically less than 4 hours (chronic paroxysmal hemicrania, primary stabbing headache, hypnic headache, chronic cluster headache, and short-lasting unilateral neuralgiform headache attacks with conjunctival injection and tearing [SUNCT]).

Signs and symptoms

Chronic migraine most often develops in a person who has a history of episodic migraine headache. Certain patients with episodic migraine pattern may experience a transformation to a chronic migraine pattern ($\geq$ 15 headache days a month, each headache lasting more than 4 hours per day). Chronic migraine sufferers commonly experience near-daily or daily headaches of low to moderate severity with intermittent severe exacerbations as well.

Chronic tension-type headache. Tension-type headache is a bilateral, non-throbbing headache with gradual onset, with or without pericranial muscle tenderness, that is mild to moderate in intensity. Individuals experiencing more than 15 days of tension-type headaches each month are diagnosed with chronic tension-type headache.

Medication-overuse headache (MOH). Other terms used to describe this CDH type include analgesic-rebound headache and drug-induced headache. MOH is diagnosed when a primary headache, e.g., migraine, markedly worsens (more common) or develops for the first time during medication overuse.

New daily persistent headache. This daily headache type begins suddenly in a person without a prior history of headache and is unrelenting often from onset or within several days of onset. The symptoms tend to be quite variable pain: mild to moderate in intensity, sometimes bilateral with pressing pain features, and at other times unilateral with migrainous symptoms.

Hemicrania continua. This is often described as indomethacin-responsive headache, because of its unique response to this medication. It is a continuous and always unilateral headache combined with superimposed paroxysms of moderate to severe intensity and accompanied by autonomic features and/or migrainous symptoms.

Chronic paroxysmal hemicrania. People who experience paroxysmal hemicrania have unilateral, brief, severe attacks several times daily of cranial pain associated with autonomic features. Attacks may occur between 10 and 14 times daily and last usually between 2 and 30 minutes. Approximately 80% of the people experiencing paroxysmal hemicrania experience the chronic form, i.e., no remission occurs.

Primary stabbing headache is characterized by intermittent, sharp, jabbing pains lasting 1–10 seconds occurring over a localized scalp area predominantly over the territory of the first division of the trigeminal nerve. This occurs with variable frequency throughout the day.

Hypnic headache. Sometimes referred to as alarm-clock headache, hypnic headache is associated with frequently bilateral episodes of dull head pain that awaken the patient from sleep. It most commonly occurs in those over 50 years old.

Chronic cluster headache. Cluster headache is associated with attacks of severe unilateral orbital, supraorbital, or temporal pain. Unilateral autonomic symptoms are ipsilateral to the pain and may include ptosis, mitosis, lacrimation, conjunctival injection, rhinorrhea, and nasal congestion. Attacks are of short duration, lasting from 15 minutes to no more than 3 hours. For those experiencing **episodic cluster headache**, attacks occur daily, but in clusters of time allowing for long periods of remission. In the chronic form, there is no period of meaningful remission.

Short-lasting unilateral neuralgiform headache attacks with conjunctival injection and tearing (SUNCT) is characterized by up to 200 attacks per day of brief (5–120 seconds), severe, unilateral pain around and behind the eye accompanied by ipsilateral conjunctival injection and lacrimation.

Laboratory tests and diagnostic investigations

The diagnosis of primary CDH is made after reviewing the headache history. A diagnosis of CDH is made when there is a pattern of frequent headaches that fulfill diagnostic criteria for one of the forms of CDH characterized by prolonged headaches, as described above. A diagnosis of CDH may also be made when there is persistence of daily or near-daily headache associated with shorter durations such as chronic cluster headache, chronic paroxysmal hemicrania, hypnic headache, or primary stabbing headache, for at least 1 year without remission.

Secondary headaches, e.g., those caused by a specific medical condition and/or structural lesion, must be considered and must be excluded. This is based upon a careful medical and headache history, a comprehensive physical and neurologic examination, and assessing the need as described previously for laboratory tests, neuroimaging (brain, cervical spine, intracranial arteries, venous sinuses, cervical spine imaging), lumbar puncture, and other tests as deemed appropriate.

Consistent with many of the primary headache disorders, patients with CDH are likely to demonstrate normal physical and neurologic examinations. One must keep in mind, however, that certain headache types associated with CDH may have specific examination findings to look for and recognize.

For those with chronic migraine, the skin overlying the affected area during a headache may demonstrate allodynia (pain from a normally non-painful stimulus) and hyperalgesia (more pain than would be normally expected from a noxious stimulus).

Patients with chronic cluster headache, chronic paroxysmal hemicrania, or SUNCT may demonstrate autonomic symptoms such as conjunctival injection and lacrimation.

For those with chronic tension-type headache, pericranial muscle tenderness may be noted on examination. New focal neurological findings and many other new abnormalities on examination should prompt one to consider the possibility of a secondary headache diagnosis. Further investigations should be considered on an individualized basis.

Troublesome signs and symptoms that should prompt further evaluation include (but should not be considered limited to) the new onset of headache, the acute onset of a "thunderclap" headache type, a significant change in the reported headache characteristics compared to prior report, new focal neurological findings (especially if not typically associated with the headache type experienced), onset of headache after 50 years of age, signs or symptoms of a systemic illness such as cancer, known infection (HIV), new fever or weight loss, headaches that only occur with increased or decreased intracranial pressure (e.g., occurring with Valsalva maneuver or only with orthostatic changes).

Differential diagnosis

The differential diagnosis is quite extensive and includes infections, structural lesions, changes in intracranial pressure, post-traumatic headache, cerebral venous sinus thrombosis, vasculitis, and cervicogenic headache, as well as numerous other medical conditions.

Pharmacotherapy, non-pharmacologic approaches, and interventional procedures

The management of each of the headache types leading to CDH may be different. This treatment section is therefore organized by type of headache, not treatment type. In particular, the effective treatment of CDH depends not only on the specific headache type but also on recognizing the presence or absence of medication overuse and assertively addressing this.

The treatment of chronic migraine should include appropriate prophylactic therapy and advising the patient to avoiding migraine triggers. Effective prophylactic interventions may include pharmacotherapy, behavioral therapy, physical therapy, botulinum toxin A (Botox) injections, and other interventions. It is vital to successful treatment that the use of acute/symptomatic headache medications be limited to prevent the development of MOH. Multimodal therapy is often needed to optimize outcomes.

The treatment of chronic tension-type headache may include the use of daily prophylactic medications (e.g., tricyclic antidepressants), behavioral therapies, and physical therapy. Interventional therapies are not typically used for this form of CDH, and a multimodal approach may also be best for many patients.

The treatment of MOH depends upon seemingly simple and basic steps being implemented. These include patient education and withdrawal of the overused medication(s). The patient at the same time must be supported with bridge therapy: treatment directed towards providing symptomatic relief during discontinuation of the overused medication(s), and in addition the establishment of a headache treatment regimen appropriate for the underlying headache type, to prevent MOH relapse. The patient with MOH may need to be hospitalized in order to accomplish these steps.

New daily persistent headache is difficult to treat, and there is little high-quality evidence to support a particular treatment, although some advocate using an approach similar to that taken for chronic tension-type headache.

Verapamil is considered first-line treatment for chronic cluster headache. In addition, topiramate, lithium carbonate, and corticosteroid medications may be considered.

Indomethacin is considered the most appropriate treatment for chronic paroxysmal hemicrania.

There is only limited evidence for the treatment of hypnic headache, with bedtime use of caffeine, indomethacin, and lithium carbonate among the treatments studied with limited success.

SUNCT tends to be more refractory to treatment than other primary headaches, with only weak evidence for the use of various anticonvulsants such as gabapentin, valproic acid, and lamotrigine, as well as for corticosteroids.

Primary stabbing headache has been treated successfully with indomethacin or melatonin.

Follow-up

All patients with CDH, regardless of the headache subtype but especially those with MOH, need to be followed regularly to monitor progress, to adjust the treatment regimen, and to attempt to ensure adherence to the treatment plan.

Given the easy availability of many over-the-counter (OTC) analgesic preparations whose inappropriate use can result in MOH, and the difficulty of monitoring their use, ensuring that patients with MOH do not relapse can be challenging.

Prognosis

For all patients with CDH, regardless of the headache subtype, the prognosis is guarded. Patients with MOH who refrain from use of offending agents can do well.

REFERENCES AND FURTHER READING

Dodick DW. Clinical practice. Chronic daily headache. *N Engl J Med* 2006; **354**: 158–65.

Halker RB, Hastriter EV, Dodick DW. Chronic daily headache: an evidence-based and systematic approach to a challenging problem. *Neurology* 2011; **76** (7 Suppl 2): S37–43.

Stewart WF, Ricci JA, Chee E, Morganstein D, Lipton R. Lost productive time and cost due to common pain conditions in the US workforce. *JAMA* 2003; **290**: 2443–54.

5

Post-lumbar-puncture headache

Clinical presentation

Since headache is so common following lumbar puncture, affecting approximately 10–30% of patients undergoing this procedure, the clinician performing a lumbar puncture must not only be aware of this, but must be prepared to reduce the risk of such an occurrence as well as to treat it aggressively.

It has been proposed, and maintained for many years, that following a lumbar puncture, ongoing leakage of cerebrospinal fluid (CSF) via the dural puncture site exceeds the rate of CSF production, resulting in low CSF volume and pressure as well as subsequent traction on pain-sensitive structures within the dura.

Most commonly, patients with post-lumbar-puncture headache will note the onset of either a frontal or an occipital headache within 12–24 hours of the procedure. The headache is clearly and overtly exacerbated when the patient is in an upright position, and equally clearly and overtly diminished when the patient changes to the supine position. Known risk factors for the development of post-lumbar-puncture headache include previous headache history, younger age (with a peak incidence at 20–40 years old), and being female. According to several reports, the volume of fluid removed does not appear to alter the risk of developing this syndrome.

Much thought has been given to attempting to determine means to reduce the risk of the occurrence of this condition. Use of a higher-gauge needle (the higher the gauge, the smaller the needle bore) and orientation of the needle bevel parallel to the longitudinal fibers of the dura have been associated with reduced incidence of post-lumbar-puncture headache. Since using a higher-gauge needle (e.g., 27-gauge) may make the procedure itself more difficult to complete, many use a 22-gauge needle to balance the ability to complete the procedure while reducing the risk of post-procedure headache.

Whenever possible, one should use an atraumatic spinal needle so that a smaller dural defect occurs. Examples of atraumatic needles include the Whitacre and Sprotte needles. Of interest is that various studies of patient positioning during the lumbar puncture have not shown one position to be superior with respect to reducing the likelihood of developing post-lumbar-puncture headache. Also of interest, and perhaps contrary to what many clinicians have practiced, longer bed rest following the procedure does not lessen the chances of post-lumbar-puncture headache compared to no bed rest or shorter periods of bed rest.

Signs and symptoms

In addition to the post-lumbar-puncture headache itself, other commonly reported symptoms include visual changes, dizziness, tinnitus, nausea, and emesis.

Laboratory tests and diagnostic investigations

No specific laboratory tests are routinely recommended for patients with post-lumbar-puncture headache. However, laboratory tests would be recommended if, for example, an infection were suspected (e.g., fever and concern for meningitis) as a consequence of the lumbar puncture.

Imaging studies

Imaging studies are not typically ordered during the evaluation and treatment of post-lumbar-puncture headache. However, because a lumbar puncture can rarely result in a cerebral venous thrombosis, the clinician must recognize this as a possible cause of post-lumbar-puncture headache. If there is concern for the development of a cerebral venous thrombosis, then appropriate imaging studies for that patient including MRI, MRV, or CTV, depending upon the patient and the clinical setting, need to be completed urgently.

Differential diagnosis

There is truly a limited differential diagnosis for this condition, given its close relationship, by definition, to the procedure that apparently causes it. As already noted, one must be concerned about the development of an infection following the procedure, as well as the development of a cerebral venous thrombosis. In contrast to post-lumbar-puncture headache, the headache associated with a cerebral venous thrombosis does not typically change with posture, and the severity is usually greater sooner after the procedure.

Pharmacotherapy and non-pharmacologic approaches

Fortunately post-lumbar-puncture headache is often mild, with quick and seemingly spontaneous resolution. A conservative approach, including bed rest, oral analgesics (acetaminophen, non-steroidal anti-inflammatory drugs, rarely opioids), and hydration are typically recommended for the first 24 hours in most cases.

Without treatment, the headache typically lasts 2–14 days, with an average of 4–8 days. However, if the headache is more severe and/or prolonged, other measures need to be considered including triptans, oral theophylline and gabapentin, intravenous adrenocorticotropic hormone (ACTH), steroids, and ketoralac (if not otherwise contraindicated).

Interventional procedures

For patients with moderate to severe prolonged headache refractory to conservative measures, intravenous caffeine and epidural blood patch are important considerations.

Intravenous caffeine infusions have been used in the treatment of this condition, and some would advocate completing this prior to using an epidural blood patch. The efficacy of this procedure has also been demonstrated in a randomized controlled study, with reduced headache more likely to be reported in patients treated with caffeine infusions at 2 hours compared with saline. Its mechanism of action is thought to be vasoconstriction of the cerebral vasculature. One suggested regimen is to give caffeine 500 mg diluted in 1000 mL of normal saline as a slow intravenous infusion over 1 hour, followed by 1000 mL of normal saline alone infused over 1 hour. A second dose of caffeine can be given in 4 hours if headache pain is unrelieved. Oral caffeine has been studied, but there is a high likelihood of headache recurrence.

Epidural saline is thought to transiently compress the subarachnoid space and allow the dural defect to seal. This procedure, however, is associated with a high recurrence rate.

The results of three randomized controlled trials as well as clinical experience suggest that an epidural blood patch is effective compared with conservative treatment. There are instances in which more than one epidural blood patch may need to be given, usually no more than two. This should be considered for patients who initially fail to respond to conservative treatment, and it is uniformly considered the treatment of choice in this setting. It is a simple procedure in which the patient's own blood (autologous) is drawn via sterile technique and then injected epidurally at or near the prior lumbar puncture site. It is believed that the epidural blood patch works by causing a dural tamponade, thus helping to stop the fluid loss rather quickly; in addition, the patch is believed to seal the leak. Infection, nerve injury, and increased low back pain are among the adverse effects to be mindful of.

Follow-up and prognosis

As previously mentioned, without treatment the post-lumbar-puncture headache typically lasts 2–14 days with an average of 4–8 days. For patients with moderate to severe prolonged headache refractory to conservative measures, epidural blood patch and intravenous caffeine are important considerations. There is a very favorable prognosis when available measures are used to treat this condition.

REFERENCES AND FURTHER READING

Armon C, Evans RW. Addendum to assessment: prevention of post-lumbar puncture headaches. Report of the Therapeutics and Technology Assessment Subcommittee of the American Academy of Neurology. *Neurology* 2005; **65**: 510–12.

Evans RW, Armon C, Frohman EM, Goodin DS. Assessment: prevention of post-lumbar puncture headaches: report of the therapeutics and technology assessment subcommittee of the American Academy of Neurology. *Neurology* 2000; **55**: 909–14.

Morewood GH. A rational approach to the cause, prevention and treatment of postdural puncture headache. *CMAJ* 1993; **149**: 1087–93.

Raskin NH. Lumbar puncture headache: a review. *Headache* 1990; **30**: 197–200.

Vallejo MC, Mandell GL, Sabo DP, Ramanathan S. Postdural puncture headache: a randomized comparison of five spinal needles in obstetric patients. *Anesth Analg* 2000; **91**: 916–20.

6

Trigeminal neuralgia

Clinical presentation

Trigeminal neuralgia (TN) is often referred to as *tic douloureux*, which is French for "painful spasm." The three main divisions of the trigeminal nerve (cranial nerve V) are the ophthalmic (V_1), maxillary (V_2), and mandibular (V_3), which supply sensation to the face. The ophthalmic division supplies sensation from the eyebrows to the coronal suture. The sensory innervation stops at the corona, not at the hairline, and this fact may help one to differentiate a true abnormality from a factitious one, since people who are "faking" sensory loss more often lose sensation at the hairline. Innervation of the cornea is divided, being supplied by V_1 in its upper half and V_2 in its lower half. The cheek bones and the inside of the nostrils are supplied by V_2. The mandibular branch supplies the lower jaw. However, the angle of the jaw is supplied by a cervical root rather than by the trigeminal nerve, and knowledge of this helps the clinician with anatomic differentiation. The motor functions of the trigeminal nerve include the muscles of mastication: temporalis, masseters, and pterygoids. The first two are involved in vertical closing of the jaw, and the third is involved in lateral motion of the jaw (grinding).

Patients with trigeminal neuralgia fall into two major categories: those with idiopathic trigeminal neuralgia and those with symptomatic (secondary) trigeminal neuralgia. As the terms suggest, patients with idiopathic TN have no clearly identified cause, whereas in those with symptomatic TN there is an identifiable cause. In so-called idiopathic TN abnormal blood vessels may be found compressing the trigeminal nerve as it exits the brainstem, and this observation is often used to aid in treatment (see below). Symptomatic TN is generally associated with either a compressive or a demyelinating lesion. Keep in mind that the pain experienced by patients with idiopathic TN is not different from that experienced in symptomatic TN. Frank loss of sensation in the V_1, V_2, or V_3 trigeminal distribution, or actual motor impairment, may occur in patients with symptomatic TN. Pretrigeminal neuralgia is an uncommon prodromal type of pain whose onset precedes trigeminal neuralgia. It is often described as a dull toothache, and it often prompts visits to the dentist and possibly dental treatments before trigeminal neuralgia is diagnosed.

The exact etiology of trigeminal neuralgia is unknown. Both peripheral and central nervous system mechanisms have been hypothesized, with the central nervous system theory suggesting that there is an abnormally hyperexcitable group of neurons in the brainstem (pons), and spontaneous discharge in these neurons results in the pain. The peripheral nervous system theory hypothesizes that trigeminal nerve compression by an aberrant blood vessel as it exits the brainstem results in abnormal spontaneous discharges. This theory has led to treatment of some patients with trigeminal neuralgia by surgical decompression of the nerve.

Signs and symptoms

Patients with trigeminal neuralgia complain of a sharp, shooting, lightning- or electric-shock-like sensation usually lasting seconds to minutes within the distribution of one or more branches of the trigeminal nerve. The V_2–V_3 distribution is the most common location; the ophthalmic division is involved in only 5% of patients. The attacks, which are intensely painful, are followed by pain-free periods. For patients with idiopathic trigeminal neuralgia, the pain is most often unilateral.

The physical and neurological examinations are generally without objective sensory or motor abnormalities. The pain in patients with the symptomatic form can be bilateral in up to 4%, and one is more likely to observe objective sensory loss or other clear findings on examination. Painful attacks of trigeminal neuralgia have common triggers including everyday activities such as brushing teeth, chewing, eating, drinking, shaving, and even lightly touching the face. Triggers (anatomic areas or functions that, when activated or "triggered," bring on paroxysms of pain) are key clinical features of trigeminal neuralgia for which patients must be screened. The most common triggers are located around the upper lip and nose. Chewing, brushing teeth, or even a breeze or any moving air can trigger such a painful event. In contrast, swallowing, a feature of glossopharyngeal neuralgia, does not trigger pain in trigeminal neuralgia.

Laboratory tests and diagnostic investigations

There are no specific laboratory tests to order for idiopathic trigeminal neuralgia. For patients for whom the diagnosis of secondary trigeminal neuralgia is being considered, the choice of laboratory tests depends upon what condition the clinician feels may be responsible for the neuralgia.

Imaging studies

Failure to properly assess for secondary trigeminal neuralgia should not occur. A careful examination of the cranial nerves and an MRI of the brain, especially in individuals under age 60, is necessary to evaluate for structural lesions (e.g., tumor, cerebral aneurysm, acoustic neuroma). MRI of the brain with gadolinium (unless otherwise contraindicated) with special attention to Meckel's cave, an indentation in the petrous bone where the gasserian ganglion (the sensory ganglion for the trigeminal nerve) is located, may identify specific structural or other abnormalities that could result in compression, inflammation, or dysfunction of the trigeminal nerve.

Differential diagnosis

Trigeminal neuralgia needs to be distinguished from migraine, cluster headache, chronic paroxysmal hemicrania, glossopharyngeal neuralgia, atypical facial pain, temporomandibular joint dysfunction, other dental problems, occipital neuralgia, and hemifacial spasm. Additional investigation may reveal multiple sclerosis (MS), a tumor in the posterior fossa, or a tumor on the trigeminal nerve.

Acoustic neuromas, cerebral aneurysms, trigeminal neuromas, and meningiomas are structural lesions that produce pain and other symptoms similar to idiopathic trigeminal neuralgia. These conditions must be considered in individuals younger than 40 with onset of symptoms, and in those with predominant forehead and/or orbit pain or with bilateral facial pain. Granulomatous inflammation (e.g., tuberculosis, sarcoidosis, Behçet syndrome, collagen vascular diseases, vasculitis) may also affect the trigeminal nerve and result in symptomatic/secondary trigeminal neuralgia.

Pharmacotherapy

Carbamazepine is first-line therapy for trigeminal neuralgia, with a recommended starting dose of 100 mg twice a day, increasing by 100 mg every day or two until the patient is pain-free or side effects occur. The common maintenance dose is 600–1200 mg/day (serum levels of 4–10 mg/mL). The half-life of carbamazepine decreases with chronic dosing because of auto-induction of enzymes. Carbamazepine is effective in 80% of patients with idiopathic trigeminal neuralgia. If individuals are pain-free for 3 months, a gradual taper of this agent can be considered, keeping in mind that the patient may become symptomatic again at a later date.

Aplastic anemia, fortunately an uncommon occurrence, is the most feared side effect of carbamazepine. Commonly, however, mild depression of the white blood cell count may occur. Other common side effects include drowsiness, dizziness, diplopia, and dyspepsia, which are dose-related. A complete blood count and hepatic and renal profiles should be performed before starting treatment with carbamazepine, after the first 2 months, then every 3 months. After the first year, blood counts should be performed every 6–12 months. The prescriber must be aware of the drug interactions of carbamazepine.

The following are additional, less rigorously studied pharmacological options for the treatment of trigeminal neuralgia. Oxcarbazepine is probably as effective as carbamazepine at doses of 900–1200 mg/day. Its side-effect profile is better than that of carbamazepine. Serum testing for agranulocytosis and blood levels is not necessary, but the possibility of hyponatremia needs to be monitored.

Lamotrigine at doses of 150–400 mg/day may be effective. Its side-effect profile is also favorable compared to carbamazepine. One major side effect to be concerned about is rash, which, although uncommon, can evolve into the Stevens–Johnson syndrome.

Gabapentin in doses ranging from 300 to 3600 mg in divided doses may be considered, as there is some evidence of benefit. Pregabalin, a medication with a presumed similar mechanism of action to gabapentin, may also be considered.

Baclofen may show benefit for those patients who do not respond to, or are unable to take, carbamazepine. The starting dose is 5 mg three times/day, with an increase of 5–10 mg every other day, depending on the patient's response. Maintenance dose is 50–60 mg/day in divided doses, with a recommended maximum of 80 mg/day. Side effects include sedation and nausea. When baclofen and carbamazepine are taken together, side effects are more common.

Phenytoin has been used in trigeminal neuralgia, and it can be effective in up to 60% of patients. However, it should only be considered in patients who did not respond to baclofen or carbamazepine. The initial starting dose is 200–300 mg/day, with a target of 300–500 mg/day. One advantage of phenytoin over the other agents is that it can be given intravenously if a patient presents with severe, intractable trigeminal neuralgia.

In refractory cases, short- or long-acting opioids may be considered, but only with proper assessment and monitoring by a properly trained prescriber.

Non-pharmacologic approaches

There are no specific non-pharmacologic approaches recommended for trigeminal neuralgia.

Interventional procedures

Surgical and other procedures for trigeminal neuralgia can be considered. A common decompressive technique is based on the hypothesis that an aberrant vessel, often one of the cerebellar arteries or veins, compresses the trigeminal nerve near its brainstem exit/entry zone. Following a posterior fossa craniotomy, the suspected "offending" vessel is lifted and a cushion is placed between the nerve and the vessel to decompress the nerve. While success rates of over 90% have been reported, there have been no double-blind studies and pain has been reported to recur.

In a destructive technique, the offending branches of the nerve may be lesioned percutaneously, either with radiofrequency devices or with alcohol injection. The latter procedure involves inserting a needle through the skin, into the foramen of the nerve where it exits the skull. Anesthesia dolorosa (pain in the numb area previously supplied by the nerve) is a bothersome complication. Percutaneous injection of glycerol around the gasserian ganglion is also effective. While these destructive lesions are less invasive than a craniectomy for decompression, they have a higher incidence of side effects and failures.

Gamma knife surgery, a form of radiotherapy, has become more widely available. This treatment is less technically demanding, less operator-dependent, and less invasive than the percutaneous procedures. It is certainly less invasive than a craniotomy. Gamma knife surgery appears to be about as effective as the percutaneous procedures (80% of patients), but it may be weeks to months before patients feel better, and this may not be acceptable for some patients. A handful of small studies have described potential benefit of the use of botulinum toxin for trigeminal neuralgia.

Follow-up and prognosis

Trigeminal neuralgia most often is associated with an exacerbating but remitting course. Over 50% of individuals will have at least a 6-month remission during their lifetime. There may be months or years when the patient is pain-free. Thus, drug holidays should be attempted to see if the patient is indeed responding to the drug, or simply having a remission of the disease. In some patients, the attacks become more frequent and may become nearly continuous, resulting in the need to modify treatment approaches. For those individuals with secondary trigeminal neuralgia, the prognosis will also depend upon the underlying condition.

REFERENCES AND FURTHER READING

Cutrer FM, Moskowitz MA. Headaches and other head pain. In Goldman L, Ausiello D, eds., *Cecil Medicine*, 23rd edn. Philadelphia, PA: Saunders Elsevier; 2007; Chapter 421.

Goetz CG, ed. *Textbook of Clinical Neurology*, 3rd edn. Philadelphia, PA: Saunders; 2007.

Gronseth G, Cruccu G, Alksne J, *et al.* Practice parameter: the diagnostic evaluation and treatment of trigeminal neuralgia (an evidence-based review). Report of the Quality Standards Subcommittee of the American Academy of Neurology and the European Federation of Neurological Societies. *Neurology* 2008; **71**: 1183–90.

Manzoni GC, Torelli CP. Epidemiology of typical and atypical craniofacial neuralgia. *Neurol Sci* 2005; **26** (Suppl 2): s65–7.

Sindrup SH, Jensen TS. Pharmacotherapy of trigeminal neuralgia. *Clin J Pain* 2002; **18**: 22–7.

7

Temporomandibular joint syndrome and orofacial pain

Clinical presentation

The term temporomandibular joint (TMJ) syndrome is often used to describe a wide variety of painful conditions, second only to headache as a cause of facial pain. The more common form of the syndrome has also been referred to as an extracapsular disorder, and it is known by a variety of terms such as myofascial pain affecting the TMJ. The less common or intracapsular form of the TMJ syndrome is associated with specific conditions such as osteoarthritis, articular disc displacement, or rheumatoid arthritis.

TMJ syndrome may develop as a result of stress, trauma, dental work, jaw malocclusion, jaw clenching, TMJ derangements, or the unconscious repeated use of the muscles of mastication. Almost all individuals with TMJ syndrome will experience nighttime bruxism.

TMJ syndrome occurs more frequently in patients with articular disc displacement than in those without. Ongoing muscle tightness, with its impact on the TMJ, may lead to or enhance jaw malocclusion. Since certain other musculoskeletal pain conditions can be associated with or lead to TMJ syndrome, it is important to be aware of these; they include scoliosis, pronounced cervical and/or lumbar lordosis, fibromyalgia, and increased joint laxity. TMJ syndrome most frequently affects women in the third or fourth decade.

Unlike TMJ syndrome or other more specific facial pain syndromes such as trigeminal neuralgia, persistent idiopathic facial pain (also known as atypical facial pain) is less well defined. Persistent idiopathic facial pain is not well localized and is present for most of each day. It is not associated with any specific signs on physical examination.

Signs and symptoms

Presenting signs and symptoms are most often unilateral, and they commonly initially appear after a stressful event. Symptoms include dull pain in the muscles of mastication which is worsened by chewing. The pain may radiate to the posterior neck, the head, the jaw, or the ear – and in fact, for some patients, headache is the symptom of TMJ syndrome that they report first.

Patients will often complain of clicking of the TMJ when moving the jaw, and this may be a sign of articular disc displacement. However, many people with articular disc displacement are asymptomatic, and not all patients with clicking experience other symptoms associated with the TMJ syndrome.

When the patient is examined, the examiner should look for signs of facial asymmetry. The patient is asked to open and close the mouth to evaluate for restriction of mouth opening as well as for evidence for jaw displacement. Typically there is no joint swelling, but the patient may report pain with jaw opening and closing.

When examining the patient, the examiner should place the fingers behind the tragi of the external acoustic meatus pulling slightly forward as the patient is asked to open his/her mouth. A symptomatic patient will likely experience reduced jaw motion with this maneuver. The examination also involves an evaluation of the muscles of mastication. These are palpated bilaterally to compare the degree of tenderness between the symptomatic and asymptomatic side in patients with unilateral TMJ syndrome.

To assess the temporal muscles, they should be palpated while the patient opens and closes the jaw. The pterygoid muscles can be assessed by palpating them in between the tonsillar pillars in the posterior aspect of the mouth on the inner side of the mandible. The masseter muscle can be assessed by palpation over the mandibular angle.

Laboratory tests and diagnostic investigations

No specific laboratory testing is recommended to make the diagnosis of TMJ syndrome. However, the clinician may choose to consider such tests when a comorbid condition such as rheumatoid arthritis is believed to be associated with the complaint.

Imaging studies

Unless the patient is suspected of also experiencing dental disease, plain x-rays of the TMJ are not considered to be useful. MRI of the TMJ is the imaging procedure of choice when evaluating a patient with TMJ syndrome. This should be considered when the pain is severe and/or when the patient is experiencing pain as well as joint clicking, or when there is obvious joint displacement upon examination. Disc desiccation, other degenerative changes, and disc displacement may be seen in MRI studies.

Differential diagnosis

Many other medical conditions can result in pain over the temporomandibular joints. These include but are not restricted to trigeminal neuralgia, disorders of the parotid gland, glossopharyngeal neuralgia, various lesions of the oral cavity including neoplasms or lymphoproliferative disorders, carotidynia, Eagle syndrome, various dental problems, rheumatoid arthritis, and temporal arteritis.

Pharmacotherapy

If appropriate use of non-prescription medications has not resulted in adequate benefit, one could consider the use of various pharmacologic agents as one component in the treatment of pain related to the TMJ syndrome.

Non-steroidal anti-inflammatory drugs (NSAIDs) are typically not beneficial enough if used in the absence of any other treatment. However, proper use of NSAIDs in combination with jaw muscle exercises may be more helpful. In this context, one study found that naproxen at an oral dose of 500 mg twice daily was particularly helpful when combined with exercise.

The tricyclic antidepressant amitriptyline at a low dose (10–25 mg at bedtime) may also provide pain relief to many with TMJ syndrome. The structurally related compound cyclobenzaprine, marketed not as an antidepressant but as a muscle relaxant, has also been shown to be of potential benefit at doses ranging from 10 to 30 mg daily in divided doses. Given the similarity of these two agents, the prescriber should consider avoiding their co-administration to the same patient, even though one is marketed as an antidepressant and the other as a muscle relaxant, because the risk of serious side effects could be significantly magnified.

Non-pharmacologic approaches

A significant benefit for the patient with TMJ syndrome may be recognizing and avoiding, if at all possible, the provocative factors that increase the symptoms associated with the condition. These may include avoiding or reducing activities that promote jaw muscle spasm, and attempting to reduce nighttime jaw clenching through the use of an appropriate oral bite plate appliance.

In addition, some have advocated the avoidance of coffee, tea, chocolate, various colas, diet pills, and other stimulants in an attempt to reduce stress, which may be associated with the symptoms of TMJ syndrome.

Since dental problems may lead to TMJ syndrome symptoms, proper general dental care itself is advised. Jaw-opening exercises may be of particular benefit and may be even more beneficial if combined with certain pharmacologic therapies.

A TMJ syndrome education program used in combination with a home exercise program resulted in better jaw opening than education alone but did not necessarily result in greater pain relief.

Many different occlusal appliances have been considered for TMJ syndrome, with the idea that these may reduce nocturnal joint loading and muscle hyperactivity. In more than one study, including those that compared a true appliance to a sham appliance, many patients experienced short-term benefit. In one study in particular an occlusal appliance was found to be more helpful than TMJ syndrome patient education or the use of relaxation techniques.

Stabilization splints may also be considered, although there is debate about whether hard or soft splints are superior. The TMJ syndrome patients who are most likely to respond to appliances appear to be those with difficulties with occlusion, as evidenced by mandibular deviation, and those with pterygoid muscle spasm.

Low-level laser therapy has been studied in TMJ syndrome and may be worth considering for some patients. Improvements not only in pain relief but also in jaw opening and overall jaw motion have been noted with this modality in a formal study comparing laser to placebo treatment.

Interventional procedures

Various interventional approaches to the management of TMJ syndrome can be considered, especially if more conservative approaches, including the management of any dental problems that may be contributing, have been optimally addressed.

The TMJ can be injected with a combination of a corticosteroid combined with a local anesthetic, e.g., 40 mg of methylprednisolone combined with 1% preservative-free lidocaine. Prior to the injection, the patient is examined and the joint to be injected is palpated during jaw movement. The area to be injected is properly cleaned and the patient observed after the injection for approximately 30 minutes. Infection, bleeding, and adverse reaction to any of the medications used, as well as increased pain, are among the adverse events to advise the patient of before treatment, and to monitor for after.

A randomized controlled study has demonstrated that botulinum toxin A (Botox) injected into the muscles of mastication may significantly reduce pain in patients with TMJ syndrome.

For patients who have failed to respond adequately to any of the above interventions or any of the previously discussed measures, surgical management may need to be considered. This may be more likely to occur in a patient with TMJ syndrome associated with a significant internal joint derangement, including severe degenerative joint changes.

Surgical procedures that may be considered include arthroscopic lysis of adhesions, and a partial or total meniscectomy. Patients should be referred only to surgeons with experience and demonstrated competence performing these procedures, with successful outcomes. Some patients may be also considered for arthrodesis surgery.

TMJ disc replacement surgery has mixed results in terms of benefit, and again emphasis is placed not only on the current limits of this treatment but also on recognizing that the surgeon's experience with it must be factored in to deciding if it should be offered to the patient.

Follow-up

Fortunately, the majority of patients with TMJ syndrome will respond to conservative measures including pharmacotherapy. Follow-up is advised not only to address treatment outcome but also to continue to address potentially correctable mechanical factors that may contribute to the symptoms associated with TMJ syndrome.

Prognosis

The prognosis is variable. Most patients with TMJ syndrome will experience a relapsing and remitting course, and this point should be discussed with the patient at the onset of evaluation and treatment, to assist with appropriate patient expectations. Only a minority of patients with TMJ syndrome will become "permanently" asymptomatic, regardless of the treatment(s) utilized.

REFERENCES AND FURTHER READING

Chen H, Slade G, Lim PF, *et al*. Relationship between temporomandibular disorders, widespread palpation tenderness, and multiple pain conditions: a case control study. *J Pain* 2012; **13**: 1016–27.

De Laat A, Stappaerts K, Papy S. Counseling and physical therapy as treatment for myofascial pain of the masticatory system. *J Orofac Pain* 2003; **17**: 42–9.

Freund BJ, Schwartz M. Relief of tension-type headache symptoms in subjects with temporomandibular disorders treated with botulinum toxin-A. *Headache* 2002; **42**: 1033–7.

Fricton JR. Clinical care for myofascial pain. *Dent Clin North Am* 1991; **35**: 1–28.

8

Occipital neuralgia

Clinical presentation

Occipital neuralgia is the term used to describe sudden, paroxysmal pain, often jabbing, in the distribution of the greater occipital, the lesser occipital, or the third occipital nerve. Occipital neuralgia results in occipital headaches and is at times associated with abnormal sensation or loss of sensation in the area affected by the neuralgic pain.

Occipital neuralgia can occur as a result of referred pain from cervical myofascial trigger points, or from the upper zygapophyseal or atlantoaxial joints. The diagnosis of occipital neuralgia can therefore be made only if these processes have been ruled out.

The true incidence of occipital neuralgia is unknown, and it has been suggested that occipital neuralgia is often overdiagnosed, since not uncommonly clinicians incorrectly refer to any pain in the occipital region as occipital neuralgia. Many investigators believe that neck injuries following a motor vehicle accident predispose an individual to developing occipital neuralgia.

Signs and symptoms

The onset of pain associated with occipital neuralgia is sudden, beginning in the nuchal region and traveling to the vertex of the head. It is most often unilateral, but bilateral presentations are not rare. Patients describe the pain as severe shooting, stabbing, or shock-like. Although many painful episodes may begin without a specific trigger, several recognized triggers of occipital neuralgia include neck movement and hair brushing.

The physical examination may reveal a restricted range of motion of the neck, as well as active painful spasm. During the examination, palpation or pressure over the occipital nerve trunks may trigger a neuralgic episode, cause abnormal dysesthesias in the nerve's distribution, or increase the overall pain.

The neurological examination is generally unremarkable except for occasional diminished or abnormal sensation over the nerve's distribution; in fact, a clearly abnormal neurologic examination should prompt the clinician to evaluate for a more specific cause of the symptoms other than occipital neuralgia.

The diagnosis of occipital neuralgia should be considered when the above clinical features are noted, and it can be aided when the pain is temporarily relieved by an occipital nerve block performed with a local anesthetic.

The current classification scheme of the International Headache Society (IHS) indicates that in order to make the diagnosis of occipital neuralgia the following must be present: (1) paroxysmal stabbing pain in the distribution of the greater, lesser, and/or third occipital nerves, with or without aching in between the paroxysmal pain, (2) tenderness over the affected occipital nerve(s), (3) pain that is temporarily diminished by a local anesthetic occipital nerve block.

Laboratory tests and diagnostic investigations

For typical occipital neuralgia, there are no specific laboratory tests to order. For patients for whom the diagnosis of secondary occipital neuralgia is being considered, the choice of laboratory tests would clearly depend upon what condition the clinician feels is responsible for the condition.

Imaging studies

Clear guidelines regarding the use of neuroimaging for the evaluation of occipital neuralgia are not currently available. However, given the myriad of structural and other medical conditions, including infiltrative processes, that can result in occipital neuralgic pain, it is reasonable to obtain an MRI of the cervical spine and of the brain during the initial evaluation.

Differential diagnosis

Many medical conditions are associated with cervical spine pain and radiation to the head; thus, the differential diagnosis of occipital neuralgia is extensive.

True occipital neuralgia should be distinguished from pain in the occiput that is referred from another source that is innervated by the upper three cervical spinal nerves. Such structures include various muscles, including trapezius and sternocleidomastoid, as well as other posterior cervical and suboccipital muscles, the vertebral arteries, the C2–C3 intervertebral disc and zygapophyseal joint, the dura surrounding the posterior fossa and upper cervical spine, and the atlantoaxial and atlanto-occipital joints.

Multiple other structural causes of occipital neuralgia-like pain have been identified, including vascular compression and vascular structural anomalies including arteriovenous fistula, myelitis, multiple myeloma, schwannoma, and meningioma.

Cervicogenic headache is a not uncommon headache type whose pathophysiology, although often debated, is nevertheless believed to be associated with referred pain from the upper cervical spine. The common sources of cervicogenic headache include the atlantoaxial joint and the C2–C3 zygapophyseal (facet) joint. The third occipital nerve (TON) is the superficial medial branch of C3 dorsal ramus. TON supplies the C2–C3 facet joint, the semispinalis capitis muscle, and the cutaneous area below the occiput. The pain associated with cervicogenic headache may overlap the symptoms of occipital neuralgia, and thus it is part of the differential diagnosis of occipital neuralgia.

If the pain is not noticeably improved after an occipital nerve block, then the diagnosis of occipital neuralgia should be reconsidered and other sources of the patient's pain evaluated.

Pharmacotherapy

There are no clear data to support the use of any specific pharmacologic approach to the management of occipital neuralgia. Various reports have suggested the potential benefits of carbamazepine, gabapentin, or tricyclic antidepressants; however, the data are scant. Others have reported the potential benefit of topical local anesthetics as well as topical non-steroidal anti-inflammatory drugs, although the true benefit of these is unclear.

Non-pharmacologic approaches

Many patients with occipital neuralgia may benefit from the use of conservative approaches to treatment including the application of heat (dry or moist) or cold.

Interventional procedures

Undoubtedly, the treatment that most practitioners will offer patients with occipital neuralgia is greater and/or lesser occipital nerve block. The greater occipital nerve is the terminal branch of the dorsal ramus of C2, with contribution from C3. The lesser occipital nerve is a branch of the dorsal ramus of C3, with contribution from C2. The landmarks for nerve block are mastoid, occipital protuberance, and occipital artery.

This procedure is considered potentially diagnostic, as well as therapeutic, and should only be performed by a practitioner who is trained to do it. Generally a local anesthetic alone, or local anesthetic in combination with a glucocorticoid, is used during the injection.

Care must be taken to avoid intravascular injection of the anesthetic and/or glucocorticoid. When performed by a practitioner who is experienced with the procedure, occipital nerve blocks have a good safety record, especially with ultrasound guidance.

The pain relief associated with an occipital nerve block is nearly immediate in most instances. As is the case with many nerve blocks, it has a variable duration of benefit ranging from hours to days to weeks or months, as well as variable benefit with respect to degree of pain reduction (none to complete).

Either cryoneurolysis or radiofrequency ablation can be considered if there is only temporary improvement despite repeated nerve blocks.

Neuromodulation may be used as an alternative to neuroablation for occipital neuralgia. A percutaneous trial of peripheral nerve stimulation is usually done first. If a percutaneous trial provides satisfactory pain relief, then convert to permanent implant with an electrode lead connected to a pulse generator.

Occipital nerve stimulation is by no means routinely used for the treatment of occipital neuralgia, and clinical studies have shown variable success.

Unfortunately, intractable instances of occipital neuralgia do occur. In such cases, neuroablation such as rhizotomy at C1–C3 may provide benefit, though it should be performed only by experienced surgeons, and again the success rate is variable.

Follow-up and prognosis

Patients who benefit from occipital nerve blocks may experience months or more of pain relief. However, many patients will require repeated treatment at some point. The precise incidence of recurrence and long-term outcomes are not known for occipital neuralgia. Intractable instances do occur, and their true incidence is also unknown. In general, the practitioner can expect a treatment response for most patients with occipital neuralgia, but one should also expect recurrence at some point and the likely need for additional treatment.

REFERENCES AND FURTHER READING

Ashkenazi A, Levin M. Three common neuralgias. How to manage trigeminal, occipital, and postherpetic pain. *Postgrad Med* 2004; **116**: 16–18, 21–4, 31–2.
Bogduk N. The anatomy of occipital neuralgia. *Clin Exp Neurol* 1981; **17**: 167–184.
Bogduk N. The neck and headaches. *Neurol Clin* 2004; **22**: 151–71, vii.

Neck and shoulder

9

Neck strain/sprain

Clinical presentation

Cervical sprains and strains are a common disorder of the musculoskeletal system. Acute sprains and strains may occur as a result of strenuous lifting and pulling activities, or not uncommonly after relatively low-speed/low-energy impact-type injuries. They can occur in the recreational as well as vocational arenas. Acute sprain/strain syndromes are self-limiting and generally resolve in days to several weeks.

Acute and chronic sprain/strain syndromes can also be referred to as whiplash-associated disorders (WAD), when the mechanism of injury includes a component of rapid acceleration/deceleration or eccentric muscle loading of the posterior as well as anterior cervical paraspinal musculature. WAD can be divided into four categories:
- WAD type 1 – neck pain complaints with normal exam
- WAD type 2 – neck pain complaints in conjunction with limited range of motion and trigger points
- WAD type 3 – neck pain complaints, limited cervical range of motion, trigger points, radiating paresthesias
- WAD type 4 – associated with cervical fracture/dislocation

WAD becomes a chronic issue when symptoms last longer than 6 months. WAD, as diagnosed and categorized by the Quebec Task Force, generally resolves within 3 months of the inciting event. Beyond the 3-month window there is little if any improvement, and associated chronic pain and pain-related disability and dys-function affect 15–20% of people with whiplash-associated injuries. This chapter will focus on the challenging area of chronic WAD.

Signs and symptoms

Common complaints noted in WAD include neck pain, both localized and radiating to the shoulders. Additionally, posterior region headaches, fatigue, dizziness, jaw pain, photophobia, and complaints of impaired ability to concentrate are all commonly noted. Subjective sensation of numbness and tingling in the hands has also been described. As one can see, the above symptom complex is neither specific nor focal. The diffuse and somewhat vague nature of the complaints presents unique challenges in the evaluation and ultimately the management of this syndrome.

During the course of history taking not only must the above complaints be targeted, but specific questions relating to bladder function, such as urgency and frequency of urination, should be asked. Urinary urgency/frequency and occasional accidents may be the herald of a more significant issue, such as cervical myelopathy, which can be seen in older patients who were involved in relatively low-speed, low-energy, and cervical muscle eccentric loading-type injuries.

The physical examination should start with a general visual inspection of the patient. Observe the spontaneous range of motion of the patient's cervical spine during the course of the interview. Assess visually the range in flexion and extension, as well as rotation to right and left. By moving around the room and changing position during the course of the interview, the examining physician can easily assess all cervical ranges during the non-formal part of the examination. Also look for obvious deformity. Asymmetry of shoulder height may be secondary to trapezius spasm. Look for unilateral atrophy of the shoulder girdle musculature or biceps, which may indicate a C5–C6 level radiculopathy.

Once a complete observation has been made, a more hands-on examination can now be undertaken. Palpation of upper extremity musculature to assess muscle contour and bulk may reveal more subtle issues of atrophy not appreciated on inspection.

Assessment of muscle stretch reflexes with a reflex hammer is critical. Side-to-side comparison should be carried out, and lower extremity reflex assessment is critical as well. The biceps reflex assesses C5 function, wrist extensor C6 function, and triceps C7 level function. Unilateral absence of a reflex may represent a radiculopathy. Lower extremity hyperreflexia with findings of ankle clonus, crossed adductor responses, and Hoffmann's sign in the upper extremities is diagnostic of cervical myelopathy until proven otherwise, and requires in-depth imaging of the cervical spine with MRI to assess for canal stenosis and potential cord compression.

Motor testing should include manual muscle testing of the deltoid/biceps to assess C5 function, wrist extensors for C6, triceps for C7, and hand intrinsics for C8, T1. The grading system is on a 0–5 scale as determined by the American Spinal Injury Association (ASIA), with 0 being no activity, 1 visible contraction but no movement, 2 full range of motion with gravity eliminated, 3 full range of motion against gravity but no other resistance, 4 movement against partial resistance, and 5 movement against full resistance from the examiner (normal).

Sensory function to light touch should be assessed as well, with the axillary patch representing C5, thumb C6, long finger C7, small finger C8, and medial arm T1.

Lastly, palpation of the cervical musculature should be performed. Appreciation of tone, trigger points, and reproduction of symptoms with palpation should be noted.

Spurling's maneuver, which is a combination of extension and lateral rotation, can be helpful in evaluation for possible radiculopathy. The abduction tension release sign, resolution of shoulder or upper arm pain with placement of the affected arm over the patient's head, resting the forearm on the top of the head, is strongly suggestive of a C5 level radiculopathy.

Laboratory tests and diagnostic investigations

Electromyography (EMG) testing to evaluate cervical root function can be a helpful adjunctive test in the patient with multilevel findings on cervical MRI, when cervical epidural injections are being considered.

Imaging studies

Radiographs of the cervical spine, including flexion and extension views to assess for segmental instability, are important to ensure that structural and mechanical causes for ongoing pain and dysfunction are not missed. Cervical MRI is appropriate in the setting of clinical findings of cervical radiculopathy or myelopathy.

Differential diagnosis

The differential diagnosis grows from the history and physical. It includes WAD, with and without associated neurologic findings, namely radiculopathy and/or myelopathy. The complaints of headache and photophobia can be associated with cervicogenic headache as well as post-traumatic migraine.

Pharmacotherapy

Pharmacologic options include non-steroidal anti-inflammatory drugs (NSAIDs), neuromodulators such as serotonin–norepinephrine reuptake inhibitor (SNRI) antidepressants, and anti-seizure medications. To date no randomized studies have shown efficacy of these interventions above placebo. NSAID use should be approached cautiously, as long-term exposure can be associated with significant gastrointestinal as well as renal toxicity.

Non-pharmacologic approaches

These can include physical therapy, acupuncture, massage, and behavioral intervention strategies. Neither acupuncture nor massage therapy has been shown to be efficacious for pain management in chronic WAD.

Randomized control group data suggest that in the chronic WAD group, cognitive behavioral therapies can be associated with improvements in pain cognition, cervical pain pressure threshold, and pain-free cervical movement. The emphasis in these forms of therapy is on retraining the proprioception and movement control of the cranial or cervical region, as well as addressing cognitive–emotional sensitization.

Classical strengthening and range of motion exercises have not been shown to be helpful in chronic WAD associated with a motor vehicle accident, and in fact they may exacerbate symptoms. Exercise has been shown to be helpful in chronic cervical pain of etiology other than motor vehicle accident.

Interventional procedures

Interventions can include radiofrequency procedures to the cervical facet joints. Recent studies have confirmed the utility of this intervention in chronic WAD, further confirming that in a subset of chronic WAD patients the cervical facet capsule is a probable source generator of chronic pain.

Epidural steroid injections can have utility in the subset of chronic WAD patients with clearly demonstrable radiculopathy, namely physical exam findings, with concordant MRI imaging and EMG findings of radiculopathy.

Botulinun toxin injections have been proposed and used for the management of pain from tender muscular trigger points. Although few randomized studies are available, and the studies that are available have methodological flaws, it appears that botulinum toxin may result in short-term pain reduction.

Cervical spine surgery should be limited to the subset of patients with demonstrable segmental instability with associated neurological findings, most significantly myelopathy. In this group the goal is stabilization of the cervical spine to prevent further spinal cord injury from such things as future falls or other low-speed, low-energy impact-type injuries.

Surgery for radiculopathy can be cautiously approached in the patient who has failed conservative management, who has concordant physical exam, imaging, and electrodiagnostic studies, and who has had at least a transiently positive response to cervical epidural steroid injection.

Follow-up

The management of chronic WAD presents unique challenges. The follow-up should focus on function and maintenance of activity. Utilization of behavioral models should be emphasized for long-term management, and pharmacologic intervention should be limited.

Prognosis

The majority of patients with WAD resolve their issues within 3 months. The 10–20% who persists with symptoms after 6 months present the greatest challenge, and require a thorough and detailed evaluation to ensure that treatable issues have not been overlooked.

REFERENCES AND FURTHER READING

Berg HE, Berggren G, Tesch PA. Dynamic neck strength training effect on pain and function. *Arch Phys Med Rehabil* 1994; **75**: 661–5.

Geisser ME, Roth RS. Knowledge of and agreement with chronic pain diagnosis: relation to affective distress, pain beliefs and coping, pain intensity and disability. *J Occup Rehabil* 1998; **8**: 73–88.

Nijs J, Van Oosterwijck J, De Hertogh W. Rehabilitation of chronic whiplash: treatment of cervical dysfunction or chronic pain syndrome? *Clin Rheumatol* 2009; **28**: 243–51.

Rodriguez AA, Barr KP, Burns SP. Whiplash: pathophysiology, diagnosis, treatment, and prognosis. *Muscle Nerve* 2004; **29**: 768–81.

Spitzer WO, Skovron, ML, Salmi LR, *et al.* Scientific monograph of the Quebec Task Force on Whiplash-Associated Disorders: redefining " whiplash" and its management. *Spine (Phila Pa 1976)* 1995; **20**: S1–73.

10

Cervical radiculopathy

Clinical presentation

Patients with cervical radiculopathy may suffer from intermittent and deteriorating neck pain prior to abrupt onset of radicular pain, numbness, tingling, and weakness. In theory, cervical radiculopathy could be due to either irritation or inflammation of nerve roots at various levels.

The common causes of cervical radiculopathy may include disc protrusion, herniation, and spondylosis linked to nerve root compression; less likely are degenerative disc disease, spinal canal stenosis, foraminal narrowing, cervical facet arthropathy, and spondylolisthesis.

The most frequent sites of cervical disc herniation are at the C5–C6 and C6–C7 levels, with the manifestation corresponding to the 6th and 7th cervical nerve roots.

Signs and symptoms

Cervical radiculopathy describes neck and upper extremity pain associated with demonstrable motor and/or sensory deficit. The radicular symptoms are aggravated by movement of the neck, coughing, sneezing, or strenuous activities. Spurling's (neck compression) test is performed by passive lateral flexion and compression of the head. A positive Spurling's test may mimic the patient's clinical presentation of radicular symptoms and confirm the diagnosis of cervical radiculopathy.

The common signs and symptoms are correlated with the cervical nerve roots as follows, demonstrating the distribution of the nerves and the different possible sources of the cervical radiculopathy:

- Pain distribution: C5 = neck, shoulder, anterior and lateral arm; C6 = neck, shoulder, lateral arm; C7 = neck, shoulder, lateral arm, dorsal forearm; C8 = ulnar forearm

- Sensory changes: C4 = shoulders; C5 = deltoid region; C6 = dorsal and lateral aspects of thumb and index finger; C7 = less index, more middle finger, and dorsum of hand; C8 = fourth and fifth finger, medial forearm
- Reflex changes: C4 = none; C5 = biceps; C6 = brachioradialis; C7 = triceps reflex; C8 = none
- Nerve involvement: C4 = dorsal scapular; C5 = musculocutaneous lateral arm (C5–C6); C6 = radial (C5–C6); C7 = radial (C6–C8); C8 = anterior interosseous (median) (C7–C8)
- Action of nerve root: C4 = shoulder shrug; C5 = attempt further flexion against resistance; C6 = maintain extension against resistance; C7 = extend forearm against gravity; C8 = flexion of middle finger
- Motor weakness: C4 = levator scapulae; C5 = deltoid and biceps muscles; C6 = biceps, wrist extensors, pollicis longus; C7 = triceps muscle; C8 = flexor digitorum profundus, and hand muscles in general

When the distribution of paresthesia, weakness, and hyporeflexia associated with radicular pain is concordant with the dermatomal chart, the level of cervical radiculopathy may then be established as the working diagnosis.

Laboratory tests and diagnostic investigations

Inflammatory diseases or neoplasms may present with systemic symptoms, signs of fever, and malaise, with elevated blood count and erythrocyte sedimentation rate.

Electromyography (EMG) and nerve conduction studies (NCS) can be considered in the identification and differential diagnosis of cervical radiculopathy, peripheral nerve involvement, or entrapment neuropathy and other pathology.

Discography should be reserved to confirm the symptomatology of discogenic pain as a prelude to surgical intervention, and should not be routinely used to establish the diagnosis of either cervical disc herniation or radiculopathy.

Imaging studies

Standard radiography with additional flexion and extension views may identify spondylosis and help to rule out instability due to spinal spondylolisthesis. CT scan and myelography are valuable in documenting any cervical disc protrusion and/or bony impingement of nerve roots. MRI with and without contrast are the imaging modality of choice to verify cervical nerve root compression or other non-bony pathology, e.g., infection or neoplasm.

Differential diagnosis

Cervical radiculitis usually refers to radicular pain without any demonstrable neurologic dysfunction such as motor or sensory deficit.

Cervical facet arthropathy, inflammatory arthritis, bursitis, or common pathology of shoulder joint must always be included in the differential diagnosis of cervical radiculopathy. Myofascial trigger-point and referral pain, cervicobrachial syndrome, brachial plexopathy, and thoracic outlet syndrome may all mimic the clinical picture of cervical radiculopathy.

Cervical myelopathy is a "red flag" whenever a patient presents with radicular symptoms in the upper extremities and additional long-tract (extrapyramidal) signs or dysfunction affecting the lower extremities and trunk. The presence of spastic weakness, hyporeflexia, clonus, and extensor plantar reflexes helps to distinguish cervical myelopathy from cervical radiculopathy. Upper motor neuron disease can be evaluated by Hoffmann's reflex, illustrating passive snapping flexion of the middle finger distal phalanx and resulting in flexion–adduction of the ipsilateral thumb and index finger.

Pulmonary masses and apical tumors may present with Horner's syndrome and involvement of C8 or T1 spinal nerves, which rarely occurs in the presentation of cervical radiculopathy.

Please refer to other chapters regarding the comprehensive evaluation and treatment of coexisting shoulder, wrist, or hand conditions.

Pharmacotherapy

Acetaminophen, non-steroidal anti-inflammatory drugs (NSAIDs), cyclooxygenase-2 (COX-2) inhibitors, and skeletal muscle relaxants may help to provide symptomatic relief of mild to moderate radicular pain and muscle spasm, especially in the acute phase of cervical radiculopathy. Anticonvulsants, tricyclic antidepressants (TCAs), and serotonin–norepinephrine reuptake inhibitors (SNRIs) have all been proposed for off-label application in the modulation of assumed neuropathic pain associated with the more chronic phase of cervical radiculopathy. A methylprednisolone (Medrol) dose package with both loading and tapering-off doses can be prescribed in severe cases of intractable acute pain when there is contraindication for NSAIDs or specific COX-2 inhibitors. A methylprednisolone dose package may also be indicated in patients who are not candidates for any interventional procedure such as cervical epidural steroid injection (e.g., because of infection or because they are unable to be off anticoagulation safely).

Although opioids are prescribed in acute moderate to severe pain, their efficacy in chronic pain management of cervical radiculopathy has not been supported by evidence-based studies.

Non-pharmacologic approaches

Bed rest, a cervical collar, physical therapy, traction, transcutaneous electrical nerve stimulation (TENS), and an exercise program under supervision could all be considered in cervical radiculopathy.

Interventional procedures

Cervical interlaminar (translaminar) epidural steroid injection under fluoro-scopic guidance is usually indicated for radicular and axial pains that are refrac-tory to conservative treatments. There is modest support regarding the benefit of cervical epidural steroid injection as part of non-surgical treatment. A series of three epidural steroid injections at 3–4-week intervals every 6–12 months has become a common recommendation in moderate to severe cervical radiculopa-thy. Case studies have suggested that patients with radicular pain may respond better to epidural steroid injection.

Cervical transforaminal epidural steroid injections aimed toward the specific level of the nerve roots have been linked to more vascular-related adverse events than the regular translaminar approach. Ultrasound-guided scanning with vas-cular Doppler option in conjunction with fluoroscopic epidural injection may minimize any intravascular injection and subsequent complications.

The outlook on disc procedures and minimally invasive surgery seems promis-ing, but there is still a need for more well-designed and long-term outcome studies. Surgical exploration and decompression is usually recommended in cases of myelopathy or progressive sensory and motor dysfunction due to compromise of a cervical nerve root despite ongoing conservative non-surgical management.

Neuromodulation therapy, such as spinal cord stimulation, could be a sup-portive modality in cases of cervical radiculopathy that remain intractable despite surgical intervention and comprehensive pain management.

Follow-up

The level of pain relief, the extent of progress in reducing neurologic dysfunction, and the improvement in functional capacity should be key indicators in the follow-up of cervical radiculopathy.

Prognosis

There may be spontaneous recovery or improvement with non-surgical treatment of mild to moderate cervical radiculopathy. Although the natural course of severe cervical radiculopathy may lead to deterioration of neurologic deficit and agon-izing pain, spinal surgery should still be reserved for selected candidates after careful decision making.

REFERENCES AND FURTHER READING

Bronfort G, Evans R, Anderson AV, *et al.* Spinal manipulation, medication, or home exercise with advice for acute and subacute neck pain: a randomized trial. *Ann Intern Med* 2012; **15**: 1–10.

Hey HW, Lau PH, Hee HT. Short-term results of physiotherapy in patients with newly diagnosed degenerative cervical spine disease. *Singapore Med J* 2012; **53**: 179–82.

Kim SH, Lee KH, Yoon KB, Park WY, Yoon DM. Sonographic estimation of needle depth for cervical epidural blocks. *Anesth Analg* 2008; **106**: 1542–7.

Manchikanti L, Malla Y, Cash KA, McManus CD, Pampati V. Fluoroscopic epidural injections in cervical spinal stenosis: preliminary results of a randomized, double-blind, active control trial. *Pain Physician* 2012; **15**: E59–70.

McLean JP, Sigler JD, Plastaras CT, Garvan CW, Rittenberg JD. The rate of detection of intravascular injection in cervical transforaminal epidural steroid injections with and without digital subtraction angiography. *PM R* 2009; **1**: 636–42.

11

Cervical facet syndrome

Clinical presentation

Cervical facet syndrome (CFS) indicates axial neck pain due to involvement of posterior spinal column structures. Degenerative change of the facet (zygapophyseal) joint such as hypertrophic arthropathy or osteophytes may impinge on nerve roots and irritate any surrounding posterior and lateral structures. Degenerative changes at the level of the C2–C3 facet joint have been well documented.

CFS is a common cause of chronic neck pain after whiplash injury, with frequent involvement of C2–C3 and C5–C6 levels. Whiplash injury has been linked with acceleration of degenerative cervical facet arthropathy.

Signs and symptoms

Patients with CFS may complain of a dull ache in the neck that originates from the facet joint(s), which may also cause a prospective referred pain pattern to the head, mid back, shoulder, and even upper extremity.

The diagnosis of CFS involves a thorough history and physical examination in addition to imaging studies. Patients may have headache and limited range of motion of the cervical spine. The provocation of pain associated with extension and lateral rotation of neck, tenderness on palpation of facet joints or spinal muscles, and absence of neurologic deficit support the clinical impression of CFS. Patients may have coexisting upper extremity pain, although CFS is not usually associated with radicular symptoms.

Pain referral patterns have been well correlated between injection of contrast medium and electrical stimulation of medial branches. The potential referred and usually overlapping pain patterns due to CFS are as follows:
- C1–C2: posterior auricular and occipital region
- C2–C3: nuchal ridge, forehead, and orbital regions
- C3–C4: suboccipital posterior and lateral neck

- C4–C5: lower part and base of neck
- C5–C6: shoulders and suprascapular regions
- C6–C7: supraspinous and infraspinous fossa and in between scapulae

Laboratory tests and diagnostic investigations

Electromyography (EMG) and nerve conduction studies (NCS) need to be considered in a working diagnosis of CFS only to rule out cervical radiculopathy or other peripheral nerve neuropathy or pathology.

Laboratory tests may be ordered to rule out infection or other autoimmune disease affecting the cervical facet joints, or other systemic conditions.

Imaging studies

Standard radiography with additional flexion and extension views is indicated for the diagnosis of degenerative changes, spondylosis, and spondylolisthesis. CT and MRI may help to verify any imaging diagnosis but cannot rule out a clinical diagnosis of CFS. Although any of the imaging studies may reveal degenerative changes indicating facet arthropathy, there is no definite correlation between severity of pain due to CFS and the radiologic findings.

Differential diagnosis

Cervical radiculopathy at the C4 and C5 levels may have more localized neck and shoulder pain, with reduced radicular extremity symptoms, and may therefore mimic CFS. Case studies have reported coexisting degenerative changes in cervical discs and facet joints that both contribute as pain generators in the clinical presentation. It would be beneficial to formulate a comprehensive treatment plan that engages both cervical disc and facet joint.

Myofascial pain, fibromyalgia, inflammatory or degenerative arthritis, tendinitis, and bursitis of the shoulder may present with overlapping symptoms similar to CFS. In cases of persistent neck, shoulder, and upper back pain that are refractory to myofascial release and treatment of arthritis, the diagnosis of CFS needs to be entertained as soon as possible.

Cervicobrachial syndrome, brachial plexopathy, and thoracic outlet syndrome involving part of the brachial plexus should be considered in the differential diagnosis of CFS.

Pharmacotherapy

Acetaminophen, non-steroidal anti-inflammatory drugs (NSAIDs), cyclooxygenase-2 (COX-2) inhibitors, and skeletal muscle relaxants may offer symptomatic relief of mild to moderate pain and muscle spasm, especially in the acute phase of CFS. A topical patch of a sodium channel blocking agent such as lidocaine may be considered in the management of CFS. Anticonvulsants may be used off-label to alleviate numbness and tingling related to any neuropathic pain component of CFS; these agents may be more advantageous in cervical radiculopathy than in the more inflammatory and nociceptive process in the pain generators associated with CFS.

Although opioids are commonly prescribed in moderate to severe acute pain, their efficacy in chronic pain management of CFS has not been supported by evidence-based studies.

Non-pharmacologic approaches

Physical modalities (e.g., heat, cold, ultrasound, electrical stimulation, manual therapy, joint mobilization, massage, water therapy, and low-impact exercise programs) and complementary and alternative therapies (e.g., acupuncture) may all be valuable for different phases of CFS with or without concomitant degenerative disc disease and radiculopathy.

Interventional procedures

Cervical facet joint intra-articular injection with local anesthetics can serve as a diagnostic tool to verify the specific pain generator, and can result in clinical improvement in the range of motion of the neck in CFS. However, studies have shown wide variation regarding the duration of pain relief after intra-articular cervical facet joint injection, and thus the evidence is poor.

Neural blockade of the medial branch (of the dorsal ramus) may denervate muscle, ligament, and periosteum in addition to the facet joint. Radiofrequency neuroablation (neurotomy) of the facet medial branch may provide more lasting pain relief (estimate of nerve regeneration up to 6–9 months) than local anesthetic block, and it may facilitate physical therapy and functional restoration in CFS.

Candidates selected for radiofrequency thermal neurolysis must undergo informed consent, which should include adverse events such as worsening of baseline pain, procedure site pain and neuritis, burning pain and dysesthesia, sensory or motor deficit, and headache.

Neuromodulation therapy, such as spinal cord stimulation, may not be as effective in the management of CFS as it is in alleviating the more radicular pain commonly seen in cervical radiculopathy.

Follow-up

Rather than merely gauging the level of pain, follow-up in CFS should focus on assessing improvements in range of motion of the neck and in functional capacity.

Prognosis

Although the natural course of cervical facet arthropathy leads to deterioration of joint condition and agonizing pain, any spinal surgery, instrumentation, or fusion should be reserved for selected candidates only, and should be based on thoughtful decision making. The outcome after spinal fusion in CFS may not be as hopeful as is the symptomatic relief of radicular pain associated with disc disease and radiculopathy.

REFERENCES AND FURTHER READING

Bogduk N. On cervical zygapophysial joint pain after whiplash. *Spine (Phila Pa 1976)* 2011; **36** (25 Suppl): S194–9.

Husted DS, Orton D, Schofferman J, Kine G. Effectiveness of repeated radiofrequency neurotomy for cervical facet joint pain. *J Spinal Disord Tech* 2008; **21**: 406–8.

Kirpalani D, Mitra R. Cervical facet joint dysfunction: a review. *Arch Phys Med Rehabil* 2008; **89**: 770–4.

Manchikanti L, Helm S, Singh V, *et al.* An algorithmic approach for clinical management of chronic spinal pain. *Pain Physician* 2009; **12**: E225–64.

Peloso P, Gross A, Haines T, *et al.* Medicinal and injection therapies for mechanical neck disorders. *Cochrane Database Syst Rev* 2007; (3): CD000319.

12

Cervicobrachial pain syndrome, cervical dystonia, and spasmodic torticollis

Clinical presentation

Myofascial pain syndrome describes a soft tissue pain with localized trigger points and referred pain following a specific pattern. Myofascial pain and trigger points may involve regions such as the neck, upper back, axilla, shoulder, and upper extremities. The term cervicobrachial pain syndrome was used to describe a clinical syndrome of neck, upper back, axilla, and arm pain without any other specific diagnosis or underlying etiology. Cervical dystonia (CD) is a common form of focal dystonia in adults that is associated with repetitive twisting movements and abnormal posture. CD is mostly due to central dysfunction and more common in women, with onset around the fourth or fifth decade. CD may have various appearances such as rotation (spasmodic torticollis), flexion (anterocollis), extension (retrocollis), lateral shift, and side tilt (laterocollis) of the neck. There may be three general types of involuntary movements in spasmodic torticollis (ST) such as tonic (turning), clonic (shaking), and both tonic and clonic.

Signs and symptoms

Cervicobrachial pain presents with focal tenderness on palpation (trigger point) and distant referral pain and muscle spasm with numbness and tingling that does not usually result in the full spectrum of dystonia. As time goes by, CD may present, with sustained abnormal postures and rigid contractures. Meanwhile, ST describes involuntary movement of the head, continuous dystonia, and obvious laterocollis. ST may be associated with progressive aching pain, which often alerts the patient to call for medical attention. ST is usually less prominent while the patient is just awakening, but it deteriorates as the day progresses and activity goes on. The muscle spasm may involve the whole neck; the involvement of paraspinal muscles and sternocleidomastoid, and an escalating level of pain, are all striking features of ST.

Neurologic examinations are typically within normal limits in cervicobrachial syndrome. There is usually no focal neurologic deficit, even in the easily noticeable dystonic status of CD and ST.

Laboratory tests and diagnostic investigations

Common laboratory tests, e.g., complete blood cell count, erythrocyte sedimentation rate, and chemistry profiles, are ordered while establishing the diagnosis of cervicobrachial pain, CD, and ST to rule out any conditions such as inflammation, infection, illness, or neoplasm.

Electromyography (EMG) may help to distinguish CD from psychogenic torticollis. EMG may provide additional assistance and confirmation of involuntary contracture of deeper muscle, as a target for the injection of botulinum toxin.

Imaging studies

Standard imaging studies are indicated to rule out underlying pathology in the cervical spine, brachial plexus, shoulder and upper extremity. MRI of the brain and brainstem are indicated in CD and ST to detect any other underlying pathology such as tumors and demyelinating disease. Magnetic resonance angiography (MRA) may help to confirm that there is no aneurysm or other vascular abnormality. A CT scan serves as an alternative if there is a contraindication for MRI and MRA in the process of work-up.

Differential diagnosis

It is prudent to differentiate cervicobrachial pain syndrome from both brachial plexopathy and thoracic outlet syndrome. Fibromyalgia is a more widespread pain syndrome associated with multiple comorbidities and systemic dysfunctions. Cervical facet arthropathy or spondylosis could present with localized pain and spasm that mimic cervicobrachial syndrome and CD.

The characteristic feature of CD is the continuous active movement of the neck versus only a fixed contracture. The involuntary nature of the movement disorder is the hallmark of ST, distinguishing it from tics and habit spasms that are voluntary and exacerbate whenever patients are tense. Hysteric conversion needs to be cautiously evaluated if there is any suspicion regarding any background of behavior disorder associated with ST. The differential diagnosis of CD may also include essential tremor, cerebral palsy, multiple sclerosis, myasthenia gravis, tardive dyskinesia, and adverse effects of psychopharmacology.

Pharmacotherapy

There is no standard of care on pharmacotherapy of inflammatory, nociceptive, or neuropathic pain components in cervicobrachial pain syndrome, CD, and ST. Acetaminophen, non-steroidal anti-inflammatory drugs (NSAIDs), cyclooxygenase-2 (COX-2) inhibitors, and skeletal muscle relaxants are commonly used. Although the skeletal muscle relaxants may sound more logical as a means of suppressing the CNS mechanism of CD and ST, yet the clinical outcome is not always promising. Various anticonvulsants have been prescribed as adjuvant analgesics in cervicobrachial pain syndrome, CD, or ST without any convincing advantage in either clinical course or prognosis.

Although opioids are prescribed in moderate to severe acute pain, their efficacy in the management of chronic cervicobrachial pain, CD, and ST has not been supported by evidence-based studies.

Non-pharmacologic approaches

Hands-on techniques such as massage, myofascial release, manipulation, stretch and spray, or adjustments are all popular in acute and chronic pain management of neck, axilla, and shoulder pain. Comprehensive physical therapy and an ongoing active exercise program in addition to pharmacotherapy are advisable for cervicobrachial pain, CD, and ST. Cognitive behavioral therapy (CBT), relaxation, biofeedback, and neurofeedback may also form part of a multidisciplinary approach together with pharmacotherapy.

Interventional procedures

A variety of needling techniques are popular in cervicobrachial pain, CD, and ST, including local anesthetic injection, acupressure, and acupuncture for trigger-point and specific referral pain. However, these procedures may only provide temporary benefit without any progress, especially in CD and ST versus cervicobrachial pain syndrome.

Botulinum toxin injection over the affected side in CD has been an effective treatment in refractory cases, according to the evidence-based literature. Dysphagia after botulinum toxin injection in CD may result from weakening of the laryngeal muscles, leading to a risk of aspiration. Swallowing studies should be an essential step in evaluation prior to the decision and consent for botulinum toxin injection in the treatment of CD. Botulinum toxin injections are well documented in the dystonia disorders (e.g. CD and ST), supported by a precise disease model that allows for the assessment of cost, risk, and benefit ratios; they are more warranted in CD and ST than as a treatment for the pain and dysfunction of the cervicobrachial and myofascial pain syndromes.

Follow-up

Cervicobrachial syndrome, CD, and ST may all benefit from interdisciplinary and multimodal approaches in order to achieve the most favorable outcome in both pain management and functional restoration.

Prognosis

Early diagnosis and timely intervention in cervicobrachial syndrome, CD, and ST may result in superior prognosis and functional restoration. In ST and CD the outcome may also depend on the availability of dedicated neurology, physical medicine, and rehabilitation services, and on expertise with botulinum toxin.

REFERENCES AND FURTHER READING

Benecke R, Heinze A, Reichel G, Hefter H, Göbel H; Dysport Myofascial Pain Study Group. Botulinum type A toxin complex for the relief of upper back myofascial pain syndrome: how do fixed-location injections compare with triggerpoint-focused injections? *Pain Med* 2011; **12**: 1607–14.

Crowner BE. Cervical dystonia: disease profile and clinical management. *Phys Ther* 2007; **87**: 1511–26.

Esquenazi A, Novak I, Sheean G, Singer BJ, Ward AB. International consensus statement for the use of botulinum toxin treatment in adults and children with neurological impairments–introduction. *Eur J Neurol* 2010; **17** (Suppl 2): 1–8.

Hefter H, Kupsch A, Müngersdorf M, *et al.*; Dysport Myofascial Pain Study Group. A botulinum toxin A treatment algorithm for de novo management of torticollis and laterocollis. *BMJ Open* 2011; **1**: e000196. doi: 10.1136/bmjopen-2011-000196.

Zetterberg L, Halvorsen K, Färnstrand C, Aquilonius SM, Lindmark B. Physiotherapy in cervical dystonia: six experimental single-case studies. *Physiother Theory Pract* 2008; **24**: 275–90.

13

Brachial plexopathy

Clinical presentation

Brachial plexopathy may present with moderate or severe pain over axilla, shoulder, and arm. It is commonly associated with a history of contusion, gunshot or traumatic avulsions, and over-stretch injury of the axillary region. Birth injuries may cause brachial plexopathy in newborns. There are also idiopathic or non-specific viral or inflammatory causes (e.g., Parsonage–Turner syndrome) as uncommon etiologies of brachial plexopathy. In any oncology patient who complains of severe neck, axilla, shoulder, and arm pain, with Horner's syndrome, brachial plexopathy could be caused by primary or metastatic invasion of the lower plexus by neoplasms (e.g., Pancoast tumor, other lung or breast cancer). Post-radiation fibrosis and brachial plexopathy usually involve the upper plexus, and present with lymphedema and gradual onset of paresthesia without significant pain.

Brachial plexopathy can be classified according to the part (e.g., cord, trunk, root), or anatomic level (e.g., supraclavicular, infraclavicular, interscalene).

Signs and symptoms

Patients usually complain of significant numbness and weakness in addition to significant pain, commonly involving the axilla, the supraclavicular or infraclavicular region of the shoulder, and the ipsilateral arm. Exacerbations of the pain level may prohibit further movement of neck and shoulder, which usually results in progressively worsening dysfunction of the neck, chest wall, shoulder, and upper extremity.

Nerve injuries and involvement of the sympathetic nervous system are possible, and this may result in manifestation of complex regional pain syndrome II (CRPS II, causalgia). The presentation may start with neuropathic pain, vasomotor and sudomotor changes, and then motor weakness that may correspond to nerve root, trunk, cord, or a specific nerve.

Laboratory tests and diagnostic investigations

Electrodiagnostic studies may help to determine the level of injury and the specific sites of involved nerve or roots. Electromyography (EMG) and nerve conduction studies (NCS) can outline the specific findings a few weeks after the injury. An EMG of the affected arm and shoulder muscles may show any fibrillation potentials and positive waves (evidence of denervation) in case of neoplastic brachial plexopathy. Somatosensory evoked potentials (SEPs) may help to confirm axonal continuity and determine whether lesions are preganglionic or postganglionic.

Imaging studies

Sonography studies may offer preliminary screening without radiation exposure. MRI and CT of the cervical spine and brachial plexus are characteristic choices for neuroradiologic evaluation of brachial plexopathy. Although MR neurography has been proposed recently to assist in the evaluation of injury over the peripheral nervous system, there is no solid scientific evidence yet. Bone scan and imaging studies with and without contrast are indicated for a working diagnosis of CRPS or where there is suspicion of malignancy or infection.

MRI with gadolinium will enhance recurrent neoplasm as compared to an area of radiation brachial plexopathy. Nevertheless, fluorodeoxyglucose positron emission tomography (FDG-PET) CT scanning is potentially valuable when metastatic cancer is suspected in a case of brachial plexopathy, especially when other imaging studies are inconclusive.

Differential diagnosis

The differential diagnosis includes spinal pathology such as cervical disc diseases, radiculopathy, facet arthropathy, and spondylosis. Osteoarthritis or bursitis of the shoulder joint may need further work-up in the differential diagnosis. Myofascial pain, cervicobrachial syndrome, cervical dystonia, spasmodic torticollis, and thoracic outlet syndrome can present with some overlapping clinical pictures just like that of brachial plexopathy. CRPS should always be evaluated, since it is frequently secondary to brachial plexopathy.

Pharmacotherapy

Anticonvulsants, tricyclic antidepressants (TCAs), serotonin–norepinephrine reuptake inhibitors (SNRIs), and local anesthetics have been proposed for modulation of the neuropathic pain associated with brachial plexopathy. However, acetaminophen, non-steroidal anti-inflammatory drugs (NSAIDs), cyclooxygenase-2 (COX-2) inhibitors, and skeletal muscle relaxants may alleviate mild to moderate pain with a nociceptive etiology. All these adjuvant analgesics require vigilant follow-up throughout the course of pain management, during titration, maintenance, and tapering off.

Although opioids are prescribed in moderate to severe acute pain, their efficacy in chronic pain management for brachial plexopathy has not been well supported by evidence-based studies.

Non-pharmacologic approaches

Physical and occupational therapy are essential components of comprehensive management in brachial plexopathy. Hands-on modalities such as massage, manipulation, adjustments, ultrasound, and transcutaneous electrical nerve stimulation (TENS) are prevalent in both acute and chronic management of neck, axilla, shoulder, and arm pain. The psychosocial impact of a traumatic injury that resulted in brachial plexopathy can never be overestimated; hence patient support groups, cognitive behavioral therapy (CBT), biofeedback, and neurofeedback could all be reasonably beneficial as part of an interdisciplinary and multimodal approach.

Interventional procedures

Brachial plexus block with local anesthetic and corticosteroid can be used as both a diagnostic and a therapeutic approach. Cervicothoracic sympathetic (stellate ganglion) block is indicated for alleviation of either sympathetic overlay with brachial plexopathy or CRPS as a working diagnosis. Radiofrequency ablation of the brachial plexus has been reported in cases of avulsion or tumor invasion. Neuromodulation therapy, such as a trial of spinal cord, peripheral nerve, or deep brain stimulation, may be an alternative modality to minimize adverse events, avoiding any denervation or destruction of structure.

In traumatic brachial plexopathy, surgical exploration and repair of the lesion should be carried out as soon as possible. Tendon transfer and osteomy have also been reported in selected candidates. Neurosurgical intervention, for example dorsal root entry zone (DREZ) lesioning, can be considered for the palliative care of intractable brachial plexopathy.

Follow-up

Interdisciplinary and multimodal approaches, with vigilant follow-up guiding every step of treatment, are mandatory in brachial plexopathy.

Prognosis

The prognosis of brachial plexopathy really depends on the underlying disease (e.g., birth injury, idiopathic, trauma, or neoplasm). In general, upper brachial plexus injury may have a better prognosis than lower plexus injury. It is still possible to work on improving the patient's functional capacity and quality of life despite the deteriorating course of brachial plexopathy.

REFERENCES AND FURTHER READING

Aichaoui F, Mertens P, Sindou M. Dorsal root entry zone lesioning for pain after brachial plexus avulsion: results with special emphasis on differential effects on the paroxysmal versus the continuous components. A prospective study in a 29-patient consecutive series. *Pain* 2011; **152**: 1923–30.

Ali M, Saitoh Y, Oshino S, *et al.* Differential efficacy of electric motor cortex stimulation and lesioning of the dorsal root entry zone for continuous vs. paroxysmal pain after brachial plexus avulsion. *Neurosurgery* 2011; **68**: 1252–7.

Chen HJ, Tu YK. Long term follow-up results of dorsal root entry zone lesions for intractable pain after brachial plexus avulsion injuries. *Acta Neurochir Suppl* 2006; **99**: 73–5.

Lai HY, Lee CY, Lee ST. High cervical spinal cord stimulation after failed dorsal root entry zone surgery for brachial plexus avulsion pain. *Surg Neurol* 2009; **72**: 286–9.

Pagni CA, Canavero S, Bonicalzi V, Nurisso C. The important role of pain in neurorehabilitation. The neurosurgeon's approach or (neurorehabilitation: the neurosurgeon's role with special emphasis on pain and spasticity). *Acta Neurochir Suppl* 2002; **79**: 67–74.

14

Thoracic outlet syndrome

Clinical presentation

Thoracic outlet syndrome (TOS) is attributed to compression of the neurovascular structures (brachial plexus, subclavian artery and vein) where they exit the narrow space between the shoulder girdle and the first rib. TOS may be noticed in cases of congenital or abnormal cervical rib, contracted scalene muscles, or trauma and malunion of clavicular fracture. The most common – and controversial – type is neurogenic or non-specific TOS, which is usually associated with numbness, tingling, and pain, but without any obvious vascular compromise or recognized neurologic dysfunction. Neurogenic TOS is more prevalent in women aged 20–60.

Signs and symptoms

Numbness and tingling, in addition to a vague aching pain over the neck, chest wall, supraclavicular shoulder, and upper extremity, are a common spectrum of symptoms in TOS. Patients may also present with signs of arterial or venous insufficiency.

Physical examinations may reveal dysesthesia and subjective or objective motor weakness. However, the range of provocative tests, checking for diminished radial pulse and for either reproduction or aggravation of baseline symptoms, may provide high sensitivity but relatively low specificity in the clinical differential diagnosis of TOS.

- The Adson or scalene maneuver is performed with the affected arm held extended, externally rotated, and slightly abducted. The ipsilateral wrist pulse is palpated and monitored to see if it diminishes or may reproduce the symptoms while the head is turned toward the same side with a sustained inspiration.
- The Wright or shoulder brace position, or military maneuver, is used to flex the elbow, retract the shoulder backward and downward, then check for reduction of radial pulse or aggravation of baseline symptoms of TOS.

. In the Roos stress test, or abduction and external rotation (AER) or hands-up test, the arms are held at 90 degrees at the shoulders with the elbows flexed at 90 degrees and the hands are contracted repeatedly for up to 3 minutes. A test positive for TOS will demonstrate paresthesia, fatigue, and pain over the affected upper extremity after usually much less than 3 minutes.

Laboratory tests and diagnostic investigations

Electromyography (EMG) or nerve conduction studies (NCS) are useful to identify injury to the nerve root, brachial plexus, or peripheral nerves, e.g., ulnar or median nerve. EMG and NCS have been frequently normal in "non-specific" neurogenic TOS. The demonstrable or "true" neurologic (axonal) TOS may reveal abnormal EMG over the C8 or T1 myotomes.

Ulnar nerve somatosensory evoked potentials (SEPs) have been proposed to assist in the diagnosis of neurogenic TOS versus vascular or other non-specific etiologies.

Imaging studies

The role of imaging studies in the confirmation of TOS has not been clearly defined, and more investigations are needed to establish the standard protocol. Chest or cervical spine radiography may catch the congenital or abnormal cervical ribs, if they exist. CT scan may evaluate either bony or vascular structures but is not as specific for soft tissue. MRI of neck, shoulder, and brachial plexus may detect possible pathology and/or distortion or displacement of the brachial plexus or subclavian veins. However, vascular compression may be observed in the normal population without TOS. MR neurography may help to delineate any pathology over the course of the brachial plexus trunks as they pass through the scalene triangle, with signal change of any hypothetically affected nerve structures.

Differential diagnosis

Spurling's test may help to confirm cervical radiculopathy by demonstration of radicular pain and numbness and tingling dysesthesia with lateral flexion of the neck toward the affected side, due to protrusion or herniation of cervical discs. Carpal tunnel syndrome and ulnar entrapment neuropathy are potential differential diagnoses.

Diffuse pain, muscle tenderness, and spasm are commonly seen in patients with cervical facet arthropathy, myofascial pain, cervicobrachial syndrome, fibromyalgia, and brachial plexopathy.

Acute whiplash injury or neck strain and sprain related to trauma, especially in a motor vehicle accident, could mimic TOS. However, TOS may transpire later as a consequence of compromise of vascular or neurogenic structures or significant contracture of scalene muscles.

Nerve injuries and involvement of the sympathetic nervous system may result in manifestation of complex regional pain syndrome I (CRPS I, reflex sympathetic dystrophy, RSD). The presentation may start with neuropathic pain, vasomotor and sudomotor changes, and then motor weakness without specific nerve lesion or correspondence to a specific dermatome.

Pharmacotherapy

Acetaminophen, non-steroidal anti-inflammatory drugs (NSAIDs), cyclooxygenase-2 (COX-2) inhibitors, and skeletal muscle relaxants have all been frequently prescribed for both acute and chronic management in a working diagnosis of TOS. However, there is no strong support from evidence-based studies for their use in the treatment of TOS.

Anticonvulsants, tricyclic antidepressants (TCAs), and serotonin–norepinephrine reuptake inhibitors (SNRIs) have been frequently prescribed for modulation of the presumed neuropathic pain component associated with TOS. This is an off-label use of anticonvulsants and antidepressants in TOS according to all previous efficacy studies on chronic pain management.

However, all these non-opioid adjuvant analgesics may provide an opioid-sparing effect in TOS, especially in cases of the controversial non-specific neurogenic TOS.

Although opioids are prescribed in moderate to severe acute pain, their efficacy in the management of chronic pain in TOS has not been supported by evidence-based studies.

Non-pharmacologic approaches

Physical modalities (e.g., heat, cold, ultrasound, electrical stimulation, massage) and complementary and alternative medicine (e.g., acupuncture) may all be valuable at different stages of TOS.

Physical therapy with water exercises, postural training, and stretch and strengthening programs may be considered in TOS. Psychosocial counseling and a support group are crucial. Meditation, relaxation, biofeedback, and neurofeedback of scalene muscles and all other involved structures may be appreciated in the management of TOS.

Interventional procedures

Brachial plexus block with local anesthetic and corticosteroid can be used as both a diagnostic and a therapeutic approach in work-up and pain management of TOS. Ultrasound- and EMG-guided intrascalene muscle injection of bupivacaine, and subsequent injection of botulinum toxin, has been studied for both diagnostic and therapeutic approaches in neurogenic TOS, prior to a decision concerning surgical intervention.

Cervicothoracic sympathetic (stellate ganglion) block is indicated for the alleviation of sympathetic overlay with TOS or when CRPS I is emerging as a working diagnosis. Neuromodulation therapy, such as a trial of spinal cord or peripheral nerve stimulation, may be an alternative modality to avoid any denervation or destruction of structure and to minimize adverse events.

Surgery is indicated in cases of vascular compromise, wasting of muscle, and loss of function. Surgery may consist of supraclavicular decompression of the compromised subclavian vessels, and/or radical excision of the anterior and middle scalene muscles, and removal of any abnormal cervical rib. Transaxillary exploration of the first rib and lysis of adhesions in the brachial plexus, exploration of the malunion of a clavicle fracture, and decompression of pectoralis minor muscle are among numerous techniques reported in case studies of TOS, with variable outcomes.

Follow-up

The disease model and definitive diagnostic criteria are still controversial, especially in cases of non-specific neurogenic TOS. Vigilant follow-up in the working diagnosis and management of TOS should always be the standard of care.

Prognosis

The prognosis of TOS really depends on whether there is any identified etiology or pathology correlated with the clinical presentation. Whether timely medical and surgical interventions are available via an interdisciplinary and multimodal approach may also affect the outcome of an assumed case of TOS.

REFERENCES AND FURTHER READING

Chandra V, Olcott C, Lee JT. Early results of a highly selective algorithm for surgery on patients with neurogenic thoracic outlet syndrome. *J Vasc Surg* 2011; **54**: 1698–705.

Chang K, Graf E, Davis K, *et al.* Spectrum of thoracic outlet syndrome presentation in adolescents. *Arch Sur* 2011; **146**: 1383–7.

Finlayson HC, O'Connor RJ, Brasher PM, Travlos A. Botulinum toxin injection for management of thoracic outlet syndrome: a double-blind, randomized, controlled trial. *Pain* 2011; **152**: 2023–8.

Jordan SE, Ahn SS, Gelabert HA. Differentiation of thoracic outlet syndrome from treatment-resistant cervical brachial pain syndromes: development and utilization of a questionnaire, clinical examination and ultrasound evaluation. *Pain Physician* 2007; **10**: 441–52. Erratum in *Pain Physician* 2007; **10**: 599.

Nichols AW. Diagnosis and management of thoracic outlet syndrome. *Curr Sports Med Rep* 2009; **8**: 240–9.

15

Shoulder arthritis

Clinical presentation

Shoulder pain is a non-specific complaint that can be due to multiple etiologies. An understanding of shoulder anatomy is imperative for understanding the causes of shoulder pain. The shoulder is made up of multiple articulations, including the glenohumeral, acromioclavicular, and sternoclavicular joints, as well as a scapulothoracic articulation.

Functionally, the shoulder is a ball and socket joint. Unlike the hip, which is also a ball and socket joint, the shoulder is not intrinsically stable. The shallow nature of the glenoid cup allows for increased range of motion but sacrifices stability. The cup is augmented by a labrum, which serves to deepen the glenoid cup. Ultimately, the stability and function of the glenohumeral joint is dependent upon the surrounding musculature.

The muscles of the rotator cuff, comprising the supraspinatus, infraspinatus, teres minor, and subscapularis, in addition to the deltoid, long head of biceps, pectoralis major, and latissimus dorsi, all serve to stabilize and mobilize the shoulder. Additional muscles of importance include the trapezius, rhomboid, and serratus anterior, all of which control scapular motion, which in turn impacts on glenohumeral function.

Degenerative joint disease (DJD) of the shoulder can involve the glenohumeral (GH) joint, as well as the acromioclavicular (AC) joint, either in isolation or in combination. The challenge is trying to determine the source generator for the shoulder pain. Intra-articular, musculotendinous, bursas, and neurogenic are all potential causes.

The focus of this chapter is on assessment of the shoulder with DJD.

Signs and symptoms

Typical complaints in shoulder DJD include limitations in range of motion. Commonly both internal and external rotation are limited, with internal rotation more affected. Pain is characteristically noted with range of motion, and lessened with rest. Crepitus, both audible and palpable, is a common manifestation in shoulder joint DJD.

Patients will note impairment in functional activities, such as the ability to reach over the head, tuck their shirt into their pants, reach into a rear pocket for a wallet, don and doff a bra, and comb and wash their hair. Lying on the affected shoulder may also be poorly tolerated secondary to GH joint compression with side lying.

Obtaining the above-noted complaints during the history-taking part of the examination is critical.

Observation during history taking is imperative. Patients with DJD of the shoulder will subconsciously guard the spontaneous movement of the shoulder and without realizing it keep all ranges of motion below shoulder height and within a restricted pain-free arc.

Additionally, observe for atrophy of the deltoid, supraspinatus, infraspinatus, and biceps muscles. Atrophy involving all of the above muscles could be secondary to cervical root level issues at C5–C6, or may be secondary to disuse atrophy from pain. Focal atrophy of the deltoid may be secondary to axillary nerve neuropathy. Focal atrophy of rotator cuff musculature can be neurogenic in etiology as well as secondary to rotator cuff tear.

In assessing the shoulder with DJD, it is critical to determine if there is an underlying cervical radiculopathy or isolated axillary nerve neuropathy, as this will complicate both management and prognosis.

Range of motion (ROM) assessment should be done both passively and actively. Elicitation of pain with the examiner ranging the shoulder joint through internal and external rotation is consistent with shoulder DJD. This is less likely to be seen in a rotator cuff tendinitis, which is typically more painful on volitional patient activation. Crepitus on ROM testing is also a common feature of shoulder DJD.

Manual muscle testing of the internal and external rotators of the shoulders should be carried out with the arm at the side and with the elbow flexed at 90 degrees. In this way GH rotation can be tested without placing the arm in an abducted position, which will be poorly tolerated if there is DJD involving the GH joint. Shoulder abduction can be assessed in an isometric manner with the arm at the side and having the person attempt active abduction at the GH joint while resistance is applied. Once again this allows for strength assessment while avoiding painful arcs of motion. Biceps function is assessed by having the person flex the elbow against resistance applied to the volar forearm. Subscapularis function can be assessed by having the patient press the palm of the hand into the belly using internal rotation at the shoulder. A positive test is noted if the elbow drops to the side or behind the trunk. The lift-off test evaluates the lower fibers of the subscapularis and is performed by having the patient place the dorsum of the hand at the position of the mid lumbar spine. The test is considered positive if the patient is unable to lift off the hand utilizing internal rotation at the GH joint, but rather substitutes shoulder extension or elbow extension to perform the maneuver. Rotator cuff function must be fully appreciated, as an incompetent rotator cuff allows for superior migration of the humeral head within the glenoid, causing impingement, which in turn further exacerbates the functional deficits of the shoulder with DJD. The grading for strength testing is on the 0–5 scale, with 0 being no activation, 1 a flicker of activity without motion, 2 full range of motion gravity eliminated, 3 full range of motion against gravity only, 4 full range of motion against greater than gravity resistance (able to take partial resistance), and lastly 5, which is full range of motion against full resistance.

Critical elements of sensory testing include the axillary patch or sergeant's patch to assess C5 as well as axillary nerve function, and the lateral forearm to check lateral antebrachial cutaneous nerve function (this is the sensory continuation of the musculocutaneous nerve, which in turn supplies motor function to the biceps, coracobrachialis, and brachialis muscles). Sensory function to the thumb and index finger allows for evaluation of C6 level root function. Detailed evaluation of C5–C6 level root function is imperative, as the major nerve supply to the shoulder musculature derives from the C5–C6 roots.

The resolution of shoulder pain with placement of the affected arm on top of the head, a positive abduction tension release sign, is highly suggestive of a C5 level radiculopathy and for all practical purposes rules out GH DJD, subacromial bursitis, or impingement syndrome as the source of the shoulder pain. The complaint of deep gnawing aching-type pain at the level of the rhomboid major muscle, just medial to the medial scapular border, is also highly suggestive of C5 level root involvement.

A simple test for AC joint pathology is the scratch test. The patient is asked to reach across his or her anterior chest to touch the posterior aspect of the contralateral shoulder, as if scratching the shoulder. A positive test will elicit pain over the ipsilateral AC joint, with an audible and palpable clunk being appreciated many times. This is classically seen in the face of a history of previous AC joint separation.

Laboratory tests and diagnostic investigations

Physical examination is the mainstay in the evaluation of the shoulder. Electrodiagnostic testing, in the form of electromyography (EMG) and nerve conduction studies (NCS), can have utility if one suspects radiculopathy, brachial plexopathy, or an isolated axillary or suprascapular nerve neuropathy.

Imaging studies

Radiographs to look at the overall architecture of the shoulder are important in the evaluation of the painful shoulder. They allow one to observe loss of GH joint space, AC joint arthritis changes, and Hill–Sachs deformities in the humeral head consistent with old shoulder dislocation injury. Subacromial spurring can also be seen on shoulder radiographs. A high-riding humeral head may be suggestive of rotator cuff tear.

MRI imaging allows for the detailed evaluation of the rotator cuff as well as the labrum.

MR arthrography can be helpful in the assessment of possible SLAP (superior labral anterior to posterior) lesions of the labrum, and can also have utility in the evaluation for intra-articular loose bodies.

Differential diagnosis

The major mimics in shoulder DJD include rotator cuff pathology, labral tears, subacromial bursitis, impingement syndrome, and AC joint arthritis/dysfunction in association with GH joint DJD.

Pharmacotherapy and non-pharmacologic approaches

Non-steroidal anti-inflammatory drugs (NSAIDs) can be utilized, but with caution, as their side-effect profile can be problematic for long-term use.

The treatment of shoulder (GH) arthritis presents several challenges. Ultimately the status of the rotator cuff and scapular stabilizer/mobilizer muscles is critical. Strengthening of cuff muscles within a pain-free arc is appropriate under physical therapy guidance. This can be accomplished with limited range of motion exercises or isometric exercises.

Diagnostic and potentially therapeutic intra-articular corticosteroid injections mixed with local anesthetic can be very helpful. The injection allows for the potential isolation of the pain generator. If an intra-articular injection with local anesthetic does not result in several hours of pain relief, it is unlikely that the GH joint is the primary source generator for the pain. In this scenario, other injections into the subdeltoid bursa region may be helpful in localization.

If all injections fail, strong consideration should be given to a non-structural/ mechanical cause for the pain. Neurogenic sources clearly become more likely, and strong consideration should be given to cervical radiculopathy involving the C5–C6 level roots. Additionally, axillary nerve neuropathy as well as suprascapular nerve neuropathy should be considered.

Interventional procedures

Shoulder arthroscopy for the treatment of subacromial spurs, causing impingement, can be of utility. Additionally, distal clavicle resection or AC joint resection may have a role in the management of the painful arthritic shoulder. In each case the goal is to increase the subacromial space to allow for a greater pain-free arc of motion.

Total shoulder arthroplasty has been demonstrated to be very efficacious for pain control. However, it does result in significant functional limitations, in that activities above shoulder height are not well tolerated, nor is weight bearing or pushing and pulling activities. It does provide for excellent pain relief in the refractory shoulder, however, and should be one of the treatment options available for consideration in the appropriate patient.

Follow-up and prognosis

The long-term prognosis of shoulder DJD is one of progression. The major thrust of intervention in early shoulder DJD would be to develop all the surrounding musculature. This may optimize joint motion and glenohumeral and scapulothoracic rhythm, decreasing the transmission of abnormal forces across the joint surfaces.

REFERENCES AND FURTHER READING

Ellman H, Harris E, Kay SP. Early degenerative joint disease simulating impingement syndrome. *Arthroscopy* 1992, **8**: 482–7.

Green S, Buchbinder R, Hetrick S. Physiotherapy interventions for shoulder pain. *Cochrane Database Syst Rev* 2003; (**2**): CD004258.

Guyette TM, Bae RF, Craig E, Wickiewicz TL. Results of arthroscopic subacromial decompression in patients with subacromial impingement and glenohumeral degenerative joint disease. *J Shoulder Elbow Surg* 2002; **11**: 299–304.

Johnson TS, Mesfin A, Farmer KW, *et al.* Accuracy of intra-articular glenohumeral injections: the anterosuperior technique with arthroscopic documentation. *Arthroscopy* 2011; **27**: 745–9.

Tokish JM, Decker MJ, Ellis HB, Torry MR, Hawkins RJ. The belly press test for the physical examination of the subscapularis muscle: Electromyographic validation and comparison to the lift-off test. *J Shoulder Elbow Surg* 2003; **12**: 427–30.

16

Shoulder bursitis and tendinitis

Clinical presentation

Bursitis and tendinitis can be common causes of shoulder dysfunction and pain. Two of the more significant bursas in the shoulder region are the subacromial and the subdeltoid bursa. The subacromial bursa is the more frequent source of pain of the two.

Tendinitis can occur at any tendon attachment to bone or at any myotendinous junction. Common locations for tendinopathies involving the shoulder region include rotator cuff tendinitis and biceps tendinitis.

As the names imply, both bursitis and tendinitis are associated with inflammation, and can be secondary to acute trauma, repetitive overuse, or possible underlying inflammatory disorders, such as rheumatoid arthritis and other associated inflammatory arthropathies.

Signs and symptoms

Common to both shoulder bursitis and tendinitis is the complaint of pain, particularly with activity.

With subacromial bursitis the patient will frequently note pain with both active and passive glenohumeral abduction. Patients will note poor tolerance for overhead activities and may note a subjective sense of arm weakness. Minimal pain is noted when the arm is held at the side, and patients will preferentially limit abduction. Lying on the symptomatic side may be poorly tolerated, but this is somewhat variable.

Subdeltoid bursitis will commonly present with complaints of aching-type pain in the deltoid region. Pain on active shoulder abduction will be a common feature, particularly with resistive abduction. Passive abduction is typically well tolerated, as there is no compromise of the subacromial space. Pain may also be elicited with palpation over the insertion of the deltoid on the humeral tubercle. Lying on the symptomatic side is commonly poorly tolerated.

Rotator cuff tendinitis commonly presents with many features that are similar to subacromial bursitis. Pain will be noted with both active and passive glenohumeral abduction. Additionally, rotator cuff tendinitis will also manifest with pain during resistive external rotation of the shoulder when the arm is held at the side with the elbow flexed to 90 degrees with resistive external rotation being tested. This is in contradistinction to subacromial bursitis, where this maneuver is generally reasonably well tolerated. Patients will note poor tolerance for abduction, overhead activities, and throwing activities. Falling asleep with the symptomatic arm overhead will predictably result in the patient being awakened by shoulder pain. With rotator cuff tendinitis, lying on the asymptomatic side with the symptomatic side up will result in pain when the symptomatic arm is left unsupported, allowing it to cross in front of the chest, placing the rotator cuff on stretch.

Biceps tendinitis will frequently manifest with complaints of pain on forward flexion of the shoulder, as this requires activation of the long head of the biceps. Resistive elbow flexion with supination is also poorly tolerated and will commonly localize pain to the anterior shoulder at the level of the bicipital groove. Forward flexion with resistance will augment the pain secondary to strong activation of the long head of the biceps. Patients will also note anterior shoulder pain, on palpation of the proximal biceps tendon.

In all instances the physical starts with visual inspection during the history-gathering part of the examination. Subconscious restriction of shoulder range of motion may be observed, and avoidance of reaching beyond shoulder height is a typical finding.

The muscle contour of the shoulder girdle should be assessed. Look for focal versus diffuse atrophy. Diffuse atrophy of the shoulder musculature may be neurogenic in etiology, but more commonly is secondary to disuse atrophy from pain inhibition. Focal atrophy raises the specter of a neurogenic cause, radicular versus possible focal peripheral nerve entrapment, such as an axillary nerve neuropathy.

Radiculopathies may manifest with loss of muscle strength and mass in a root distribution. Additionally, hyporeflexia may be noted on testing of the biceps (C5 root level innervation) or wrist extensor (C6 root level innervation). These two reflexes must always be tested in shoulder pain complaints, as they supply innervation to the major shoulder and scapular stabilizer and mobilizer musculature.

Manual muscle testing of the primary and secondary shoulder muscles is imperative. Primary muscles of the shoulder are those that directly control glenohumeral range of motion. Specifically, the deltoid, biceps, triceps, and rotator cuff muscles need to be tested, Additionally, the secondary shoulder muscles or scapular mobilizers, which include the serratus anterior, rhomboid, and trapezius, need to be tested. The serratus anterior is tested by having the patient actively protract the shoulder against resistance. If the serratus is weak, scapular winging will be noted. The scapular will pull away from the posterior thorax, making the medial border very prominent. A simple way to observe this is have the patient perform a push-up against the wall. Subtle weakness may require the patient to perform a full push-up on the floor. Rhomboid weakness will result in lateral winging of the scapula. Trapezius weakness will manifest with impaired shoulder shrug.

Focal testing of the rotator cuff muscles can be accomplished in several ways. The belly press and lift-off tests can evaluate the function of the subscapularis muscle. The tipped can test can isolate supraspinatus function. Passively placing the involved arm in an abducted, internally rotated position at the shoulder, with the arm aligned in the plane of the scapular, allows one to assess supraspinatus function. In essence one mimics the posture of pouring out a cup of water. Pain with resistance applied to the arm in this position can be secondary to rotator cuff tendinitis. Inability to hold this position can be seen with rotator cuff tear.

Sensory testing to evaluate specifically the C5–C6 roots is paramount to avoid missing a radiculopathy, which can complicate the treatment of shoulder bursitis and tendinitis.

Palpation of the subacromial space and subdeltoid region will be painful in the patient with bursitis. Bicipital tendinitis will manifest with pain on palpation of the proximal biceps tendon as it courses through the bicipital groove.

Laboratory tests and diagnostic investigations

Utilization of ancillary tests is guided by the history and physical examination, which in turn helps formulate the differential diagnosis. Concern for a cervical radiculopathy or brachial plexopathy necessitates additional investigation. This may include electrodiagnostic testing, in addition to appropriate imaging studies.

If the patient is noted to have inflammation involving multiple joints or bursas, consideration should be given to more systemic disorders. Blood work to check erythrocyte sedimentation rate (ESR), rheumatoid factor, antinuclear antibody (ANA), and C-reactive protein (CRP) are reasonable first steps in the work-up of a possible inflammatory arthropathy. Depending on the results of the blood work, referral to rheumatology may be appropriate.

Imaging studies

Radiographs are helpful in the evaluation of shoulder pain. They allow for simple inexpensive imaging of the glenohumeral (GH) joint, acromioclavicular (AC) joint, and subacromial space. Glenohumeral degenerative joint disease (DJD), AC joint arthritis, or subacromial spurs can all mimic subacromial bursitis or rotator cuff tendinitis-type complaints. Of equal importance is that all of these issues can augment and potentiate the pain complaints of shoulder bursitis and rotator cuff tendinitis.

MRI has utility, particularly in the patient where pain limits the ability to perform an adequate physical examination. MRI may reveal a cuff tear or possibly a labral tear.

Ultrasound can be helpful in finding small tears that are not large enough to be seen on MRI, but remains an operator-dependent tool.

Differential diagnosis

Cervical radiculopathy involving the C5–C6 roots, rotator cuff tears, and gleno-humeral DJD are common masqueraders. AC joint arthritis can also mimic subacromial bursitis. A positive scarf or scratch test is commonly seen in AC joint pathology. The test is performed by having the patient reach across his/her anterior chest with the symptomatic arm, while the arm is maintained in a horizontal position. Pain is elicited as the patient reaches across in an attempt to scratch or touch the contralateral posterior shoulder. Cervical radiculopathy should be recognized based upon findings noted on manual muscle testing, sensory testing, and evaluation of muscle stretch reflexes.

Pharmacotherapy and non-pharmacologic approaches

Initial first-line treatments should focus on controlling inflammation. Cautious use of non-steroidal anti-inflammatory drugs (NSAIDs) is appropriate, and can be supplemented with the application of ice. Ice is not only a potent anti-inflammatory agent but also has analgesic potential. Activity modification during the acute phase of inflammation is reasonable. Overhead activities should be limited, as should significant lifting and pulling activities.

Once the acute inflammation has been quieted, enrollment in physical therapy (PT) is appropriate. Premature utilization of PT may exacerbate the patient's pain complaints, especially if strengthening is started too quickly and progressed too aggressively. If started early, PT should focus on pain control, with utilization of modalities to decrease pain. Use of ice or steroid iontophoresis may be helpful. Ultimately, a slow progressive strengthening program can be undertaken. Initial strengthening should be done below shoulder height to avoid flaring of symptoms. Range of motion activities are important as well, and, as with strengthening, these should be progressed slowly to avoid exacerbations. Ultrasound can be helpful in more chronic bursitis and tendinitis issues as a source of heat.

Interventional procedures

Injections of the subacromial space as well as the intra-articular space have both diagnostic and potentially therapeutic efficacy. All injections should be done with a local anesthetic to assess for a local anesthetic response. This is critical, as localization of the source generator of the patient's shoulder pain is essential before one can hope to treat it.

Refractory subacromial bursitis and rotator cuff tendinitis may require arthroscopic intervention for subacromial decompression. However, before considering this, diagnostic injections should be performed. This can be done with local anesthetic to assess response. A positive response allows for localization of the pain generator. This is paramount before contemplating orthopedic referral.

Refractory biceps tendinitis can also potentially be approached and managed arthroscopically, with the above caveats noted and satisfied.

Follow-up and prognosis

Treatment of shoulder bursitis and tendinitis is episodic, and the prognosis is for remissions and episodic flares.

REFERENCES AND FURTHER READING

Elser F, Braun S, Dewing CB, Giphart JE, Millett PJ. Anatomy, function, injuries, and treatment of the long head of the biceps brachii tendon. *Arthroscopy* 2011; **27**: 581–92.

Friedman DJ, Dunn JC, Higgins LD, Warner JJ. Proximal biceps tendon: injuries and management. *Sports Med Arthosc* 2008; **16**: 162–9.

Hossain S, Jacobs LG, Hashmi R. The long-term effectiveness of steroid injections in primary acromioclavicular joint arthritis: a five-year prospective study. *J Shoulder Elbow Surg* 2008; **17**: 535–8.

Ottenheijm RP, Jansen MJ, Staal JB, *et al.* Accuracy of diagnostic ultrasound in patients with suspected subacromial disorders: a systematic review and meta-analysis. *Arch Phys Med Rehabil* 2010; **91**: 1616–25.

Serafini G, Sconfienza LM, Lacelli F, *et al.* Rotator cuff calcific tendonitis: short-term and 10-year outcomes after two-needle us-guided percutaneous treatment–nonrandomized controlled trial. *Radiology* 2009; **252**: 157–64.

17

Rotator cuff tear

Clinical presentation

Rotator cuff tears can present with a spectrum of complaints. Partial tears may present primarily with complaints of pain and volitional restriction of range of motion. Most commonly the patient with a partial cuff tear will restrict overhead activities and abduction activities.

Complete massive tears typically manifest with profound weakness in abduction as well as internal and external rotation. Scapular substitution is frequently seen in patients with massive tears. This can manifest as early activation of the trapezius to rotate the scapula to a more favorable position, to get around an incompetent rotator cuff. This can be seen with attempted abduction activities. The patient with a significant rotator cuff tear may therefore complain of upper trapezius ache, secondary to overuse.

Incomplete tears are usually secondary to chronic wear and tear, with fraying of the rotator cuff acquired over time. Complete tears are commonly associated with acute trauma and present with abrupt onset of weakness in abduction and shoulder rotation.

Signs and symptoms

Observation of the patient will reveal volitional restriction of shoulder range of motion. Motion may be limited by pain in incomplete tears or by marked weakness in full-thickness or complete tears.

Diffuse atrophy of shoulder girdle musculature may be manifest with incomplete tears secondary to long-term restriction of activities from pain.

Massive tears do not present with associated atrophy if they are acute in nature, as the sudden onset of profound weakness with abduction and shoulder rotation activities generally results in early evaluation. Massive tears that have been ignored for extended periods of time will be associated with shoulder girdle muscle atrophy.

Evaluation of rotator cuff strength can be assessed with the belly press test and lift-off test. As noted in Chapter 15, these tests are an excellent test of subscapularis muscle function, a major internal rotator cuff muscle.

Supraspinatus muscle strength is easily assessed with the tipped can test. A positive test is inability to assume the tip-can posture, seen in massive tears, or inability to tolerate resistive loading, seen in incomplete tears.

Shoulder impingement symptoms frequently occur with partial rotator cuff tears. Therefore, classic impingement signs will not uncommonly be noted. These include pain with passive glenohumeral abduction, as well as positive Neer and Hawkins tests. A positive Neer is seen with reproduction of shoulder pain with full forward flexion at the glenohumeral joint. A positive Hawkins is noted with reproduction of pain with passive forward shoulder flexion to 90 degrees with passive internal rotation at the glenohumeral joint. The elbow should be at 90 degrees of flexion as well.

In addition to the above-noted "special" tests, formal strength testing of the biceps and wrist extensors must be performed to ensure that a concomitant C5–C6 level radiculopathy is not being overlooked.

Additionally, sensory testing of the axillary (sergeant's patch), as well as the lateral antebrachial cutaneous and radial thumb, should be evaluated to assess not only for possible C5–C6 level radiculopathy, but also for possible upper trunk plexopathy in the patient with an acute traumatic rotator cuff tear.

Testing of the sergeant's patch also allows for the exploration of a possible isolated or superimposed axillary neuropathy.

Weakness of external rotation should always raise the question of possible suprascapular nerve neuropathy. Visual inspection of the infraspinatus fossa is critical to observe for possible atrophy of the infraspinatus muscle. Therefore a thorough examination of the shoulder requires that the patient remove all outer garments and wear an examination gown. Failure to adopt this simple measure will dramatically hamper the examiner's ability to establish the correct diagnosis.

Laboratory tests and diagnostic investigations

Electrodiagnostic testing is not needed to confirm a rotator cuff tear, but should be strongly considered if the examination points towards a possible neurogenic component. Cervical radiculopathy, brachial plexopathy, suprascapular nerve neuropathy, and axillary nerve neuropathy can all cause functional limitations that mimic primary rotator cuff dysfunction. Failure to appreciate these neurogenic causes will predictably result in a less than favorable outcome for all interventions, conservative as well as invasive. Not uncommonly, failure to respond to surgical repair of the rotator cuff is due to an unappreciated superimposed C5–C6 level radiculopathy. The success of a rotator cuff repair is low if the cuff musculature is partially enervated.

Imaging studies

Clinical examination is the mainstay for diagnosing rotator cuff pathology.

Imaging studies, such as MRI and MR arthrogram, allow for in-depth evaluation of the anatomy. This helps to confirm the clinical suspicion and also rule out other intra-articular pathology such as a SLAP (superior labral anterior to posterior) lesion, or a biceps tendon lesion, which can be difficult to discern in the patient with an acutely painful shoulder.

Ultrasound allows for the dynamic evaluation of the shoulder, and may pick up small tears not seen on MRI. However, interpretation is very much operator-dependent, and as such it is not the gold-standard evaluation tool to assess the rotator cuff.

Differential diagnosis

Based upon a focused yet detailed examination, the common mimics of a rotator cuff tear should be relatively easy to discern.

Common mimics include C5–C6 radiculopathy with partial denervation of the C5–C6 innervated musculature. This will result in a pattern of weakness in a radicular distribution. This includes not only all of the rotator cuff muscles, but also the deltoid and biceps, which receive significant innervation from the C5 nerve root. Additionally, the extensor carpri radialis longus and pronator teres may be weak, as they are innervated primarily by the C6 nerve root. This pattern of weakness is not seen with isolated rotator cuff pathology, as the biceps, extensor carpi radialis longus, and pronator teres are clearly not part of the rotator cuff.

An isolated suprascapular nerve neuropathy will manifest with weakness of external rotation, as the infraspinatus is a major external rotator of the glenohumeral joint. Early atrophy will be noted as well. Isolated infraspinatus atrophy is typical of suprascapular nerve compression at the level of the spinoglenoid notch, usually associated with a degenerative cyst.

Atrophy of both the supraspinatus and infraspinatus places the suprascapular nerve injury more proximal, and consideration for brachial plexopathy versus cervical radiculopathy should now be entertained.

Impingement syndromes may mimic rotator cuff tears, as pain may limit volitional activation of the cuff musculature, resulting in functional weakness. However, strength will be maintained if testing is performed in a pain-free arc.

SLAP lesions can also be confused for rotator cuff problems. However, SLAP lesions more commonly present with a catching type of sensation in the shoulder, usually associated with overhead throwing activities. SLAP lesions also commonly present with a complaint of deep aching pain in the shoulder that is poorly localized. Many times they are also associated with biceps tendinitis issues. Complaints of biceps tendon pain with palpation of the tendon at the level of the anterior shoulder, in concert with deep aching shoulder pain, should therefore raise the suspicion of labral pathology as opposed to rotator cuff issues.

Pharmacotherapy and non-pharmacologic approaches

Treatment depends to some degree on the extent of the rotator cuff tear. Small partial tears can be conservatively managed with a combination of initial activity modification, followed by physical therapy to work on strengthening of the rotator cuff and scapular stabilizers.

Initial pain management includes the use of ice and non-steroidal anti-inflammatory drugs (NSAIDs).

Interventional approaches

Acute massive tears respond best to surgical intervention. The goal in this case is to restore the structural integrity of the cuff and the mechanics of the shoulder. Early repair is recommended to avoid issues of retraction and contracture of the cuff musculature, which will complicate the repair and negatively impact on the long-term recovery.

Once there has been significant retraction and contracture of the rotator cuff musculature it is impossible to bring the cuff out to length, negating the possibility of a primary repair. At that point salvage procedures such as subacromial decompression may give pain relief, but will not result in functional gains. Physical therapy in this case may be of utility for strengthening of the scapular stabilizers, as well as the pectoralis major, deltoid, biceps, and latissimus dorsi. Strengthening these muscles can result in functional improvement in range of motion, because the deltoid is a potent shoulder abductor. The pectoralis major and latissimus dorsi are powerful internal rotators of the shoulder, and the biceps and anterior deltoid are potent forward flexors of the shoulder. The posterior deltoid can assist with eternal rotation. As one can see, strengthening of the musculature around the shoulder joint can result in improved function for the patient with a non-repairable rotator cuff tear.

Follow-up and prognosis

Patients with small partial tears may experience exacerbations of symptoms with repetitive activities of the shoulder, particularly overhead activities. Activity modification, with continued strengthening of the shoulder girdle musculature, can be helpful in decreasing the frequency and intensity of flairs by maintaining more normal shoulder kinematics.

Acute massive tears are best managed with surgical repair, followed by specific postoperative rehabilitation. Long-term maintenance of shoulder function is dependent upon continued range of motion and strengthening activities to avoid the complication of adhesive capsulitis.

REFERENCES AND FURTHER READING

Carbone S, Gumina S, Arceri V, *et al.* The impact of preoperative smoking habit on rotator cuff tear: cigarette smoking influences rotator cuff tear sizes. *J Shoulder Elbow Surg* 2012; **21**: 56–60.

Kluger R, Bock P, Mittlböck M, Krampla W, Engel A. Long-term survivorship of rotator cuff repairs using ultrasound and magnetic resonance imaging analysis. *Am J Sports Med* 2011; **39**: 2071–81.

Mihata T, Watanabe C, Fukunishi K, *et al.* Functional and structural outcomes of single-row versus double-row versus combined double-row and suture-bridge repair for rotator cuff tears. *Am J Sports Med* 2011; **39**: 2091–8.

Pedowitz RA, Yamaguchi K, Ahmad CS, *et al.* Optimizing the management of rotator cuff problems. *J Am Acad Orthop Surg* 2011; **19**: 368–79.

Singisetti K, Hinsche A. Shoulder ultrasonography versus arthroscopy for the detection of rotator cuff tears: analysis of errors. *J Orthop Surg (Hong Kong)* 2011; **19**: 76–9.

18

Elbow degenerative joint disease and elbow bursitis

Clinical presentation

The true elbow joint is composed of an articulation between the distal humerus and olecranon (proximal ulna).The humero-olecranon articulation represents a true hinge joint. The range of motion measured from the anatomic position is from full extension, zero degrees, to approximately 140 degrees of flexion.

Other motions frequently associated with elbow function, besides flexion and extension, include supination and pronation of the forearm. These are not motions of the true elbow joint, but rather represent a radio-ulnar articulation. However, these motions are critical to the biomechanical function of the elbow, because limitations in supination mechanically limit the ability of the biceps to work as an elbow flexor, and restrictions in pronation limit the biomechanical function of the brachioradialis muscle as an elbow flexor.

Common causes of elbow degenerative joint disease (DJD) are traumatic arthritis and rheumatologic disorders such as rheumatoid arthritis (RA).

Olecranon bursitis is an inflammation of the bursa overlying the bony olecranon. Bursitis may be acute or chronic in nature. Common causes of acute olecranon bursitis include direct trauma and infection. Skin flora is a common infectious source, but in immunocompromised patients infections can be secondary to fungal infections as well as tuberculosis. Chronic bursitis can be secondary to repetitive low-grade trauma, as well as such disorders as RA and gout. Infection of the olecranon bursa requires management with appropriate antibiotics, and possible surgery for recalcitrant infections.

Signs and symptoms

True elbow joint arthritis or DJD will commonly present with complaints of pain and limitations of joint range of motion. Classically patients will note loss of terminal extension as well as possible loss of flexion. Anterior arthritic spurs at the humero-olecranon joint will typically result in loss of flexion. Loss of elbow extension should raise concerns of varus or valgus elbow joint deformity and malalignment.

Weakness noted during elbow flexion and extension activities will commonly occur secondary to pain. Complicating the clinical manifestation of weakness in elbow flexion and extension is the not uncommon finding of biceps and/or triceps atrophy. The atrophy in this case is from disuse, as opposed to a neurogenic etiology, and it is most likely secondary to reflex pain inhibition. Disuse atrophy most commonly presents with diffuse loss of muscle mass in the involved muscle without loss of general muscle contour. In contrast, neurogenic atrophy commonly manifests with scalloping out and wasting away of the muscle with associated loss of the general muscle contour. Observation of varus or valgus malalignment should raise the question of previous trauma, with a history of supracondylar humeral fracture being a common cause.

Radio-ulnar joint dysfunction will not usually result in limitations in elbow range of motion or dramatic loss of function. However, weakness of elbow flexion may be noted as a complaint, as the biceps is the major functional supinator of the forearm, in addition to being a powerful elbow flexor. Functional complaints are generally uncommon, as a loss of supination or pronation at the forearm level can easily be compensated for by internal or external rotation at the shoulder.

Acute olecranon bursitis commonly presents with pain localized to the olecranon with associated swelling and erythema. Patients will complain of pain with leaning on the elbow. Concerns with acute to subacute olecranon bursitis include infection of the bursa, versus possible presentation for gout, rheumatoid arthritis, or lupus. Chronic olecranon bursitis, or idiopathic, is typically painless, and without erythema or warmth.

History is vital in the evaluation of the arthritic elbow joint. History of an old supracondylar fracture of the humerus increases the risk of a tardy ulnar palsy. The term *tardy ulnar palsy* is commonly misused. It does not refer to the slowing of ulnar conduction velocities on EMG studies across the elbow, but rather refers to the late onset of ulnar nerve symptoms, many years after the supracondylar fracture.

Findings that increase the likelihood of a tardy ulnar palsy include cubitus valgus or varus deformity. The deformity at the elbow places the ulnar nerve on stretch. Additionally, one should look for wasting of the first dorsal interosseous (FDI) muscle, as this is the most distal muscle that is innervated by the ulnar nerve and commonly shows evidence of atrophy early in ulnar neuropathy.

RA can also be a cause of elbow deformity and loss of range of motion. Common physical exam findings that should trigger an investigation for possible underlying RA includes arthritic changes, swelling of the synovium of the metacarpophalangeal joints (MCPs), and ulnar rift of the MCPs. Swelling and pain of the small joints of the hands and feet should trigger an RA work-up in addition to evaluation for other spondyloarthropathies.

Observation of biceps and triceps bulk can also be helpful in appreciating the duration of the patient's complaint. Long-standing elbow DJD, with associated pain, will commonly result in diffuse loss of both triceps and biceps bulk. To rule out the possibility of neurogenic atrophy, assessment of the biceps and triceps reflexes is mandatory. Preservation of reflexes would argue against neurogenic causes for the atrophy and would support the diagnosis of atrophy secondary to pain inhibition from underlying elbow DJD.

The sensory examination should focus on ulnar nerve distribution sensation. Preserved ulnar sensation to the small finger and in the distribution of the dorsal ulnar cutaneous nerve would argue against ulnar nerve entrapment at the elbow. Altered sensation in the small finger and the dorsal ulnar cutaneous distribution would be consistent with ulnar nerve dysfunction at the elbow.

In elbow DJD, strength testing should include an assessment of elbow flexor and extensor strength. One must bear in mind that the patient's ability to give a full effort may be pain-limited. Muscle strength testing of ulnar-innervated muscles should include assessment of the flexor digitorum profundus (FDP) to the small and ring finger as well as the FDI.

FDP weakness in concert with FDI weakness would place the ulnar nerve dysfunction at the elbow. Isolated FDI weakness could be secondary to ulnar nerve dysfunction at the elbow or wrist.

Olecranon bursitis can be divided into two broad categories, acute and chronic. Acute olecranon bursitis may be secondary to acute focal trauma, such as falling on the elbow, or can be due to infection. Traumatic acute olecranon bursitis is usually obvious on history taking. Range of motion of the elbow should be assessed, and radiographs of the elbow and shoulder should be obtained to rule out concomitant fractures.

An infected olecranon bursa will typically present with pain in the elbow region and swelling of the bursa, with erythema, warmth, and sometimes drainage. Chronic olecranon bursitis presents several challenges. It may be secondary to systemic disorders such as RA, gout, or lupus or it may be idiopathic. The typical presentation in this case is one of a boggy olecranon bursa that is non-painful to palpation. It is not associated with warmth, erythema, or drainage. The imperative in chronic olecranon bursitis is determining if there is an underlying source generator. Once again, history and physical will be of paramount importance.

Laboratory tests and diagnostic investigations

Eletrodiagnostic testing should be considered in a patient with historical findings and physical examination consistent with a tardy ulnar palsy, or ulnar nerve dysfunction in general.

Blood work to evaluate for RA, lupus, gout, and infection is appropriate when clinical suspicion warrants.

Imaging studies

Plain film x-rays should be obtained as part of the evaluation of the arthritic elbow joint. They should also be obtained for instances of acute traumatic olecranon bursitis, to rule out olecranon fracture.

For the arthritic elbow, x-rays allow for evaluation of the true elbow joint space, proximal radio-ulnar joint, and presence of loose bodies within the elbow joint.

In general, MRI studies are not necessary.

Differential diagnosis

If elbow flexor weakness is noted one must consider a C5–C6 radiculopathy as the etiology of weakness. Triceps weakness may be secondary to a C7 level radiculopathy. Tendinitis of the distal biceps tendon may also present with complaints of elbow pain and weakness. Ulnar neuropathy at the elbow can cause medial elbow region pain.

Pharmacotherapy and non-pharmacologic approaches

Treatment for DJD of the elbow should be stratified based upon pain, dysfunction, and patient desires. First-line management of the pain should include a trial of ice and non-steroidal anti-inflammatory drugs (NSAIDs). Care should be exercised in the use of NSAIDs in patients with a history of ulcers, renal insufficiency, hypertension, and coronary artery disease.

Physical therapy may be helpful. Gentle strengthening of the elbow flexors and extensors may increase function. If range of motion is limited by pain, isometric strengthening can be done, and will even be tolerated in an acutely inflamed joint. Bracing for issues of valgus/varus instability can be helpful and should be considered for patients who note pain with valgus or varus stressing.

The management of olecranon bursitis depends upon whether or not it is acute or chronic. Acute traumatic bursitis can be managed with ice, compression, and NSAIDs. Management of chronic olecranon bursitis is somewhat controversial. If it is secondary to underlying gout or RA, treatment of the systemic disorder is the treatment of choice. No clear-cut treatment algorithms are noted for the management of chronic idiopathic olecranon bursitis. In general ice, compression, activity modification, and the use of an elbow pad are common and appropriate interventions.

Interventional procedures

An infected olecranon bursa needs treatment with antibiotics, to cover skin flora, with orthopedic referral for possible surgical management.

Orthopedic referral for possible elbow arthroplasty may be necessary for patients with issues of severe refractory pain and deformity.

Follow-up and prognosis

Aspiration of the bursa followed by corticosteroid injection can be considered, but this is clearly controversial as it can increase the risk for infection, sloughing of the overlying skin, or the development of a chronic sinus track. This is generally, therefore, a last resort. To date there are no randomized trials showing efficacy for this intervention compared to conservative management. An increased incidence of infection has been noted.

REFERENCES AND FURTHER READING

Hattori Y, Doi K, Sakamoto S, Hoshino S, Dodakundi C. Capsulectomy and debridement for primary osteoarthritis of the elbow through a medial trans-flexor approach. *J Hand Surg Am* 2011; **36**: 1652–8.

Smith DL, McAfee JH, Lucas LM, Kumar KL, Romney DM. Treatment of nonseptic olecranon bursitis: a controlled, blinded prospective trial. *Arch Intern Med* 1989; **149**: 2527–30.

Stewart NJ, Manzanares JB, Morrey BF. Surgical treatment of aseptic olecranon bursitis. *J Shoulder Elbow Surg* 1997; **6**: 49–54.

Wada T, Isogai S, Ishii S, Yamashita T. Debridement arthroplasy for primary osteoarthritis of the elbow: surgical technique. *J Bone Joint Surg Am* 2005; **87** Suppl 1: 95–105

Weinstein PS, Canoso JJ, Wolgethen JR. Long-term follow-up of corticosteroid injection for traumatic olecranon bursitis. *Ann Rheum Dis* 1984; **43**: 44–6.

19

Tennis and golfer's elbow: lateral and medial epicondylitis

Clinical presentation

The exact etiology of lateral and medial epicondylitis is unclear. Several mechanisms have been proposed, including repetitive overuse with resultant microtrauma, eccentric muscle loading, awkward positioning during performance of activities, and lastly underlying weakness of forearm musculature.

Lateral epicondylitis, or tennis elbow, typically presents with pain in the lateral epicondylar region or proximal dorsal forearm. Pain is commonly accentuated with resistive wrist extension activities. Pain on palpation of the mobile extensor mass and lateral epicondylar region is typical. Pain will commonly refer along the anatomic course of the extensor carpi radialis longus muscle. Stretching of the wrist extensors will also elicit pain. Functionally, patients may complain of pain with use of screwdrivers, or with forceful closure of bottles or valves.

Medial epicondylitis, or golfer's elbow, commonly presents with pain on active or resistive wrist flexion. Pain will also be noted on palpation of the medial epicondylar region as well as along the anatomic distribution of the flexor carpi ulnaris (FCU). Patients will complain of pain with gripping activities and hooked-finger grasp activities, as well as with the use of hammers and sometimes screwdrivers.

Signs and symptoms

History will be very important in establishing the diagnosis of lateral or medial epicondylitis. Certain occupations and recreational activities are associated with increased risk for these disorders. Carpenters, electricians, machinists, and mechanics are at risk for lateral epicondylitis, as are golfers and tennis players. Softball and baseball players are at risk for medial epicondylitis.

Visual inspection of the forearm is typically unremarkable. Side-to-side asymmetry can be seen in patients who chronically use one arm disproportionally.

This can be seen in high-caliber tennis players and golfers, as well as electricians, carpenters, and mechanics. Unbalanced forearm musculature, for example increased flexor mass relative to extensor mass, can increase the risk for development of lateral epicondylitis.

Range of motion (ROM) evaluation should assess the shoulder, elbow, and wrist joints. The development of medial or lateral epicondylitis can occur when limitations in shoulder, elbow, or wrist range of motion results in an alteration of upper extremity mechanics, placing more stress on the wrist extensors or flexors. Forearm supination and pronation should be assessed as well, for the same reasons. Side-to-side comparison is the best way to appreciate a range of motion limitation.

Manual muscle testing should include evaluation of the wrist extensors, wrist flexors, long finger extensors and flexors. Pain with resistive activation of the wrist extensors and finger extensors is typically seen in lateral epicondylitis. Pain with resistive wrist flexion or resistive activation of the long finger flexors is commonly seen with medial epicondylitis.

Sensory examination should be unremarkable. Careful evaluation of the C6, C7, and C8 dermatomes is critical to make sure there is no evidence of an underlying C6, C7, or C8 radiculopathy. Important to realize is that a C6, C7 radiculopathy will result in wrist extensor weakness and increase the risk for lateral epicondylitis. Similarly, a C8 level radiculopathy will result in weakness of the FCU and flexor digitorum profundus (FDP) and medial epicondylar region pain.

Atrophy of the first dorsal interosseous (FDI) may be an early indicator for C8 radiculopathy or ulnar neuropathy, and should raise an index of suspicion if seen.

If a cervical radiculopathy is suspected, additional testing by trying to elicit a Spurling's sign is appropriate. A Spurling's sign is reproduction of radicular pain with cervical extension and lateral flexion to the involved side. A positive abduction tension release sign can be seen in a C6 radiculopathy.

Testing of muscle stretch reflexes (MSRs) emphasizing the wrist extensor reflex is critical as part of the assessment for a possible C6 radiculopathy masquerading as a lateral epicondylitis.

Unfortunately no reflex is readily testable for the C8 root, though sometimes blunting of the triceps reflex can occur in a C8 level radiculopathy. For C8 level dysfunction, manual muscle testing of the FDP to the small and ring fingers is imperative, in addition to strength testing of the FDI and the extensor indicis proprius (EIP). The determination of weakness in the above-noted muscle groups is consistent with a C8 level radiculopathy, as all share C8 level innervation.

Laboratory tests, diagnostic investigations, and imaging studies

Plain x-rays can be useful if calcific tendinitis is suspected.

MRI in refractory cases of medial or lateral epicondylitis can be of utility to assess for possible partial muscle tears, especially in patients with a history of repetitive eccentric loading injuries.

Refractory lateral epicondylitis should raise the question of radial tunnel syndrome. Though electromyography (EMG) testing is limited in utility for the evaluation of radial tunnel syndrome, it does have utility. Unfortunately, EMG testing for a posterior interosseous nerve (PIN) neuropathy is generally unremarkable unless the neuropathy is significant. In contrast, EMG testing for ulnar neuropathy at the elbow has more utility and a higher yield rate, even in more subtle compression.

Differential diagnosis

As noted above, a C6 level radiculopathy can masquerade as lateral epicondylitis. To a lesser degree a C7 level radiculopathy can also look like a lateral epicondylitis, as the extensor carpi ulnaris is largely C7 innervated.

Radial tunnel syndrome, compression of the PIN at the level of the supinator muscle, can result in complaints of dorsal forearm ache, wrist extensor weakness, and a sensation of arm fatigue. Additionally, pain in the lateral epicondylar region is common with a PIN neuropathy.

A C8 level radiculopathy can mimic a medial epicondylitis.

Ulnar neuropathy at the level of the elbow can cause medial elbow region pain with associated weakness and pain in the distribution of the FCU.

Pharmacotherapy

Treatment for lateral and medial epicondylitis should be stratified. Initial management should include a trial of ice, compression, and if not medically contraindicated a 7–10-day course of non-steroidal anti-inflammatory drugs (NSAIDs).

Non-pharmacologic approaches

Ice should be applied for 20 minutes 2–3 times per day. Compression or use of tennis-elbow or golfer's-elbow straps can be helpful, as the compression changes the functional origin of the wrist extensor or wrist flexor mass respectively. By doing this the stress is no longer at the bone–tendon junction. This in turn results in less stress at the level of the lateral and medial epicondylar region, resulting in less pain.

Physical therapy can be helpful for the treatment of lateral and medial epicondylitis. Ultrasound can be useful as a heating modality for chronic cases of tendinitis, and iontophoresis or phonophoresis with corticosteroid can be helpful in more acute cases. Both of these modalities allow for the local introduction of anti-inflammatory medications.

Interventional procedures

Platelet-rich plasma (PRP) is a newer form of treatment for management of tendinopathies. To date the data on PRP are controversial and inconsistent. For every study that seems to show a trend towards a positive response there are others that show no difference when compared to sham. Given the out-of-pocket cost of the procedure for the patient, without clear-cut benefit, the use of PRP remains controversial. Clearly well-designed placebo-controlled trials need to be done before the utility of PRP can be assessed.

Injections of corticosteroids at the level of the lateral or medial epicondyle can be undertaken with caution. Injections should be limited to one trial with a low concentration of steroid to decrease the risk of tendon rupture, which can occur with multiple steroid injections as a result of tendon weakening.

Orthopedic referral for refractory cases should be considered, as surgical intervention in appropriate cases can be very helpful. Refractory lateral epicondylitis may require surgical intervention. Release of the common extensor origin has been shown to be helpful and should be considered for the truly refractory case. Surgical release and advancement of the flexor mass has also been successfully used for the treatment of recalcitrant medial epicondylitis.

Follow-up and prognosis

These disorders do not require routine follow-up. Treatment is episodic.

REFERENCES AND FURTHER READING

Coonrad RW, Hooper WR. Tennis elbow: its course, natural history, conservative and surgical management. *J Bone Joint Surg Am* 1973; **55**: 1177–82.

Leach RE, Miller JK. Lateral and medial epicondylitis of the elbow. *Clin Sports Med* 1987; **6**: 259–72.

Owens BD, Murphy KP, Kuklo TR. Arthroscopic release for lateral epicondylitis. *Arthroscopy* 2001; **17**: 582–7.

Rayan F, Rao VSR, Purushothamdas S, Mukundan C, Shafqat SO. Common extensor origin release in recalcitrant lateral epicondylitis: role justified? *J Orthop Surg Res* 2010; **5**: 31.

Suresh SP, Ali KE, Jones H, Connell DA. Medial epicondylitis: is ultrasound guided autologous blood injection an effective treatment? *Br J Sports Med* 2006; **40**: 935–9.

Vangsness CT, Jobe FW. Surgical technique of medial epicondylitis: results in 35 elbows. *J Bone Joint Surg Br* 1991; **73**: 409–11.

20

Nerve entrapments at the elbow

Clinical presentation

Nerve entrapments at the elbow can include the ulnar nerve in the medial epicondylar zone, the median nerve at the supracondylar level secondary to a ligamentous attachment from a supracondylar spur to the medial epicondyle (ligament of Struthers), and the radial nerve at the supinator muscle (arcade of Frohse).

Ulnar nerve compression at the elbow is the most common of the above entrapment neuropathies. The ulnar nerve is at risk of entrapment or compression at the elbow because of its anatomic location, as it courses between the bony olecranon and the medial epicondyle in the retrocondylar groove. A shallow groove with associated mild cubitus valgus increases the risk for ulnar nerve subluxation. Even in normal anatomy, flexion at the elbow joint places the ulnar nerve in a superficial position, prone to compression.

Median nerve entrapment at the elbow is an uncommon neuropathy. Entrapment at this level can be secondary to an anatomic variant, a supracondylar spur with an associated ligamentous band that spans from the medial epicondyle to the supracondylar spur (ligament of Struthers). This can compress the median nerve just proximal to the elbow joint.

Radial nerve entrapment, if proximal to the elbow, will compress the radial nerve proper. If distal to the elbow, at the level of the supinator (arcade of Frohse), it will spare radial nerve sensation but result in weakness of the posterior interosseous nerve (PIN)-innervated muscles.

Classically, entrapment of the ulnar nerve at the elbow results in altered ulnar sensation both on the dorsal and palmar surfaces of the hand. Weakness will typically involve all ulnar hand intrinsic muscles. The flexor carpi ulnaris (FCU) will be involved if the compression is proximal to the true elbow joint, but will be spared if the compression is distal to the elbow joint at the cubital tunnel level. In contrast, the flexor digitorum profundus to the small and ring fingers will be involved in ulnar compressions proximal to the elbow, at the epicondylar level, as well as at the cubital tunnel level.

Median nerve compression at the ligament of Struthers will result in compression of the true median nerve. In this case weakness of muscles innervated by the median nerve, as well as the anterior interosseous nerve (AIN), may be noted. Equally important to realize is that impaired median nerve sensation will be noted, including in the thenar patch, which is spared in median nerve compression at the wrist. Entrapment just distal to the elbow, at the level of the pronator teres, will mimic ligament of Struthers entrapment, but with much milder symptoms. Weakness, if present, will be mild and may only be noted in the abductor pollicis brevis (APB) and flexor pollicis longus (FPL). Sensory abnormalities are not a typical complaint. More distal in the forearm, the AIN, the pure motor branch of the median nerve, can be entrapped. AIN compression can occur with mid-shaft radius fractures or radial artery aneurysm, as well as with anomalous muscular bands from the FPL. In this scenario, weakness will be noted in the FPL and pronator quadratus (PQ). The flexor digitorum profundus (FDP) to the index and long fingers will be involved if the lesion to the AIN is more proximal. However, if the lesion is more distal, only the FPL and PQ may be involved. As the AIN is a pure motor nerve, no sensory complaints should be noted.

Radial nerve compression just proximal to the elbow may result in weakness of the brachioradialis as well as forearm muscles innervated by the radial nerve and PIN. Weakness of wrist extension and finger extension will be noted, along with sensory complaints involving the thumb. More distally, compression at the arcade of Frohse will result in weakness of wrist extension and finger extension without sensory changes, because at this level entrapment involves the PIN, a pure motor branch of the radial nerve. A not uncommon complaint seen in radial nerve compression at the arcade of Frohse is one of deep forearm ache with an associated sensation of muscle fatigue.

Signs and symptoms

History, once again, is of paramount importance. Upper extremity weakness involving the forearm musculature, in concert with sensory abnormalities, should trigger consideration for ulnar, radial, or median nerve involvement depending upon the distribution of changes noted. Weakness of forearm musculature without sensory changes should immediately raise the specter of either PIN or AIN neuropathy, again depending upon the pattern and distribution of weakness.

Ulnar neuropathy at the elbow presents with certain predictable features. In all instances true compression of the ulnar nerve at the elbow will present with weakness of ulnar-innervated hand intrinsics, easily noted by weakness of the first dorsal interosseous (FDI). Additionally, weakness of the ulnar-innervated FDP will be noted. This will result in weakness of flexion of the distal finger flexors of the small and ring fingers. Sensory changes will be noted in the small finger and ring finger, and altered sensation in the dorsal ulnar cutaneous (DUC) distribution will also be present. If the compression of the ulnar nerve is just proximal to the elbow joint, all of the above findings will be noted, but now the FCU, a powerful wrist flexor, will also be weak. In contrast, ulnar nerve compression at the wrist will spare the FDP and FCU. Additionally, no sensory changes will be noted in the DUC distribution. Altered sensation in the medial forearm is not seen in ulnar neuropathy at the elbow, and when noted should trigger a work-up for lower trunk or medial cord level brachial plexopathy.

Median nerve compression at the elbow is not common. When seen, it may be secondary to compression at the ligament of Struthers. Injury to the median nerve can also occur during placement of an intravenous catheter. In this scenario the median nerve neuropathy is secondary to a partial laceration, as opposed to a compression neuropathy. Median nerve compression at the ligament of Struthers will result in weakness of the median-nerve-innervated pronator teres and flexor digitorum superficialis, as well as median-innervated hand intrinsics, with the APB being most notably involved. The AIN-innervated FDP to the distal finger flexors of the index and long fingers, FPL, and PQ will also be involved. Sensory changes will be noted in a median nerve distribution, involving thumb, index finger, long finger, and radial side of ring finger. The thenar mass will also have altered sensation. In contrast, involvement of the AIN will result in motor weakness of the AIN-innervated long finger flexors to the index and long fingers, the FPL, and the PQ, but the median-innervated pronator teres, flexor digitorum superficialis, and hand intrinsics will be spared. Additionally, no sensory complaints will be noted or demonstrated on exam. Median nerve compression at the wrist can result in median hand intrinsic muscle weakness with altered sensation, but thenar patch sensation will be maintained.

Radial nerve compression at the elbow is also relatively uncommon. When it occurs it can do so proximal to the elbow or more distally at the level of the supinator (arcade of Frohse). If the compression occurs proximal to the elbow, weakness will be noted in the brachioradialis as well as the wrist extensors and finger extensors. The brachioradialis is a powerful elbow flexor when the forearm is in a neutral posture, halfway between full supination and full pronation. In this scenario patients will note weakness of elbow flexion. Altered sensation in a radial nerve distribution will also be manifest. Compression at the arcade of Frohse will cause wrist extensor weakness, but the extensor carpi radialis longus will be spared, as it receives its nerve supply from the radial nerve proximal to the elbow joint. Additionally, the brachioradialis will be spared. Finally, no sensory complaints will be noted.

Laboratory tests, diagnostic investigations, and imaging studies

Imaging studies should include plain films of the elbow to evaluate for a supracondylar spur in suspected median nerve compression at the elbow.

MRI of the forearm, to evaluate for radial nerve aneurysm or aberrant muscle slip from the FPL, is appropriate as part of the work-up for an AIN neuropathy.

The mainstay studies for nerve compression at the elbow are electrodiagnostic tests such as electromyography (EMG) and nerve conduction studies (NCS). Even with careful testing, however, these compressions may go undiagnosed.

Differential diagnosis

Ulnar nerve neuropathy at the elbow can initially be confused for an upper trunk or medial cord level brachial plexopathy. However, ulnar neuropathy at the elbow will not be associated with sensory changes in the medial forearm in the medial antebrachial cutaneous (MABC) distribution. Additionally, with an ulnar neuropathy at the elbow there will be no findings of weakness in median-innervated thenar musculature.

A C8 radiculopathy will have similar sensory findings as an ulnar neuropathy at the elbow, but the C8 level radiculopathy will also be associated with weakness in C8 median- and radial-nerve-innervated musculature.

Median nerve neuropathy at the elbow will have sensory findings that appear to mimic carpal tunnel syndrome (CTS), but CTS does not cause sensory changes in the thenar mass region. Additionally, CTS would not be associated with weakness of the wrist flexors or flexor digitorum superficialis.

A C7 level radiculopathy can mimic median nerve compression at the elbow, but would also be associated with weakness of radial C7 innervated musculature, such as the triceps.

Radial nerve compression at the elbow should not be confused with a PIN neuropathy, as the PIN neuropathy is not associated with sensory changes. Radial nerve neuropathy at the elbow can mimic a C6–C7 level radiculopathy, but in this scenario the radiculopathy would result in weakness of the triceps, which derives radial nerve sensation well proximal to the elbow. Also, one must realize that weakness would also be present in median C6–C7 innervated muscles such as the pronator teres and flexor digitorum superficialis.

Pharmacotherapy

Initial treatment should emphasize conservative management. A brief course of non-steroidal anti-inflammatory drugs (NSAIDs), if not medically contraindicated, may be helpful for reducing inflammation.

Neuromodulators, such as antidepressants or anti-seizure medications, for control of associated neurogenic pain can have utility. The side-effect profiles of these medications should always be kept in mind.

Non-pharmacologic approaches

A trial of physical therapy is appropriate, using modalities including ultrasound for heating of soft tissue structures to facilitate stretch. Nerve glide exercises in concert with ultrasound may also have utility.

Interventional procedures

Surgical referral for refractory ulnar compression at the elbow with demonstrable axonal injury on electrodiagnostic testing is appropriate.

Radial nerve decompression at the level of the arcade of Frohse can be considered for refractory cases with demonstrable compression and axonal injury on electrodiagnostic testing.

Median nerve decompression at the ligament of Struthers can be accomplished, and is generally well tolerated. Decompression of the median nerve at the level of the pronator teres is much less predictable in terms of outcome, and should be viewed as a last resort.

Follow-up and prognosis

Follow-up will vary depending upon the intervention and response to conservative management. The prognosis for nerve entrapment at the elbow is variable. For severe ulnar entrapment with denervation noted on EMG, surgical transposition is the treatment of choice. However, the results are guarded in terms of nerve recovery. For radial and median nerve entrapment the treatment is typically conservative management with occupational therapy and trials of neuromodulators. Surgery is a last resort with guarded outcomes.

REFERENCES AND FURTHER READING

Assmus H, Antoniadis G, Bischoff C, *et al.* Cubital tunnel syndrome: a review and management guidelines. *Cent Eur Neurosurg* 2011; **72**: 90–8.

Dick FD, Graveling RA, Munro W, Walker-Bone K; Guideline Development Group. Workplace management of upper limb disorders: a systematic review. *Occup Med (Lond)* 2011; **61**: 19–25.

Lubahn JD, Cermak MB. Uncommon nerve compression syndromes of the upper extremity. *J Am Acad Orthop Surg* 1998; **6**: 378–86.

Rajabally YA, Narasimhan M. Electrophysiological entrapment syndromes in chronic inflammatory demyelinating polyneuropathy. *Muscle Nerve* 2011; **44**: 444–7.

21

Hand and wrist arthritis

Clinical presentation

Arthritis of the hand can involve multiple joints, with varying degrees of symptoms, and in a subset can show central erosive changes on radiographs. The heterogeneous nature of this disorder can make it challenging to diagnose as well as to treat.

Typically, erosive hand osteoarthritis is more commonly seen in post-menopausal women seeking evaluation and treatment in rheumatology clinics. For age-matched men and women the prevalence of hand osteoarthritis is mildly increased in women compared to men (approximately 44% vs. 38%). In distinction, women have a much greater prevalence of erosive and symptomatic arthritis compared to men (approximately 10% vs. 3.3% and 15.9% vs. 8.2%, respectively).

The prevalence of radiographic findings of arthritis of the hand is similar for men and women. Women, however, are more likely to have symptomatic arthritis of the hand, as well as erosive changes on radiographs.

Wrist arthritis can be post-traumatic as well as non-traumatic. Wrist arthritis may develop after distal radius fracture with malalignment. Carpal dislocations can also be associated with delayed onset of wrist degenerative joint disease (DJD).

The clinical presentation for hand and wrist arthritis can be very variable. Hand arthritis is not commonly associated with pain. Joint involvement may include the proximal interphalangeal (PIP) and distal interphalangeal (DIP) joints. Bouchard's nodes are the changes noted at the PIP joints, and Heberden's nodes are noted at the DIP joints. While these degenerative changes can result in significant changes in anatomy of the fingers, they are not commonly associated with pain. These changes can frequently impact on activities of daily living (ADL).

Patients may complain of decreased hand dexterity, loss of grip strength, and a sensation of hand stiffness. Symptomatic as well as erosive hand arthritis is seen in a subset of patients, and has a female predominance. This group of patients will frequently note pain as well as impairment of ADL. Limitations in power grip, three-jaw chuck type activity (opposition of the thumb to the distal finger tufts of the index and long fingers), and lateral key pinch may be noted. Weakness in lateral key pinch can be a sign of gamekeeper's thumb, laxity of the ulnar collateral ligament at the metacarpophalangeal (MCP) joint of the thumb.

Wrist DJD, whether from trauma or from underlying rheumatoid arthritis (RA), increases the risk for median nerve compression at the wrist, and careful attention should therefore be given to complaints of numbness and tingling in the hand of a patient with wrist arthritis.

Signs and symptoms

Observation is very important in the evaluation of hand and wrist arthritis. Patterns of involvement can give clues to potential underlying diagnoses.

Swelling, synovial hypertrophy of the wrist and MCP joints, ulnar deviation of the wrist, and volar subluxation of the MCP joints with associated complaints of pain can be seen in RA. Involvement of the DIP and PIP joints is classic for DJD, and is usually asymptomatic in regards to pain. Palpation of all the finger joints as well as the wrist joints is critical to assess for synovial hypertrophy or bogginess.

Range of motion (ROM) assessment must include wrist flexion, extension, and circumduction. Wrist extension to 45 degrees is functional, as is flexion to 45 degrees. Checking for crepitus with range of motion is critical, as this is commonly noted in wrist DJD.

Finger function can be assessed by looking at the range of motion of each joint for each finger. More practical is the assessment of the fingers as a functional unit. Evaluation of grip, three-jaw chuck grasp, and lateral key pinch allows for better assessment of the patient's ability to perform ADL. Grip or cylindrical grasp can be quantified by measuring the distance between the palm and finger tips in centimeters. The greater the distance the more impaired the cylindrical grip.

Appreciation of light touch and pin sensation should be checked as well. Arthritis of the wrist, whether post-traumatic or secondary to underlying RA, can be associated with an increased risk for carpal tunnel syndrome (CTS). Ulnar nerve compression at Guyon's canal can also be seen in a patient with arthritis of the wrist.

Tinel's sign over the median and ulnar nerves at the wrist, while not specific for median or ulnar nerve compression at the wrist, should raise the index of suspicion for these compressive neuropathies. A positive carpal pressure test, pressure applied over the distal carpal ligament with thumb pressure for 20–30 seconds, may be slightly more sensitive and specific than a Tinel's for median nerve compression at the wrist.

Laboratory tests and diagnostic investigations

Blood work, including erythrocyte sedimentation rate (ESR), antinuclear antibody (ANA), and complete blood count with differential (CBC with diff), should be obtained in all patients with suspected RA or erosive arthritis.

Electromyography (EMG) and nerve conduction studies (NCS) should be reserved for patients with complaints of hand numbness and tingling, particularly if there is associated wrist arthritis.

Imaging studies

Plain x-rays can be helpful in checking for erosive changes in patients with hand arthritis. Strong consideration should be given to obtaining x-rays in females with symptomatic arthritis of the hands. X-rays may also reveal post-traumatic arthritis of the wrist in patients with previous distal radius fracture and malalignment.

Differential diagnosis

The differential diagnosis for arthritis of the hand or wrist includes RA and erosive arthritis. Swelling and pain involving the MCP joints and wrist should always trigger consideration for possible RA, especially when seen in women. Additionally, complaints of significant joint stiffness in the morning that takes more than 30 minutes to "loosen up" should raise the specter of possible underlying RA.

Septic arthritis should be considered in the patient with an acutely swollen and painful wrist or finger joint. Though not common, this is an orthopedic medical emergency, and it requires prompt treatment with antibiotics and close orthopedic monitoring.

Pharmacotherapy

Non-steroidal anti-inflammatory drugs (NSAIDs) can have utility in patients with RA and symptomatic or erosive hand arthritis. Given that many patients with hand or wrist arthritis are older, careful attention should be given to issues of hypertension and renal disease before instituting NSAID treatment.

In patients with RA, referral to rheumatology for consideration of disease-modifying agents should be undertaken.

Non-pharmacologic approaches

Treatment should be targeted to the underlying issue, if a clearly demonstrable one can be identified. For the patient with arthritis of the hand, without significant symptoms, physical modalities can be very helpful.

The use of a paraffin bath as a source of heating for the wrist and finger joints can provide symptomatic relief. Twenty minutes of paraffin bath use twice a day can provide pain modulation as well as skin lubrication, as the paraffin bath is a mixture of paraffin and mineral oil. In older patients with fragile skin the moisturizing quality of the mineral oil can also help maintain skin integrity.

Wrist bracing can be useful for resting and protecting the acutely inflamed wrist joint. Bracing can also provide stability for the arthritic unstable wrist. A thumb spica component to a wrist brace can stabilize a gamekeeper's thumb and improve function of the thumb.

Interventional procedures

Orthopedic referral should be considered for patients with refractory wrist pain with instability. This subset of patients can benefit from wrist fusion. Thumb MCP joint fusion can also be helpful and provide good relief of pain for the patient with gross thumb instability and pain from a late-stage gamekeeper's thumb. Thumb interposition arthroplasty can give good pain relief for painful carpometacarpal (CMC) arthritis.

Follow-up and prognosis

Follow-up should be with rheumatology for patients with rheumatoid, symptomatic, and/or erosive arthritis, and with occupational therapy for instruction in joint preservation techniques when performing routine ADL. Patients on NSAIDs should have routine follow-up for monitoring of renal function, occult gastrointestinal bleeding, and worsening hypertension. The prognosis is one of slow progression.

REFERENCES AND FURTHER READING

Bassey EJ, Harries UJ. Normal values for handgrip strength in 920 men and women over 65 years, and longitudinal changes over 4 years in 620 survivors. *Clin Sci (Lond)* 1993; **84**: 331–7.

Chaisson CE, Zhang Y, Sharma L, Kannel W, Felson DT. Grip strength and the risk of developing radiographic hand osteoarthritis: results from the Framingham study. *Arthritis Rheum* 1999; **42**: 33–8.

Crosby CA, Wehbé MA, Mawr B. Hand strength: normative values. *Am J Hand Surg* 1994; **19**: 665–70.

Haugen IK, Englund M, Aliabadi P, *et al.* Prevalence, incidence and progression of hand osteoarthritis in the general population: the Framingham Osteoarthritis Study. *Ann Rheum Dis* 2011; **70**: 1581–6.

Peterfy CG. MRI of the wrist in early rheumatoid arthritis. *Ann Rheum Dis* 2004: **63**; 473–7.

22

Carpal tunnel syndrome

Clinical presentation

Carpal tunnel syndrome (CTS) refers to a constellation of signs and symptoms that results from focal compression of the median nerve at the level of the wrist. Multiple structures pass through the bony carpal tunnel: tendons of the flexor digitorum profunda, flexor digitorum superficialis, and flexor pollicis longus. The carpal bones comprise the side walls and floor of the tunnel. The roof of the tunnel is formed by a thick fibrous structure called the transverse carpal ligament.

Risk factors for median nerve compression at the wrist include, but are not limited to, rheumatoid arthritis, osteoarthritis of the wrist, pregnancy (with its attendant fluid retention), and occupations having exposure to vibratory equipment. Additionally, patients with a history of known peripheral neuropathy or underlying metabolic disorders such as diabetes, thyroid dysfunction, amyloidosis, renal failure, or liver failure are also at an increased risk for CTS specifically and compressive-type neuropathies in general. Many of the above disorders increase the risk for CTS by functionally decreasing the volume of the carpal tunnel. This can occur when degenerative structural changes decrease the actual volume of the tunnel as a result of mechanical encroachment. Edema or tenosynovitis can also result in CTS by increasing the volume of the structures that pass through the fixed architecture of the bony tunnel.

Patients with CTS will typically complain of a sensation of tingling and numbness involving the thumb, index finger, and long finger. Discomfort can radiate proximally, and patients may thus also complain of a sensation of forearm discomfort or ache with an associated decrease in grip strength. In severe cases patients may complain of proximal migration of pain to the level of the shoulder. Patients may also complain of dropping items and decreased hand dexterity.

Focused questioning will commonly reveal that patients awaken at night complaining of hand numbness. Typically "shaking out" the hands will decrease symptoms. Patients may also complain of numbness and tingling with driving, and with use of lawnmowers, leaf blowers, snow blowers, or any piece of equipment that tends to vibrate.

Signs and symptoms

Initial evaluation should focus on inspection of the involved hand. Observe for atrophy of the thenar eminence. This is not a common finding, but when seen it is highly suggestive of severe CTS, and carries with it a poor prognosis for recovery even with surgical decompression. If hypothenar eminence atrophy is also noted, CTS becomes less likely as an isolated entity, and a C8 level radiculopathy or possible lower trunk brachial plexopathy starts to increase as a possibility.

Examination must include evaluation of sensory function. Mapping out of median nerve sensory function must be assessed, and should be compared to ulnar and radial sensory function to confirm alteration in median sensation. Care should be taken to document that thenar sensation is retained in the face of decreased median nerve distribution sensation in the fingers. Thenar eminence sensation should be retained in CTS, as the median thenar branch goes over the transverse carpal ligament, rather than through the carpal tunnel.

Tinel's sign, tapping over the median nerve at the wrist, may result in tingling in a median nerve distribution. This finding is neither sensitive nor specific for CTS and can be elicited with percussion over a non-compressed nerve. A positive carpal pressure test, pressure applied for 30 seconds over the distal transverse ligament, may also result in production of numbness and tingling in the median nerve distribution. Once again, this test is neither sensitive nor specific. Phalen's test, pressing the backs of the hands together in a downward "prayer sign," is also neither sensitive nor specific.

Evaluation of the involved upper extremity must also include assessment of reflexes. A C6 or C6–C7 level radiculopathy can look like CTS. However, with a C6 level radiculopathy there will be associated blunting of the wrist extensor reflex. With a C7 radiculopathy, blunting of the triceps reflex will be noted. Additionally, a positive Spurling's sign may be noted. Spurling's sign is reproduction of radicular symptoms with cervical extension and lateral flexion to the involved side. With a C6 radiculopathy, an abduction tension release sign may be noted. This will manifest with improvement of symptoms with placement of the involved arm on top of the patient's head.

Manual muscle testing is also required to rule out a cervical radiculopathy. Weakness of biceps and wrist extensors can be seen in a C6 radiculopathy.

Weakness of the triceps and flexor digitorum superficialis can be seen with a C7 radiculopathy. A C8–T1 level radiculopathy can cause weakness of the thenar muscles, but should not be mistaken for CTS, as the sensory disturbances will be along the ulnar border of the hand.

Laboratory tests and diagnostic investigations

The gold-standard test for the evaluation of a possible CTS and quantification of the degree of median nerve compression at the wrist is electrodiagnostic testing. The electrodiagnostic test is composed of needle electromyography (EMG) and nerve conduction studies (NCS). In CTS the most useful test is an NCS of the median nerve across the wrist. Both sensory and motor function of the median nerve are evaluated.

Mild CTS is generally considered to be median nerve compression that is limited to sensory fiber involvement. Moderate CTS refers to abnormalities of both sensory and motor fiber function in the across-wrist segment of the median nerve. A severe CTS would be noted when there is involvement of both sensory and motor fibers and an element of actual sensory fiber axonal dropout is noted. Profound CTS is reserved for those cases of median nerve compression where there is complete loss of sensory axon function, as well as partial to complete loss of median motor axon function.

Imaging studies

Imaging studies may include cervical spine radiographs and MRI when the clinical picture correlates with a possible radicular etiology for the patient's complaints. MRI of the brachial plexus along with an anteroposterior chest x-ray should be obtained in a patient with clinical findings consistent with neurogenic thoracic outlet syndrome (TOS). This will allow for assessment of a possible cervical rib, as well as a possible infiltrating compressive lesion such as a Pancoast tumor. The risk for tumor invasion as the cause of a neurogenic TOS increases with a history of smoking, particularly in a patient with historical findings of unexplained weight loss, cough, with associated upper extremity weakness.

Differential diagnosis

As previously noted, CTS will typically present with numbness, tingling, and paresthesias involving the thumb, index finger, and long finger. Therefore, the differential diagnosis must include entities that can cause sensory disturbances in a similar distribution. Cervical nerve root compression involving the C6 and C7 nerve roots will give similar sensory findings. However, CTS will not result in sensory disturbances involving the dorsal radial aspect of the hand. Additionally, CTS would not result in attenuation of the wrist and/or triceps muscle stretch reflexes.

Proximal median nerve compression at the elbow region (ligament of Struthers) will result in sensory disturbances in a median nerve distribution.

However, in this scenario sensory disturbances will also be noted in the thenar mass region, an area not involved in CTS. Additionally, the proximal nature of this compression may also result in weakness of forearm musculature that is innervated by the median nerve or anterior interosseous nerve. Careful evaluation of flexor digitorum superficialis, profundus to the index and long fingers, flexor pollicis longus, and pronator quadratus function should quickly establish the proximal nature of this compressive neuropathy.

An upper trunk brachial plexopathy can result in sensory disturbances that include the thumb and long finger, and hence confusion could arise. However, an upper trunk brachial plexopathy will also have sensory disturbances in the distribution of the lateral antebrachial cutaneous nerve to the forearm, as well as weakness of the deltoid, biceps, and rotator cuff musculature.

Classic neurogenic TOS, a rare disorder, can give rise to weakness of the thenar mass musculature. At first glance this could be mistaken for CTS, but this is easily avoided if one bears in mind that neurogenic TOS involves compression of the lower trunk of the brachial plexus. Motor weakness will therefore include not only the thenar mass, but also ulnar hand intrinsics and ulnar-innervated long finger flexors and wrist flexors. Just as important is the realization that sensory disturbances will be in an ulnar distribution and not a median nerve distribution.

Pharmacotherapy

A brief course of non-steroidal anti-inflammatory drugs (NSAIDs) may have utility if the CTS is secondary to underlying inflammation such as a flare-up of wrist rheumatoid arthritis or osteoarthritis.

Non-pharmacologic approaches

Treatment of CTS relates to the degree of abnormality and pathology noted on electrodiagnostic testing. Mild to moderate cases of CTS can be managed conservatively. This can include splinting at night to maintain the wrist in a neutral posture. Additionally, activity modification may be helpful.

Interventional procedures

Injection of the carpal tunnel with corticosteroid can be diagnostic as well as therapeutic in patients with symptoms and borderline electrodiagnostic abnormalities. It can also be efficacious in patients with mild to moderate CTS.

Once median compression progresses to the point of moderate to severe, conservative management is not likely to be of utility. Corticosteroid injection can give transient relief, but this will usually be short-lived. It may have utility as a bridge to quiet symptoms while awaiting surgery.

Surgical decompression of the median nerve, either as an endoscopic or as an open procedure, is the definitive treatment for CTS of a moderate to severe degree or worse. It will predictably result in decompression of the nerve and allow for the best chance of recovery of nerve function. In patients who have an element of significant axonal injury noted on electrodiagnostic testing, resolution of symptoms may be prolonged and incomplete.

Follow-up

Follow-up is dependent upon the intervention. Patients managed conservatively should be instructed to monitor symptoms. They should also be encouraged to follow up for clinical assessment in the office 1–2 times per year to monitor their status. Worsening symptoms warrant repeated electrodiagnostic testing and comparison against previous studies. Progression of abnormalities noted on electrodiagnostic studies with worsening symptoms warrants a referral to a hand surgeon.

Prognosis

Patients who have undergone surgical release should be periodically reassessed, as a small percentage can develop late-onset recompression. Incidence of this increases in patients with known underlying inflammatory arthritis, as well as in patients whose occupations require extensive use of vibratory equipment.

REFERENCES AND FURTHER READING

Atcheson SG, Ward JR, Lowe W. Concurrent medical disease in work-related carpal tunnel syndrome. *Arch Intern Med* 1998; **158**: 1506–12.

Cho DS, MacLean IC. Comparison of normal values of median, radial and ulnar sensory latencies. *Muscle Nerve* 1984; **7**: 575.

Katz JN, Larson MG, Sabra A, *et al.* The carpal tunnel syndrome: diagnostic utility of the history and physical examination findings. *Ann Intern Med* 1990; **112**: 321–7.

Kuhlman KA, Hennessey WJ. Sensitivity and specificity of carpal tunnel syndrome signs. *Am J Phys Med and Rehabil* 1997; **76**: 451–7.

Robinson LR, Micklesen PJ, Wang L. Stratagies for analyzing nerve conduction data: superiority of a summary index over single tests. *Muscle Nerve* 1998; **21**: 1166–71.

23

Costosternal, costochondral, and costovertebral syndromes

Clinical presentation

Complaints of chest wall pain can be alarming, often prompting patients to seek medical attention because of concerns over possible pain from cardiac infarction. Chest wall pain due to musculoskeletal causes is quite common, and must be considered among the possibilities for patient presentation. Estimates suggest that, among patients presenting to emergency rooms with chest wall pain complaints, approximately 30% of them have pain that is attributable to a musculoskeletal origin.

A brief discussion of the anatomy of the chest wall may help to elucidate the nomenclature for pain conditions described herein and clarify the potential causes of chest wall pain that the clinician must consider. Seven of the 12 pairs of ribs articulate with the sternum: the first rib with the manubrium via a synarthroidal joint, while the second through seventh ribs articulate with the body of the sternum, i.e., costosternal junction, via arthroidal joints. Ribs eight through ten articulate via costochondral cartilage with one another and the adjacent superior ribs, which ultimately attach to the sternum. The remaining eleventh and twelfth ribs are floating ribs, which remain unattached to the sternum. The ribs are attached posteriorly to the thoracic vertebra. The second through tenth ribs articulate with the vertebral bodies via costovertebral joints in addition to the transverse processes of the two adjacent thoracic vertebrae via costotransverse joints. For ribs 1, 11, and 12, there is only one attachment to the vertebrae, via costovertebral joints. The intercostal muscles extend between the individual ribs. The inferior ridges of the ribs enclose the intercostal vein, artery, and nerve. The intercostal nerves emanate from the ventral branch of the thoracic spinal nerve. The latter divides into a lateral branch supplying much of the intercostal muscle, and an anterior branch supplying the intercostal region closer to the sternal margin. Pain is produced when there is impingement of the thoracic nerves in costovertebral syndrome, whereas impingement of the intercostal nerves precipitates pain in both costosternal and costochondral syndromes.

Table 23.1 Distinguishing Tietze's and costosternal syndromes

	Tietze's syndrome	Costosternal syndrome
Prevalence	Rare	Common
Age	< 40 years	> 40 years
Number of ribs	1	> 1
Affected side(s)	Unilateral	Uni- or bilateral
Affected sites	2nd or 3rd rib	2nd through 5th ribs
Signs	Inflammation, swelling, erythema	Absent

Adapted from Gregory *et al.* 2002, Stochkendahl & Christensen 2010.

Typically, costosternal and costochondral pain is localized to the anterior chest wall. Costosternal syndrome manifests as pain at the juncture of the ribs and sternum bilaterally and at multiple levels, i.e., ribs 2–7. Costochondral syndrome (costochondritis) is anterior chest wall pain that may affect one or more joints involving inflammation of the costal cartilage, i.e., ribs 8–10.

Costosternal syndrome is often confused with, but should be distinguished from, Tietze's syndrome. Distinguishing characteristics between these two conditions are summarized in Table 23.1.

Another subset of patients may present with pain originating from costovertebral origins. Costovertebral syndrome arises from inflammation or injury to the posterior joint formed by the neck of the rib as it joins the thoracic vertebra. The pain can radiate anteriorly, causing patients to misinterpret the discomfort as originating from visceral origins, e.g., cardiac, pneumonia, pulmonary embolism.

The etiological factors contributing to each of these conditions can be quite varied. Costosternal, costochondral, and costovertebral syndromes can each arise from osteoarthritis, rheumatoid arthritis, psoriatic arthritis, ankylosing spondylitis, and Reiter's syndrome. In the case of costovertebral syndrome, there can be injury sustained to the costovertebral joint by trauma, i.e., acceleration-deceleration injuries and blunt trauma. In addition, the joint can be invaded by tumor/malignancy, e.g., tumor arising from localized bone tumor, or metastasis from more distant sites, such as renal sarcoma or myeloma, among others. Costosternal syndrome may arise from primary bone malignancies and localized tumors, e.g., thymoma, or metastasis from other more distant sources. Costochondritis can arise from inflammation of the costal cartilage. Other precipitants of costochondral pain include overuse injuries, e.g., shoulder protraction, and blunt trauma to the anterior chest wall.

Signs and symptoms

The patient may present with a stiff posture, i.e., the shoulders are stiffly maintained in a neutral position so as to avoid precipitating pain. For pain arising from the costosternal/chondral joints, the pain can occur at rest in the anterior chest but is often aggravated by specific movements: shoulder retraction or protraction, deep inspiration, coughing and sneezing, and full anterior elevation of the arm. The patient may appear to splint or protect the affected joints at such times. The affected costosternal/chondral joints may be tender to palpation on physical examination.

The pain produced by costovertebral syndrome, on the other hand, is usually localized close to the thoracic spine, but it may radiate laterally to the midthorax and possibly even to the anterior chest wall. It usually occurs at the level of the sixth or seventh ribs, where they articulate with the transverse processes of the thoracic vertebrae. Costovertebral pain can, likewise, be aggravated by deep inspiration, coughing, and shoulder retraction. Palpation of the thoracic spine reveals tenderness over the affected joints; palpation over the angle of the ribs will produce localized discomfort that may radiate laterally. Various manipulations, e.g., side flexion of the thoracic spine or rotation away from or toward the painful side, may reproduce the pain to facilitate localization of the origin of pain.

Laboratory tests and diagnostic investigations

It is imperative that potentially life-threatening causes of chest pain be ruled out. A carefully derived history and physical examination can assist the clinician in determining whether further laboratory and diagnostic assessments will be warranted to establish whether the pain is arising from cardiac or other visceral origins.

Laboratory investigations may be helpful in elucidating the potential underlying causes for costosternal/chondral and costovertebral chest wall pain. A complete blood count (CBC) may reveal an underlying infection. Serological investigations, e.g., erythrocyte sedimentation rate (ESR), antinuclear antibody (ANA) testing, and other investigations to work up for potential collagen vascular diseases and rheumatologic conditions, can be helpful, particularly in situations in which the chest wall joints are affected in the context of evidence of other joint involvement.

Imaging studies

Chest radiographs are useful to identify potential sternum and/or rib fracture and to rule out occult malignancy, e.g., invasion by tumor. Magnetic resonance imaging may be necessary to establish tumor if suspected by preliminary radiographic testing. Radionucleotide bone scanning, i.e., scintigraphy, is unlikely to be helpful in the evaluation of costosternal/chondral and costovertebral pain, but it may potentially unveil evidence of rib fracture that had been previously undetected. Other imaging studies, e.g., cardiac and/or ventilation/perfusion (V/Q) scanning, may be necessary if there are concerns about pain emanating from visceral sources, e.g., coronary artery disease, cardiomyopathy, valvular disease, or pulmonary embolism.

Differential diagnosis

Other common musculoskeletal syndromes must be considered in patients presenting with anterior chest wall pain. While an exhaustive review of the origins of chest wall pain is not possible given the space limitations here, one can conceptualize focal chest wall pain as arising from several possible sources. Features differentiating these conditions from costosternal/chondral and costovertebral syndromes are delineated in Table 23.2.

In addition, among cases in which the history and physical findings suggest costosternal/chondral or costovertebral pain that cannot be attributed to repetitive movements, exertion, or trauma, it may be prudent to consider the differential diagnosis of potential causes of the joint dysfunction and resultant pain including tumor, infection, Reiter's syndrome, arthritis, and ankylosing spondylitis.

Pharmacotherapy

Costosternal/chondral and costovertebral pain is generally responsive to acetaminophen, non-steroidal anti-inflammatory drugs (NSAIDs), cyclooxygenase-2 (COX-2) inhibitors, and possibly tramadol. Although anticonvulsants, e.g., gabapentin or pregabalin, may be useful in managing neuropathic pain states, e.g., post-thoracotomy intercostal neuralgia, the utility of these agents in costosternal/chondral or costovertebral pain has not been established. There have been no clinical trials assessing the relative efficacy of weak analgesics in the control of symptoms associated with costosternal/chondral and costovertebral pain. For afflicted patients, pain can be aggravated by coughing, e.g., with upper respiratory infections. Under such circumstances, cough suppressants might be a consideration so as to avoid precipitating pain.

Non-pharmacologic approaches

Non-pharmacologic approaches to the management of costosternal/chondral pain can include application of heat compresses or heating pads. Patients should be advised to avoid, or at the very least minimize, activities that aggravate the musculoskeletal pain. Activity restrictions that are likely to be required include: not flexing or extending the shoulder beyond 90 degrees; not pushing oneself up with use of the arms when arising from a seated position; not pushing or pulling oneself when reclined; avoiding breath holding during activity; avoiding reaching across the body; avoiding lifting excess weight (beyond 4–5 kg); bracing the chest

Table 23.2 Potential sources of focal chest pain

Source	Condition	Features	Symptoms
Skeletal	Sternum fracture	After trauma, sternal fractures may co-occur with rib fractures; can also arise after extreme upper torso muscular stress, e.g., wrestling	Anterior chest pain worsened with movement or deep inspiration; associated tenderness over sternum on palpation
	Rib fracture	Arises from trauma; can also arise from repetitive high-stress activities, e.g., rowing	Localized pain over the affected rib(s); can be prohibitive of certain activities, e.g., pulling, rowing, and exacerbated by deep inspiration
	Xiphisternal syndrome	Usually a result of trauma, but can occur secondary to inflammation or systemic arthritic conditions	Severe, intermittent anterior chest wall pain, often radiates to the abdomen; aggravated by coughing and bending forward
	Slipping rib	Onset usually after trauma; loosened fibrous attachments binding lower costal cartilages to one another causing one rib to "slip" over the one above	Unilateral lower chest wall pain; a painful click is appreciated with selected movements
Muscular	Pectoral muscle strain	Pain arising after overuse injury, e.g., lifting, painting an overhead ceiling, etc.	Chest wall muscle soreness; pain is usually more lateral than that of costosternal pain
	Intercostal muscle injury	Gradual onset of discomfort arising after unaccustomed and excessive activity, e.g., lifting, rowing	Vague chest wall pain, often bilateral; associated tenderness on palpation of affected muscles
	Sternalis syndrome	Myalgia affecting the sternalis muscle	Mild to moderate deep, aching pain along the sternum which radiates laterally; not aggravated by movement but can be elicited with palpation of trigger points
	Fibromyalgia	Unexplained musculoskeletal pain,	Tender spots localized to the second intercostal

Table 23.2 (*cont.*)

Source	Condition	Features	Symptoms
		associated with multiple body-wide tender points	space, but may affect other levels, lateral to the costosternal joint; pain is reproducible with palpation
	Myalgia related to infection	Caused by acute viral infections, e.g., coxsackie B virus	Sharp, lateral chest wall pain, and possibly abdominal pain, accompanied by fever and malaise
Neuropathic	Intercostal neuralgia	Intercostal nerve injury caused by prior thoracic surgery/injury or herpes zoster infection	Constant, burning or gnawing pain; not generally aggravated by movement; associated with diminished sensation and/or allodynia
	Diabetic truncal neuropathy	Usually affects the middle to lower thoracic segments of patients with diabetes mellitus	Sharp and burning pain, associated with paresthesias, dysesthesias, and hyperpathia extending over the chest and back
Other	Precordial catch syndrome	Pain associated with a slouched position; may be pleural in origin; common in children	Brief, sharp, left-sided chest pain without prototypic cardiac-like radiation patterns

Adapted from Gregory *et al.* 2002, Proulx & Zryd 2009, Stochkendahl & Christensen 2010.

when coughing or sneezing. Physical therapy may be helpful in some cases, although much of the data is anecdotal.

Costovertebral pain can be addressed with chiropractic manipulations of the affected ribs and spine, when there is subluxation. The therapist manipulates the ribs, moving them in downward, forward, and lateral directions while the patient is lying in a prone position. The manipulation has been reportedly employed to successfully mitigate pain; the response can be immediate, but in some cases may ensue over 1–2 days.

Interventional procedures

For patients with particularly severe pain and/or cases refractory to the above measures, injection of affected joints with 0.25% bupivacaine and corticosteroid, i.e., 40 mg methylprednisolone, via a 25-gauge needle under aseptic technique may be helpful in mitigating physical symptoms. This is applied via the costo-sternal joints, in proximity to the joint where the rib attaches to the sternum. Although blind injection into the costovertebral joints is possible by the experienced clinician, arthrography may help to delineate the joint(s) requiring intervention. However, in the case of pain due to tumor/metastasis, injection would not be undertaken. Oncology consultation may assist in determining whether irradiation therapy would be beneficial.

Follow-up

The frequency of patient follow-up is targeted toward monitoring of the efficacy of, and potential adverse side effects associated with, medication use. Reassess-ment will be necessary to assess the efficacy of treatment approaches and to determine whether more aggressive interventional approaches warrant consider-ation. Failure to achieve relief should prompt consideration of the accuracy of diagnosis and whether other conditions ought to be worked up.

Prognosis

With the exception of patients afflicted with tumor or systemic rheumatologic conditions precipitating pain, most patients can usually be reassured that costo-sternal/chondral as well as costovertebral syndromes are benign conditions and will eventually resolve; a majority of cases resolve within 1 year. Generally, the clinical course is self-limiting, with many patients reporting resolution of symptoms within weeks to months.

REFERENCES AND FURTHER READING

Benhamou CL, Roux CH, Gervais T, Viala JF. Costo-vertebral arthropathy: diagnostic and therapeutic value of arthography. *Clin Rheumatol* 1988; **7**: 220–3.

Disla E, Rhim HR, Reddy A, Karten I, Taranta A. Costochondritis: a prospective analysis in an emergency department setting. *Arch Int Med* 1994; **154**: 2466–9.

Gregory PL, Biswas AC, Batt ME. Musculoskeletal problems of the chest wall in athletes. *Sports Med* 2002; **32**: 235–50.

Karlson KA. Thoracic region pain in athletes. *Curr Sports Med Rep* 2004; **3**: 53–7.

Proulx AM, Zryd TW. Costochondritis: diagnosis and treatment. *Am Fam Physician* 2009; **80**: 617–20.

Stochkendahl MJ, Christensen HW. Chest pain in focal musculoskeletal disorders. *Med Clin North Am* 2010; **94**: 259–73.

24

Intercostal neuralgia

Clinical presentation

Intercostal neuralgia refers to a neuropathic condition involving the intercostal nerves, manifesting as intense dysesthetic pain, e.g., sharp, shooting, or burning in quality. The pain is localized to one or more of the intercostal spaces. Because the pain can span the chest or upper abdomen, afflicted patients may become alarmed about the possibility of having an underlying serious condition from a visceral origin, e.g., myocardial infarction or gallbladder-related pain, and thus may be apt to solicit medical attention.

The 12 pairs of thoracic spinal nerves exit the intervertebral foramina of the thoracic vertebrae bilaterally and immediately divide into dorsal and ventral rami. The intercostal nerves are extensions of the ventral rami. The first 11 nerves are referred to as intercostal nerves; the twelfth nerve is designated as the subcostal nerve. Each of the 12 nerves travels in a groove along the inferior border of the corresponding rib, along with the intercostal artery and vein in a neurovascular bundle sandwiched between the internal and innermost intercostal muscles. The first and second intercostal nerves can send cutaneous branches that also supply the axilla and medial aspect of the arm (i.e., the intercostobrachial nerve). In addition to serving their corresponding intercostal spaces, the lower nerves, specifically intercostal nerves 7–12, subserve abdominal cutaneous sensory functions as well as supplying motor input to the abdominal muscles.

Intercostal neuropathic pain arises from irritation or injury to the intercostal and/or subcostal nerves, e.g., nerve entrapment, traumatic neuroma, persistent nerve irritation, or infection. Surgery, blunt chest wall trauma, and infection are among the most common etiological factors. Intercostal nerve injury can arise from direct trauma, compression arising from the use of retractors and excessive stretching at the costovertebral junction in the course of thoracic surgery. The precise mechanisms underlying nerve injury following thoracic surgery can be heterogeneous, and they vary depending on whether the patient has

undergone thoracotomy, sternotomy, or video-assisted thoracic surgery. Predictive factors for chronic post-thoracotomy pain include young age, more extensive
surgery, pleurectomy, and radiotherapy. It is noteworthy that other surgical
interventions can also precipitate intercostal neuralgia, including breast surgery
(e.g., augmentation) and abdominal surgery.

Dysesthesia arising in one, or few, intercostal spaces that precedes emergence
of a maculopapular rash (usually within 2–3 days) and subsequent vesicle formation signals an emerging acute herpes zoster (varicella) infection. In contrast to
acute herpes zoster infection, long-standing deafferentation and central sensitization may precipitate pain arising from post-herpetic neuralgia affecting the
intercostal nerves. Other rare causes of intercostal mononeuropathy include
intercostal neuritis, lung and mediastinum tumor invasion, and thoracic
radiculopathy.

Signs and symptoms

Evaluation of intercostal neuralgia warrants an accurate patient history with
attention to onset and course of symptoms, location, quality and intensity of
pain symptoms, as well as aggravating and mitigating factors. Characterization
of these features will assist the clinician in determining whether the chest wall
pain with which the patient presents arises from intercostal neuralgia or from
musculoskeletal origins, e.g., costochondritis or costovertebral syndromes
(see Chapter 23). Unlike the pain of musculoskeletal origins, the pain of intercostal neuralgia is characteristically constant, enduring, and typically described as
burning, shooting, or electric in nature (as opposed to sharp and primarily related
to movement). Generally, the pain is experienced as emanating from the posterior
axillary line with anterior radiation toward the sternum. The pain is not particularly aggravated by movement (e.g., deep inspiration or coughing, etc.), as would
be the case with pain associated with musculoskeletal conditions. However, it is
conceivable that patients who have postoperative pain may experience concurrent
musculoskeletal pain and, therefore, may display commensurate overt signs, e.g.,
pain with movement and splinting of affected areas.

Physical examination typically reveals minimal findings. However, it is pertinent to assess patients for surgical scars (i.e., status post prior thoracic or subcostal
surgery) or rash along thoracic dermatomes suggestive of herpes zoster.
Significant physical findings will reveal decreased sensation and/or allodynia on
neurological examination: e.g., application of light touch, cold, and heat can be
useful to test for allodynia and/or sensory deficits; pinprick to elicit hyperesthesia;
and pressure to assess for mechanical hyperalgesia. Such measures, when systematically applied, can aid in clarifying which intercostal nerves are involved.
Implementation of an intercostal nerve blockade can serve as an adjunctive
diagnostic procedure, in addition to providing therapeutic benefit (described
below).

Laboratory tests and diagnostic investigations

The diagnosis of intercostal neuralgia is based on the above clinical findings. There are no confirmatory laboratory investigations per se. However, some laboratory investigations, such as immunoassays (indirect fluorescent antibody test), serology (enzyme-linked immunosorbent assay, ELISA), viral culture, and polymerase chain reaction (PCR), can be useful in clarifying if the patient's symptoms are related to an acute herpes zoster infection.

Imaging studies

Plain chest radiography is necessary to establish that the pain experienced by the patient cannot be better accounted for by fracture, occult bony pathology, or tumor. Radionucleotide bone scanning may detect occult rib or sternal fractures, especially if there is a history of recent trauma. If tumor is suspected, CT scanning of the thorax is warranted.

Differential diagnosis

Chest wall pain presumed to be related to intercostal neuralgia must be differentiated from pain arising from other causes. It should be noted that some of these conditions can coexist with intercostal neuralgia. For example, post-thoracotomy pain can have a myofascial component, e.g., taut muscular bands within intercostal muscles or more remote sites such as the scapular muscles, which can obscure the clinical picture. Toward this end, the clinician will need to consider the following differential diagnostic possibilities:
- chondroma
- costochondral pain
- costovertebral syndrome, e.g., subluxation
- diabetic polyneuropathy
- myofascial pain
- pleural processes (infection, abscess, mesothelioma)
- rib and/or sternum fracture
- thoracic intervertebral foramen impingement
- Tietze's syndrome
- visceral sources (pulmonary embolism, lung or mediastinal tumor)

Pharmacotherapy

Patients afflicted with intercostal neuralgia can be treated initially with non-steroidal anti-inflammatory drugs (NSAIDs) and cyclooxygenase-2 (COX-2) inhibitors, and possibly tramadol. Patients with neuropathic pain may require trials of antidepressants and anticonvulsants, e.g., alpha-2-delta ligands such as gabapentin or pregabalin among other anticonvulsant agents. The proposed benefit of antidepressants and/or anticonvulsants is largely extrapolated from studies demonstrating the benefits obtained from employing these medications in other neuropathic pain states. Systematic investigation into their use in patients with intercostal neuralgia has been lacking, with data often based on anecdotal reports and small case series. Additionally, there is a dearth of investigations comparing the efficacy of one approach versus another, or determining the efficacy of combined endeavors versus those administered in isolation. Caution would naturally be required with the use of any of these agents: for example, side effects may limit tolerability and resultant utility, and in some cases may be prohibitive (e.g., during pregnancy).

Inadequate responses to the aforementioned agents may necessitate low-dose opioid analgesics, but the benefits may need to be balanced against potential risks/adverse effects. Topical lidocaine may also be helpful to mitigate neuropathic pain, such as that associated with herpes zoster; topical capsaicin may relieve itch and skin hypersensitivity as well. However, some patients may experience significant discomfort, precluding utility. Failure to respond to these agents, along with concurrent non-pharmacologic approaches, may necessitate interventional approaches.

Non-pharmacologic approaches

Symptomatic pain relief may, in some cases, be achieved through application of heat or cold, and possibly through the use of an elastic rib belt. Patients with significant allodynia may not be able to tolerate such approaches, however.

Interventional procedures

When pharmacologic modalities produce unsatisfactory relief, treatment may proceed to non-operative interventions including intercostal nerve or thoracic nerve root blockade employing local anesthetics (either 1% lidocaine or 0.25% bupivacaine) and/or 40 mg methylprednisolone. Intercostal nerve blocks are conducted with the patient lying prone. The needle is inserted at the level of the lower half of the rib, at the angle of the rib posteriorly, laterally at the posterior axillary line, or anteriorly at the axillary line. The needle is then slowly "walked off" the width of the rib until it "slips" off the rib margin. At the level of the costal groove, the needle is aspirated to ensure that there has been no inadvertent penetration of the artery or vein. If no blood is drawn up, 2–3 mL of anesthetic is administered. By contrast, with thoracic nerve root blockade, anesthetic agent administration is directed at the posterolateral aspect of the thoracic vertebrae so as to target the nerve root as it exits the intervertebral foramina.

There is overlap of thoracic dermatomes. Therefore, to achieve complete block of a particular intercostal space, it will be necessary to concurrently block either the intercostal nerves or the thoracic nerve roots immediately above and below the intercostal space for which the intended effect is desired. The demonstration of skin anesthesia over the intercostal space demonstrates that an adequate block has been achieved.

Both procedures are relatively simple, but there are noteworthy complications of which the practitioner must be aware. Although pneumothorax is a possibility, its occurrence has been reported in less than 1% of cases involving intercostal nerve blockade. Often, treatment of pneumothorax is symptomatic unless there is marked dyspnea and/or evidence of tension pneumothorax. In addition, systemic toxicity arising from intercostal nerve blockade is a potential worrisome outcome; blood levels of administered local anesthetics can be quite high, purportedly higher than that associated with administration of anesthetics in other peripheral nerve, epidural, or spinal blocks. For this reason, it is essential that the total amount of local anesthetic administered during sequential intercostal nerve blockade is limited, to reduce the potential of incurring toxic systemic effects. Patients should be closely monitored after the procedure for signs of toxicity, e.g., hypotension, nausea, and feeling faint. In addition, because of close proximity to blood vessels within the neurovascular bundle lying within the costal groove, it is imperative that the clinician first carefully perform aspiration to ensure that the anesthetic is not administered intravascularly.

Similarly, pneumothorax can be encountered in thoracic nerve root blockade, but is unlikely. Widespread anesthetic effects can be possible in this procedure as well, especially if there is a long dural sleeve over the nerve root and/or if large volumes of anesthetic (> 5 mL) are injected.

Surgical intervention is reserved for patients who fail to respond favorably to conservative treatment measures. Neurectomy of the intercostal nerve with implantation of the severed nerve into the latissimus dorsi muscle may be a consideration.

Follow-up

The frequency of patient follow-up is targeted toward monitoring of the efficacy of, and potential adverse side effects associated with, medication use and interventional approaches. Failure to achieve relief should prompt: (1) consideration of the accuracy of diagnosis; (2) assessment of alternative explanations for the persistent pain and/or coexisting conditions; (3) inquiry into patient adherence with medications; and (4) consideration of alternative interventional approaches to be undertaken.

Prognosis

Many patients can be reassured that the pain of intercostal neuralgia is often responsive to treatment. Unfortunately, in some cases, including neuralgia arising from progression and/or recurrence of mediastinum/thoracic tumor, post-herpetic, and a minority cases arising postoperatively, the intercostal neuralgia may remain recalcitrant to treatment endeavors. In such cases, continuous monitoring may be required, and it may be necessary to employ several concomitant treatment approaches to mitigate discomfort.

REFERENCES AND FURTHER READING

Karmakar MK, Ho AM. Postthoracotomy pain syndrome. *Thorac Surg Clin* 2004; **14**: 345–52.

Koehler RP, Keenan RJ. Management of postthoracotomy pain: acute and chronic. *Thorac Surg Clin* 2006; **16**: 287–97.

Rendina EA, Ciccone AM. The intercostal space. *Thorac Surg Clin* 2007; **17**: 491–501.

Sihoe ADL, Lee TW, Wan IYP, Thung KH, Yim APC. The use of gabapentin for post-operative and post-traumatic pain in thoracic surgery patients. *Eur J Cardiothorac Surg* 2006; **29**: 795–9.

25

Post-thoracotomy, post-cardiac surgery, and post-mastectomy pain syndromes

Clinical presentation

Chronic post-surgical pain after thoracotomy, cardiac surgery, and mastectomy can last for several months to years. Post-thoracotomy pain syndrome describes chronic pain conditions that last beyond the expected recovery after thoracotomy. Inadequate management of acute postoperative pain is more likely to result in chronic pain. The common causes of post-thoracotomy pain are surgical exploration and damage to ribs, retractor compression, or stretch injury of intercostal nerves and consequent formation of neuroma. The pain generators may include nociceptive pain related to injury of musculoskeletal structures and neuropathic pain of intercostal nerves.

Persistent anterior chest wall and sternal pain are common after cardiac surgery. The potential causes are sternal wires, sternal or costosternal instability, and intercostal neuralgia due to dissection of the internal mammary artery from the chest wall.

Post-mastectomy pain or post-surgical breast pain syndrome has been reported not only after radical mastectomy but also after lumpectomy and any other surgical procedures involving the breast. The onset can be either soon after surgery or a few weeks later. Post-mastectomy syndrome is commonly associated with axillary dissection and surgical injury of an intercostobrachial nerve. A neuropathic mechanism seems to play a major role in post-mastectomy pain syndrome, as compared to less input from a nociceptive source.

Signs and symptoms

Post-thoracotomy pain syndrome presents with severe chest wall pain aggravated by deep respiratory movement. There is explicit neuritis along the path of any affected intercostal nerve, as confirmed by examination. Palpation of surgical scar and previous chest tube sites may expose exquisite tenderness indicating the presence of neuroma. Post-cardiac surgery pain may consist of pain and tenderness over the costosternal region in addition to other findings similar to those of post-thoracotomy pain syndrome.

Post-mastectomy pain syndrome involves the breast, anterior chest wall, axilla, and the medial aspect of the arm. Patients complain of numbness and tingling, burning, and stabbing pain. Physical examination endorses dysesthesia, allodynia, hyperalgesia, and hyperpathia of the anterior chest wall, with characteristics of neuropathic pain.

Laboratory tests and diagnostic investigations

There is no specific laboratory test for confirmation of post-thoracotomy or post-mastectomy pain syndrome. Routine work-up, including a complete blood count, erythrocyte sedimentation rate, automated chemistry profile, and oncologic protocol are ordered according to clinical impressions.

Imaging studies

Plain radiographs are ordered as a first step to rule out bony pathology. A radionuclide bone scan can provide surveillance for any pathology of chest wall structures. A CT scan of the chest may detect a new or recurrent lesion as a latent pain generator leading to post-thoracotomy or post-mastectomy pain syndromes. MRI of the brachial plexus may outline tumor invasion as the potential cause of plexopathy.

Differential diagnosis

Please refer to Chapters 23 and 24 for differential diagnosis of costosternal, costochondral, and costovertebral syndromes, intercostal neuralgia, and potential coexisting medical conditions.

Persistent postoperative pain may not be the only cause of post-thoracotomy, post-cardiac surgery, and post-mastectomy pain syndromes. Post-surgical complications such as wound infection, hematoma or fluid retention, or re-exploration may cause more severe and persistent pain. Careful surveillance might identify tumor invasion or metastatic disease, and pathologic rib fracture as opposed to just delayed recovery from oncological thoracotomy and mastectomy. Occult fracture of ribs or sternum should always be considered in cases of trauma-related thoracotomy or cardiac surgery.

Phantom breast syndrome may occur after mastectomy, with noxious or dysesthesia complaints over the site of the missing breast. The risk factors may include significant pre-existing pain symptoms prior to the mastectomy, younger premenopausal women, and psychosocial factors such as impaired body image.

Presentation of neuropathic pain due to acute herpes zoster and diabetic polyneuropathy could be coexistent conditions in patients who have undergone thoracotomy, cardiac surgery, or mastectomy.

Myofascial pain syndrome may present deep aching pain over the anterior chest wall and tenderness on palpation of trigger points over involved muscle. Local anesthetic injection may relieve the symptoms and improve range of motion.

Pharmacotherapy

Acetaminophen, non-steroidal anti-inflammatory drugs (NSAIDs), cyclooxygenase-2 (COX-2) inhibitors, and skeletal muscle relaxants may be the first-line therapy to alleviate mild to moderate nociceptive pain after thoracotomy and mastectomy. All these adjuvant analgesics require vigilant follow-up throughout the titration and maintenance phases, and this vigilance should continue during tapering off.

Anticonvulsants, tricyclic antidepressants (TCAs), serotonin–norepinephrine reuptake inhibitors (SNRIs), and sodium channel blocking agents have all been proposed for modulation of the prevalent neuropathic pain associated with thoracotomy and mastectomy.

Although opioids are prescribed in moderate to severe acute pain after thoracotomy and mastectomy, their efficacy in chronic pain management has not been well supported by evidence-based studies.

Non-pharmacologic approaches

Physical and occupational therapy are essential components of comprehensive management after thoracotomy and mastectomy. Common hands-on and physical modalities including manipulation, adjustments, massage, ultrasound, and transcutaneous electrical nerve stimulation (TENS) are all helpful in both acute and chronic management of chest wall, axilla, shoulder, and arm pain. The psychosocial impact of injury due to thoracotomy, cardiac surgery, and mastectomy can never be overestimated; hence patient support groups, cognitive behavioral therapy (CBT), biofeedback, and neurofeedback could be implemented as part of an interdisciplinary and multimodal approach.

Interventional procedures

A thoracic epidural catheter may be placed prior to surgery and continued through postoperative care. It will provide better coverage for acute pain and may reduce the severity and incidence of chronic pain. Optimal pre-emptive and perioperative analgesia should be considered to minimize the incidence of phantom breast. Thoracic paravertebral nerve blocks may also contribute to multimodal analgesia to alleviate the acute or chronic pain related to surgery.

Intercostal nerve or brachial plexus block with local anesthetic and corticosteroid are indicated as both diagnostic and therapeutic approaches for post-thoracotomy or post-mastectomy pain. Cervicothoracic sympathetic (stellate ganglion) block is indicated for alleviation of sympathetic overlay, whether brachial plexopathy or complex regional pain syndrome (CRPS) as a working diagnosis, after thoracotomy, cardiac surgery, and mastectomy.

Cryoanalgesia offers a useful technique that does not cause any long-term histological damage to intercostal nerves and is thus without serious side effects. Cryoanalgesia is indicated to alleviate post-thoracotomy and post-mastectomy pain, and it can potentially reduce the consumption of analgesics.

Chemical neurolysis and pulsed or thermo-radiofrequency neuroablation could be considered, mostly for intractable cases of post-thoracotomy or post-mastectomy pain syndrome especially of neoplastic origin.

Neuromodulation therapy, such as a trial of peripheral nerve stimulation, spinal cord stimulation, or deep brain stimulation, may be an alternative modality to minimize adverse events, avoiding any denervation or destruction of structure.

Follow-up

Multidisciplinary and multimodal approaches and vigilant follow-up to guide every stage of treatment are mandatory to achieve the best outcome in patients with post-thoracotomy, post-cardiac surgery, and post-mastectomy pain syndromes.

Prognosis

The prognosis is really contingent on early diagnosis and treatment of underlying disease (e.g., idiopathic, trauma, or neoplasm). In general, cancer-related thoracotomy and mastectomy pain syndromes may impose both physical and psychological concerns. However, it is still encouraging to focus on improving a patient's functional capacity and quality of life despite the winding course of various post-thoracotomy, post-cardiac surgery, and post-mastectomy pain syndromes.

REFERENCES AND FURTHER READING

Alves Nogueira Fabro E, Bergmann A, do Amaral E Silva B, et al. Post-mastectomy pain syndrome: incidence and risks. Breast 2012; 21: 321–5.

Björkman B, Arnér S, Hydén LC. Phantom breast and other syndromes after mastectomy: eight breast cancer patients describe their experiences over time: a 2-year follow-up study. *J Pain* 2008; **9**: 1018–25.

Fiorelli A, Morgillo F, Milione R, *et al.* Control of post-thoracotomy pain by transcutaneous electrical nerve stimulation: effect on serum cytokine levels, visual analogue scale, pulmonary function and medication. *Eur J Cardiothorac Surg* 2012; **41**: 861–8.

Grider JS, Mullet TW, Saha SP, Harned ME, Sloan PA. A randomized, double-blind trial comparing continuous thoracic epidural bupivacaine with and without opioid in contrast to a continuous paravertebral infusion of bupivacaine for post-thoracotomy pain. *J Cardiothorac Vasc Anesth* 2012; **26**: 83–9.

Guastella V, Mick G, Soriano C, *et al.* A prospective study of neuropathic pain induced by thoracotomy: incidence, clinical description, and diagnosis. *Pain* 2011; **152**: 74–81.

Momenzadeh S, Elyasi H, Valaie N, *et al.* Effect of cryoanalgesia on post-thoracotomy pain. *Acta Med Iran* 2011; **49**: 241–5.

Mustola ST, Lempinen J, Saimanen E, Vilkko P. Efficacy of thoracic epidural analgesia with or without intercostal nerve cryoanalgesia for postthoracotomy pain. *Ann Thorac Surg* 2011; **91**: 869–73.

26

Thoracic spinal pain

Clinical presentation

Thoracic spinal pain may involve axial mid back, rib cage, chest wall, and upper abdominal regions. The common causes of thoracic spinal pain include thoracic radiculopathy, facet arthropathy, vertebral compression fracture, thoracic strain and sprain, intercostal neuralgia, herpes zoster, and post-herpetic neuralgia. The onset and sequence are determined by the underlying sources of the pain.

The etiologies of thoracic radiculopathy may consist of disc protusion or herniation, foraminal narrowing, spinal stenosis, and degenerative disc disease. Thoracic facet hypertrophy, osteophytes, and spondylosis may cause axial back pain with a specific referred pattern to the thoracic region.

Vertebral fractures could have a drastic onset due to trauma, or an insidious onset in patients with osteoporosis and primary or metastatic neoplasms. Thoracic strain or sprain could be idiopathic or related to sports injury and trauma.

Signs and symptoms

Thoracic radiculopathy may present with numbness, tingling, and radicular pain along the dermatome of a specific nerve root. Physical examination may reveal impaired sensory and motor function, or even changes in superficial abdominal reflexes. Thoracic radiculopathy may be associated with compression of the thoracic spinal cord and myelopathy resulting in motor and sensory deficit. The Brown-Séquard syndrome may be caused by compression of the thoracic spinal cord that results in spastic paralysis of the ipsilateral muscle below the lesion and loss of sensation on the contralateral side.

Thoracic facet arthropathy may cause localized aching pain and spasm that are aggravated by extension and twist movements of the spine, and relieved by flexion. There are fewer radicular symptoms, and less numbness and tingling around the rib cage and chest wall, than with radiculitis or radiculopathy.

There is tenderness on deep palpation over the facet joints, and symptoms can be reproduced by range of motion movements of the back.

The symptoms of vertebral fractures may vary from minimal displacement and only mild dull aching pain to intractable pain in severe cases. There is deformity of the spine, tenderness, and paraspinal muscle spasm on palpation of affected vertebral fractures. Burst fractures are crush fractures of the anterior and middle columns of the vertebral body that may result in neurological compromise. The extent of injury should be carefully assessed in a case of vertebral fracture related to serious trauma. The severe pain could compromise the patient's respiratory function, and this may result in subsequent atelectasis and pneumonia.

Laboratory tests and diagnostic investigations

Complete blood count (CBC), erythrocyte sedimentation rate (ESR), antinuclear antibody (ANA), and any automated blood chemistry panels can be considered as screening tests in thoracic spinal pain. Tumor markers and other oncologic tests may be indicated in a case of a vertebral compression fracture of unclear etiology.

The ESR is elevated in an estimated 85% cases of ankylosing spondylitis. HLA-B27 is a sensitive but not specific diagnostic test in ankylosing spondylitis. There is no specific laboratory test for confirmation of diffuse idiopathic skeletal hyperostosis (DISH).

Electromyography (EMG) and nerve conduction studies (NCS) can provide further neurophysiologic information regarding the extent of involvement of thoracic nerve roots and paravertebral plexus in radiculopathy, facet arthropathy, and vertebral compression fracture.

Imaging studies

MRI is indicated for work-up of thoracic radiculopathy. CT or CT myelography are alternatives whenever MRI is contraindicated. Plain radiography and radio-nuclide bone scanning are indicated for vertebral compression fractures or bony lesions including neoplasms. Bone density study is also important in patients with a history of osteopenia or osteoporosis and compression fracture.

The bilateral and symmetrical erosion and sclerosis of sacroiliac joints may be found by plain radiography in early ankylosing spondylitis. The "bamboo spine" is a characteristic late radiographic feature in ankylosing spondylitis: the vertebral bodies are fused by vertically oriented, bridging syndesmophytes formed by the ossification of the annulus fibrosus and calcification of anterior and lateral spinal ligaments.

Plain radiography and CT scans in DISH may reveal spinal hyperostosis that results in linear ossification and bridging osteophytes along the anterior and lateral aspects of vertebral bodies. The sacroiliac joints are usually normal in DISH.

Arthritis of the costovertebral and costotransverse joints may be confirmed by plain radiography in costovertebral arthritis.

Differential diagnosis

Ankylosing spondylitis and DISH may present with localized dull aching pain, tightness, or spasm of posterior paraspinal structures. There is tenderness on deep palpation, and aggravation of pain related to movements of back and chest expansion. Ankylosing spondylitis is characterized by onset of back pain prior to age 30, morning stiffness, pain that improves with activity, and bilateral sacroiliac joint pain. DISH usually affects the thoracic spine. Rheumatoid arthritis (RA) mainly disturbs the cervical spine and multiple small joints of the hands and feet. RA and DISH usually spare the sacroiliac joints.

Thoracic spinal pain of muscular origin from the posterior chest may involve rhomboid major and minor, latissimus dorsi, multifidus, serratus posterior superior and inferior, and iliocostalis thoracis and lumborum. There is deep aching pain in various parts of the back, and tenderness on identification of individual trigger points. The symptom of thoracic myofascial pain is usually aggravated by activity of certain muscles and unaffected by bodily activity.

It would be prudent to carry out a comprehensive evaluation in traumatic injury to the thoracic region to rule out cardiac or pulmonary contusion and vascular compromise in addition to vertebral compression fracture. The differential diagnosis of thoracic spinal pain in non-trauma cases may include infection, aortic aneurysm, primary or metastatic neoplasm, multiple sclerosis, syringomyelia, transverse myelitis, or other spinal cord diseases in addition to thoracic radiculopathy, facet arthropathy, and vertebral fracture.

Pharmacotherapy

Acetaminophen, non-steroidal anti-inflammatory drugs (NSAIDs), cyclooxygenase-2 (COX-2) inhibitors, and skeletal muscle relaxants may help symptomatic relief of mild to moderate pain and spasm, especially in the acute phase of thoracic radiculopathy, facet arthropathy, and vertebral compression fracture. Various anticonvulsants, sodium channel blocking agents, tricyclic antidepressants (TCAs), and serotonin–norepinephrine reuptake inhibitors (SNRIs) are commonly prescribed off-label for modulation of chronic pain that does not respond to anti-nociception treatment.

Although opioids are prescribed in moderate to severe acute pain, their efficacy in the management of chronic thoracic spinal pain has not been well supported by evidence-based studies.

Non-pharmacologic approaches

Close observation and rest are crucial in the acute phase of thoracic spinal pain. Physical modalities and agents (e.g., heat, cold, ultrasound, electrical stimulation, manual therapy, joint mobilization, massage, water therapy, and low-impact exercise programs) and complementary and alternative medicine (e.g., acupuncture) could all be valuable in the acute, subacute, and chronic phases of thoracic spinal pain. Utilizing a non-pharmacologic approach provides symptomatic relief and support while minimizing adverse events related to pharmacotherapy.

Interventional procedures

Thoracic interlaminar (translaminar) epidural steroid injection under fluoroscopic guidance is usually indicated for radicular and axial pains that are refractory to conservative treatments. There is modest support regarding the benefit of thoracic epidural steroid injection as a part of non-surgical treatment. A series of three epidural steroid injections every 6–12 months as needed, at 3–4-week intervals, is a general recommendation in moderate to severe thoracic radiculopathy. A number of case studies have suggested that patients with radicular pain may respond better than a cohort with axial pain only to thoracic epidural steroid injection.

Thoracic facet joint intra-articular injection with local anesthetic can serve as a diagnostic tool to verify the specific pain generator, and also provides clinical improvement in range of motion of the back. Neural blockade of the medial branch (of the dorsal ramus) may denervate thoracic muscle, ligament, periosteum, and facet joint. Radiofrequency thermal neuroablation (neurotomy) of the facet medial branch may provide more lasting pain relief (estimated nerve regeneration takes up to 6–9 months) and thereby facilitate timely functional restoration. The efficacy and outcome of medial branch neurotomy in the thoracic region has not been as well established as in the lumbar region.

Follow-up

The level of pain relief, reduction of neurologic dysfunction, improvement in back range of motion, and functional capacity should all be key indicators in the careful follow-up of thoracic spinal pain.

Prognosis

There may be spontaneous recovery or improvement with non-surgical treatment of mild to moderate thoracic spinal pain. Although the natural course of severe radiculopathy and facet arthropathy may lead to deterioration of neurologic deficit and agonizing pain, any spinal surgery should still be reserved for selected candidates after careful decision making.

REFERENCES AND FURTHER READING

Leininger B, Bronfort G, Evans R, Reiter T. Spinal manipulation or mobilization for radiculopathy: a systematic review. *Phys Med Rehabil Clin N Am* 2011; **22**: 105–25.

Longo UG, Loppini M, Denaro L, Maffulli N, Denaro V. Conservative management of patients with an osteoporotic vertebral fracture: a review of the literature. *J Bone Joint Surg Br* 2012; **94**: 152–7.

Manchikanti L, Cash KA, McManus CD, Pampati V, Benyamin RM. A preliminary report of a randomized double-blind, active controlled trial of fluoroscopic thoracic interlaminar epidural injections in managing chronic thoracic pain. *Pain Physician* 2010; **13**: E357–69.

Manchikanti L, Singh V, Falco FJ, *et al.* Comparative effectiveness of a one-year follow-up of thoracic medial branch blocks in management of chronic thoracic pain: a randomized, double-blind active controlled trial. *Pain Physician* 2010; **13**: 535–48.

Schofer MD, Efe T, Timmesfeld N, Kortmann HR, Quante M. Comparison of kyphoplasty and vertebroplasty in the treatment of fresh vertebral compression fractures. *Arch Orthop Trauma Surg* 2009; **129**: 1391–9.

Vanichkachorn JS, Vaccaro AR. Thoracic disk disease: diagnosis and treatment. *J Am Acad Orthop Surg* 2000; **8**: 159–69.

van Kleef M, Stolker RJ, Lataster A, *et al.* Evidence-based interventional pain medicine according to clinical diagnoses, 10. Thoracic pain. *Pain Pract* 2010; **10**: 327–38.

Abdomen and pelvis

27

Acute and chronic pancreatitis

Clinical presentation

Acute pancreatitis is an inflammatory process causing a premature release of activated pancreatic enzymes precipitating autodigestion and pain. Chronic pancreatitis refers to inflammation resulting in permanent structural damage to the pancreas. Common causes of pancreatitis are summarized in Table 27.1; the most common of these include alcoholism and biliary tract disease, which between them account for more than 80% of acute pancreatic cases.

Nociceptive information from the densely populated afferent fibers of the pancreas is relayed to the celiac plexus. The celiac plexus is a dumbbell-shaped constellation of nerve fibers located in fatty areolar tissue embedded at the origins of the celiac and superior mesenteric arteries emerging from the aorta. From here, sensory information passes via the splanchnic nerves to converge on the CNS pain pathways. The nociceptive information relayed can be triggered by mechanical (e.g., increased pancreatic duct pressure due to strictures, calculi, and pancreatic ischemia, interstitial hypertension, fibrosis, and pseudocysts); chemical (e.g., inflammatory mediators including interleukins, bradykinin, substance P, and histamine), and neurogenic stimuli (e.g., nerve entrapment, sensitized visceral nerves and receptors).

Signs and symptoms

Patients with pancreatitis report steady, deep, boring, and gnawing upper (mid-epigastric) abdominal pain. In approximately 50% of cases the pain radiates to the back. The onset can be heterogeneous: for example, the pain associated with alcoholic pancreatitis can develop gradually over several days, whereas gallstone pancreatitis pain can arise suddenly. Associated features include nausea and vomiting. The pain may be attenuated by sitting upright and leaning forward, but is aggravated by coughing, deep inspiration, and vigorous movement.

Table 27.1 Etiological factors causing pancreatitis

Alcoholism	**Autoimmune disease**
Mechanical	Sjögren's syndrome
Gallstones	Systemic lupus erythematosus
Pancreatic intraductal stones/plugs	Primary sclerosing cholangitis
Pancreas divisum	**Infection**
Pancreatic cancer	Coxsackie B virus
Periampullary cancer	Cytomegalovirus
Sphincter of Oddi stenosis	Mumps
Endoscopic retrograde cholangio-pancreatography (ERCP)-induced	**Medication**
	Angiotensin-converting enzyme (ACE) inhibitors
Trauma	Asparaginase
Metabolic disturbances	Azathioprine
Hypertriglyceridemia	Furosemide
Hypercalcemia	Sulfa drugs
Hyperparathyroidism	Valproate
Cystic fibrosis	

Patients appear acutely ill, with notable physical distress, diaphoresis, and tachycardia. The patient may be hypertensive or hypotensive. Orthostatic hypotension may be observed. Respirations are often shallow and rapid. The abdomen may be distended, possibly due to a pancreatic mass or because of ascites resulting from pancreatic duct disruption. Bowel sounds may be reduced. With palpation, the upper abdomen may reveal rebound tenderness; the lower abdomen may also be tender, but less so. There is no associated rectal pain, and the stools are occult-blood negative.

Laboratory tests and diagnostic investigations

Serum amylase and lipase are useful indicators of acute pancreatitis, although elevated serum levels of both enzymes can arise in other conditions, e.g., perforated ulcer, intestinal obstruction, and mesenteric vascular occlusion. Lipase assessments are perhaps more specific for pancreatitis than amylase, as the latter can be elevated in yet other conditions, e.g., macroamylasemia and salivary gland dysfunction (parotitis). Other useful diagnostic assessments include a complete blood count, serum calcium levels, triglycerides, and bilirubin. The white cell count is often increased in acute inflammation and may signal underlying infection. The hematocrit may increase if hypovolemia develops. Serum calcium is likely to be decreased early in the course of acute disease, due to saponification of excess free fatty acids. Bilirubin may increase if there is edema which results in compression of the common bile duct.

As the disease progresses, fibrosis of the pancreas can result in diminished capacity for the acinar cells to release pancreatic enzymes, producing falsely normal amylase and lipase levels, and thus serum assays of these enzymes may have less utility in chronic pancreatitis. An indicator of diminished pancreatic enzyme production and availability might be assessed by examination of stool for steatorrhea. Endocrine function is also likely to be impaired in chronic disease, producing laboratory parameters suggestive of diabetes mellitus, e.g., hyperglycemia, elevated hemoglobin (Hb) A1c, and impaired glucose tolerance testing. Exacerbations of symptoms and pain in the course of chronic pancreatitis may signal the need for cytological evaluation or assessment of serum markers that may unveil underlying malignancy.

Imaging studies

Abdominal x-ray may reveal pancreatic calcifications within the pancreatic ducts, signaling prior inflammation and hence chronic pancreatitis. Gallstones and localized ileus (affecting the left upper quadrant) may also be notable. Ultrasonography can be useful to detect gallstones and bile duct dilatation.

Contrast-enhanced CT scanning can reveal pancreatic necrosis, pseudocysts, and fluid collection. Bear in mind that contrast agents are useful to identify necrosis but can cause pancreatic damage and necrosis, especially in hypovolemic patients, who are at risk of incurring pancreatic ischemia. CT-guided needle aspiration may be required to collect aspirates for culture and sensitivity if infection of the pancreas is suspected.

Differential diagnosis

There are several conditions that need to be considered in the differential of pancreatitis. Among the possible etiologies, consideration must be given to:
. acute cholecystitis
. mesenteric vascular occlusion
. perforated ulcer
. intestinal obstruction
. ascending cholangitis
. myocardial infarction
. herpes zoster infection
. renal colic
Diagnostic assessments, including laboratory investigations and imaging studies, can help to decipher which of these conditions prevail.

Chronic pancreatitis is characterized by a decline in exocrine and endocrine functions, caused by permanent organ structural damage produced by fibrosis and ductal strictures. In such cases, there is evidence of malabsorption, i.e., steatorrhea. Bear in mind that similar malabsorption states can result from other conditions, such as gastric resection, celiac disease, inflammatory bowel disease, and Zollinger–Ellison syndrome. These warrant elucidation, as the treatments would necessitate other approaches.

Pharmacotherapy

In acute pancreatitis, parenteral opioids will be required to reduce the severity of pain. Initial trials can be given of weaker opioids, e.g., hydrocodone, for mild to moderate pain. If this is insufficient, transition to strong opioids, e.g., morphine, hydromorphone, fentanyl, is appropriate. Bear in mind that opioids can increase smooth muscle tone and can potentially enhance the constriction of the sphincter of Oddi, with the potential effect of exacerbating discomfort; however, the clinical significance of this propensity is uncertain.

Infection of acute necrotizing pancreatitis with commensurate sepsis is associated with significant mortality. Antibiotic prophylaxis, e.g., with imipenem, has been useful to reduce such complications, although the evidence for this remains controversial.

In chronic pancreatitis, pancreatic enzyme supplementation may reduce chronic pain. This is attributable to the reduction in the release of cholecystokinin, thereby reducing pancreatic enzyme release. Preliminary evidence suggests that use of octreotide, a long-acting somatostatic analog which reduces pancreatic enzyme secretion, may help in preventing post-ERCP pain and may mitigate pancreatic-related pain that remains refractory to opioid use in some patients with acute pancreatitis, but routine use of octreotide has not been supported in the literature. Supplementation of fat-soluble vitamins (A, D, K, E) should be provided, particularly in situations in which steatorrhea is severe. Because chronic pancreatitis can be associated with a relapsing clinical course, or persisting course of variable severity, treatment with long-term analgesics and other interventions (described below) may be required.

Non-pharmacologic approaches

Vigorous intravenous hydration will be required so as to reduce hypotension, to address sepsis, to avoid prerenal azotemia, and to avoid further pancreatic necrosis due to hypovolemia. Acutely, fasting can help assist with acute inflammation and resultant pain. Since acute pancreatitis is time-limited, fasting is likely to extend for several days, but in some cases weeks of fasting may be required. Protracted fasting, beyond 4 days, will require supplementation with total parenteral nutrition so as to avoid precipitating malnutrition. Recent research has suggested that enteral nutrition via nasojejunal tube may be more effective than total parenteral nutrition in promoting resolution of acute pancreatitis and may reduce complications, such as infection, and associated mortality.

Abstinence from alcohol is imperative to reduce the progression of disease. Psychiatric treatment, concurrent substance abuse treatment and active participation in Alcoholics Anonymous may be helpful in enhancing maintenance of sobriety in those with a history of alcoholic pancreatitis. Depression often accompanies pancreatic cancer, and this should likewise prompt psychiatric referral and treatment.

Interventional procedures

Persisting pain, poorly responsive to parenteral analgesics, is likely to warrant interventional approaches, especially as long-term opioid use on the part of the patient may raise concerns about abuse/addiction, particularly in patients with histories of alcoholism. Thoracic epidural blockade can be a consideration, using local anesthetic and/or opioid; this procedure allows for optimal analgesia while avoiding the potential for respiratory depression associated with parenteral opioids. Alternatively, CT-guided percutaneous celiac plexus block may be undertaken; however, because of its recurring and relapsing nature, the effects of celiac plexus blockade may be time-limited in chronic pancreatitis. Pain associated with pancreatic cancer may improve with neurolytic celiac plexus block with alcohol or phenol.

Surgical management of the pain of chronic pancreatitis may be undertaken if patients experience relapsing bouts of pain or persisting pain. Such measures can include endoscopic pancreatic duct stenting, pancreatojejunostomy, pancreatectomy or partial resection, and denervation procedures including chemical or endoscopic splanchnicectomy.

Follow-up

Close monitoring in the intensive care unit is required in acute pancreatitis, particularly if signs of hypovolemia and sepsis are present; this is generally not required in chronic pancreatitis. On the other hand, chronic pancreatitis can be associated with relapses and acute exacerbations. There can be a chronic, relapsing course to the pain experienced, especially if there are episodes of acute pancreatitis superimposed on chronic pancreatitis. In such cases, patients may require hospitalization and intensive monitoring. Additionally, patients need to be monitored for worsening symptoms, steatorrhea, and emerging infection. Conversely, in some cases, chronic pancreatitis can be associated with spontaneous pain remissions, due to significant reductions of cellular volume resulting in a lower propensity to develop intraductal pressure.

Prognosis

The prognosis of acute pancreatitis depends upon the extent of injury. For example, the mortality associated with pancreatitis associated with septic necrosis and hemorrhage is several times higher than that of edematous pancreatitis. The mortality of chronic pancreatitis varies widely in the literature, as there are significant confounds that obscure mortality estimates. For example, many deaths and complications arise from persistent alcohol abuse and may not be directly attributable to the pancreatitis per se. Additionally, secondary effects of chronic pancreatic insufficiency, such as diabetes mellitus, can, in turn, add to complications which subsequently increase mortality. It is noteworthy that the mortality associated with chronic pancreatitis is increased in patients with alcoholic pancreatitis as compared with those with pancreatitis arising from other causes. The literature suggests that the rate of pancreatic cancer is increased in patients with chronic pancreatitis.

REFERENCES AND FURTHER READING

Besselink MGH, van Santvoort HC, Witteman BJ, Gooszen HG. Management of severe acute pancreatitis: it's all about timing. *Curr Opin Crit Care* 2007; **13**: 200–6.

Heinrich S, Schafer M, Rousson V, Clavien PA. Evidence-based treatment of acute pancreatitis: a look at established paradigms. *Ann Surg* 2006; **243**: 154–68.

Ihse I, Andersson R, Axelson J. Pancreatic pain: is there a medical alternative to surgery? *Digestion* 1993; **54** (Suppl 2): 30–4.

Sakorafas GH, Tsiotou AG, Peros G. Mechanisms and natural history of pain in chronic pancreatitis : a surgical perspective. *J Clin Gastroenterol* 2007; **41**: 689–99.

Thuluvath PJ, Imperio D, Nair S, Cameron JL. Chronic pancreatitis: long-term pain relief with or without surgery, cancer risk, and mortality. *J Clin Gastroenterol* 2003; **36**: 159–65.

28

Functional abdominal pain

Clinical presentation

Functional abdominal pain syndromes refer to a constellation of conditions in which pain is a primary focus, along with other symptoms suggestive of gastro-intestinal disease, but for which no clear etiology can be ascertained. The mechanisms underlying these conditions are thought to be related to nociception arising from the complex interactions between psychological states, e.g., cognitive and emotional factors, leading to amplification of the pain signals relayed by sensory neurons. Although irritable bowel syndrome (IBS) will be the primary focus here, the reader should be aware of other functional gastrointestinal disorders (Table 28.1).

IBS is a syndrome characterized by bowel habit irregularity, e.g., constipation and diarrhea, associated with abdominal cramping and discomfort. It is common, affecting 10–20% of the adult population, predominantly women. The symptoms generally begin in the late teens or early twenties; for as many as 50% of IBS-afflicted patients the syndrome begins before the age of 35 years. Although there are no significant long-term physical sequelae of IBS, the symptoms can be sufficiently severe to interfere with functional capabilities and role responsibilities.

It should be noted that population-based investigations suggest that IBS is often associated with a number of comorbid conditions, including depression, anxiety, fibromyalgia, migraine headache, interstitial cystitis, chronic prostatitis, chronic pelvic pain, and chronic fatigue syndrome. The presence of such co-occurring conditions can significantly contribute to the morbidity, and adversely affect quality of life, of IBS-afflicted patients.

Signs and symptoms

The diagnosis of IBS rests on the medical history elicited from the patient and the absence of significant clinical findings on physical examination and diagnostic

Table 28.1 Functional abdominal syndromes other than IBS

Aerophagia	Abdominal bloating and pain resulting from repetitive air swallowing, brought on by carbonated beverages, eating too rapidly, chewing gum, and smoking; may also be symptomatic of depression or anxiety
Dyspepsia	Chronic and recurrent upper abdominal pain associated with subjective indigestion, postprandial fullness, epigastric gnawing or burning; associated with belching, bloating, and nausea; if associated with constipation or diarrhea, then irritable bowel syndrome is a consideration
Epigastric pain	Intermittent and recurrent pain and burning of moderate intensity, located specifically in the epigastrium, unrelieved by flatulence or defecation
Globus pharyngis	"Lump in the throat" sensation not attributable to esophageal spasm or mass, not associated with dysphagia; can be associated with unresolved grief, somatoform or mood disorders
Hiccups	Involuntary spasms of the diaphragm followed by sudden glottis closure persisting for protracted periods, e.g., beyond 2 days
Persisting nausea and vomiting	Self-induced or involuntary vomiting during periods of stress; cyclic vomiting may occur episodically with normal gastrointestinal functioning between intervals; may represent a migraine variant
Rumination	Postprandial involuntary regurgitation of small amounts of food arising 15–30 minutes after eating, which are chewed again and then re-swallowed; encountered during periods of distress

assessments. The Rome III criteria for diagnosis of IBS are symptom-based and include the presence of at least 6 months of recurrent abdominal pain or uncomfortable sensations. Additionally, at least two of the following must be present for a minimum of 3 months: (a) the abdominal pain and discomfort is relieved by defecation, and/or (b) it is associated with a change in frequency of the stool, and/or (c) it is associated with a change in stool consistency/appearance.

Although symptoms can vary among patients, and even for the same patient over the longitudinal course of the illness, the primary symptoms of IBS include abdominal pain/discomfort and bloating. Symptom exacerbation can be temporally associated with food consumption and stress; rarely are patients awakened from sleep because of symptoms. The altered defecation patterns of IBS can essentially be clustered into the constipation-predominant (IBS-C), the diarrhea-predominant (IBS-D), mixed (IBS-M), and unspecified (IBS-U) types. IBS-C is characterized by periods of constipation alternating with periods in which normal stool patterns/frequency occur. Patients may report infrequent and difficult-to-pass stools, i.e., straining and cramping during attempted defecation, only to find that they cannot eliminate any stool or that the stools are small in amount and often hard. There may be associated bouts of colicky pain or continuous dull aching sensations that are relieved with defecation. Mucus which normally moistens and protects the digestive tract may be observed in the stool. Eating can exacerbate symptoms, and bloating, flatulence and nausea are commonly co-occurring symptoms in IBS-C. The patient with IBS-D, by contrast, will report precipitous passage of stools with a loose, watery consistency associated with a sense of urgency that occurs upon awakening or immediately after eating. As with IBS-C, bloating is common. Still, some IBS-afflicted patients will report that they experience constipation alternating with diarrhea. IBS-M is generally applied to those with both hard and loose stools over periods of hours or days, whereas IBS-U refers to alternating bowel habit changes spanning periods of weeks and months.

On examination, patients generally appear to be healthy. Palpation of the abdomen may reveal mild tenderness, especially over the left lower quadrant. At times, a palpable tender sigmoid colon is appreciable, although there is no notable rebound tenderness or guarding. There is no associated rectal pain on digit examination, and the stools are occult-blood negative.

The presence of certain features such as older age of onset, weight loss, nocturnal diarrhea, rectal bleeding (not attributable to hemorrhoids), and vomiting may signal the need for more extensive diagnostic assessments for other serious conditions, including colon cancer and other conditions (see *Differential diagnosis*, below). Painless diarrhea should prompt consideration of possible malabsorption syndromes and osmotic diarrhea.

Laboratory tests and diagnostic investigations

Although there are no laboratory tests for IBS per se, several assessments may be warranted to establish that other conditions are not better accounting for symptoms. These can include complete blood count, serum electrolytes, liver function tests, serum amylase, erythrocyte sedimentation rate, thyroid-stimulating hormone level, and urinalysis. A hydrogen (H_2) breath test may be undertaken if there is a history suggestive of lactose intolerance. Analysis of stool content and stool culture, including assessments for ova and parasites, may be warranted if, based upon clinical history and physical examination findings, there is a concern about possible malabsorption syndrome or infection.

Imaging studies

Abdominal radiographs, diagnostic ultrasound, contrast-enhanced CT scans, and barium enema may be undertaken when aspects of the history and/or physical findings suggest other etiologies for the patient's symptoms. Flexible sigmoidoscopy will generally reveal normal mucosa, and bowel spasm and pain

Table 28.2 Differential diagnostic considerations for diarrhea-predominant and constipation-predominant irritable bowel syndrome

Diarrhea-predominant (IBS-D)	Constipation-predominant (IBS-C)
Carcinoid syndrome	Bowel obstruction
Hyperthyroidism	Hyperparathyroidism
Inflammatory bowel diseases	Hypothyroidism
Ischemic colitis	Pelvic floor dyssynergia
Malabsorption and osmotic diarrhea	
Microscopic colitis	
Zollinger–Ellison syndrome	

may be elicited during air insufflation. Colonoscopy is preferred for patients over 40 years of age who report changes in bowel habits, especially if there has been no history to suggest prior IBS, and it is indicated to exclude the possibility of inflammatory bowel disease, colonic polyps, and tumor. Mucosal biopsy may be undertaken to exclude microscopic colitis, celiac disease, and other malabsorption syndromes.

Differential diagnosis

There are several conditions that need to be considered in the differential of IBS. Consideration must be given to multiple conditions producing symptoms that can often mimic those of IBS, including lactose intolerance, celiac disease, diverticular disease, laxative abuse, parasitic infections, bacterial enteritis, colonic polyps and tumors, and early inflammatory bowel diseases, i.e., ulcerative colitis or Crohn's disease (Table 28.2). Evidence of steatorrhea suggests malabsorption and can include conditions that warrant identification, including chronic pancreatitis, gastric resection, celiac disease, inflammatory bowel disease, and Zollinger–Ellison syndrome, for which the treatments would differ from those for IBS. Female patients presenting with predominantly lower abdominal and pelvic pain should be evaluated for ovarian cysts or tumors and endometriosis. Diagnostic assessments, including laboratory investigations and imaging studies, can enhance deciphering which of these conditions prevail.

Pharmacotherapy

A number of pharmacological approaches can be invoked to relieve the symptoms associated with IBS (Table 28.3). The clinician must be mindful that many of these agents can potentially produce adverse effects that can mimic IBS symptoms. Some agents, e.g., anticholinergic medications, can produce a number of prohibitive systemic effects. Efforts are being directed at developing

Table 28.3 Pharmacotherapy treatment options for irritable bowel syndrome

Class (subclass)	Examples	Adverse effects	Comments
Anticholinergics	Dicyclomine 20 mg q.i.d. Propantheline 7.5–15 mg t.i.d. and 30 mg/hs Hyoscyamine 0.375–0.75 mg every 12 h	Dry mouth, reduced sweating, blurred vision, constipation, tachycardia, confusion in elderly, urinary retention in persons with benign prostatic hyperplasia	Control intestinal spasm; adjust dose in patients with renal or hepatic impairment; contraindicated in patients with closed-angle glaucoma, gastrointestinal obstruction, myasthenia gravis, paralytic ileus, toxic megacolon, thyrotoxicosis; dose reductions are required in renal or hepatic impairment
Antidepressants (selective serotonin reuptake inhibitors)	Paroxetine 10–40 mg/d	Nausea, gastrointestinal distress, tremor, sexual dysfunction	Preferred for patients with predominant constipation symptoms, can potentially exacerbate diarrhea; helpful in treating comorbid depression or anxiety
Antidepressants (tricyclic antidepressants)	Amitriptyline 10–75 mg/hs Imipramine 10–50 mg/hs	Anticholinergic side effects, sedation, constipation, orthostasis, weight gain, confusion in the elderly	Preferred for patients with diarrhea due to anticholinergic effects, can potentially exacerbate constipation; has neuromodulatory effects on pain pathways to mitigate pain; avoid if patients have significant cardiac disease; lethal if taken in overdose; helpful in treating comorbid depression or anxiety
Antidiarrheals	Loperamide 4–8 mg/d; maximum 16 mg/d	Abdominal pain, constipation, flatulence, abdominal cramps/colic	A synthetic opioid that prolongs intestinal transit time, permitting water absorption and decreasing stool frequency; may have role in IBS-D; does not cross the

Table 28.3 (*cont.*)

Class (subclass)	Examples	Adverse effects	Comments
			blood–brain barrier to produce significant CNS opioid effects
Antibiotics	Rifaximin 200–400 mg b.i.d	Nausea, flatulence, abdominal distension, constipation, abdominal pain	Used to treat traveler's diarrhea and hepatic encephalopathy; benefits in IBS may be related to antibacterial effects on colonic microflora; does not pass the gastrointestinal tract to produce systemic effects; may predispose to *Clostridium difficile*-associated diarrhea
Laxatives (stimulants)	Bisacodyl 5–15 mg/d	Abdominal pain, cramping, nausea, weakness	Stimulates enteric nerves to promote colonic mass movements; it also increases fluid and sodium chloride secretion; effects on small intestine negligible
Laxatives (prostaglandin derivatives)	Lubiprostone 8 μg b.i.d.	Nausea, abdominal distension, diarrhea, flatulence, vomiting	Useful to treat IBS-C in women; fatty acid derivative of prostaglandin E_1; affects cells by creating chloride-rich solution that lubricates the stool and facilitates stool passage; reduce the dose in patients with hepatic impairment

b.i.d., twice a day; hs, at hour of sleep; q.i.d., four times a day; t.i.d., three times a day.

anticholinergic effects that are specific to the gastrointestinal tract. For example, zamifenacin is an M_3-muscarinic receptor antagonist producing selective effects on gastric motility and contractions, which is currently in clinical trials for possible use in the treatment of IBS. Preliminary data suggest that it has the potential benefit of producing marked reduction in abdominal pain and distension in IBS patients. Antispasmodics including calcium channel blockers (e.g., peppermint oil), smooth muscle relaxants (e.g., papaverine-like agents), and antimuscarinics (e.g., hyoscine) have yielded inconsistent results regarding effectiveness in mitigating the symptoms of IBS. Studies assessing the utility of antispasmodics were generally limited in terms of quality, and had small sample sizes and high drop-out rates, impeding their ability to make definitive statements regarding efficacy.

Antidepressants can be useful in treating symptoms related to IBS. Patients with IBS-D may benefit from the use of low doses of tricyclic antidepressants (TCAs), e.g., imipramine or amitriptyline, because of their anticholinergic effects. On the other hand, patients with IBS-C may find the constipating effects of the TCAs intolerable, and may instead benefit from the use of selective serotonin reuptake inhibitors (SSRIs) such as paroxetine. Although low doses of TCAs are required to mitigate IBS symptoms, higher doses may be required to address comorbid depression and/or anxiety. It is uncertain to what extent the effectiveness of antidepressants in IBS is due to neuromodulatory effects influencing nociceptive transmission, indirect improvements from relieving depression and/or anxiety, thereby causing patients to perceive their symptoms as less distressing, the direct influences on gastrointestinal tract functioning, or some combination of these influences.

Agents with serotonergic (5-HT) effects, i.e., $5\text{-}HT_3$ antagonism (cisapride) and $5\text{-}HT_4$ agonism (tegaserod), demonstrated promise with regard to alleviating the constipation associated with IBS. However, because of concerns regarding cardiovascular adverse effects, both agents were removed from the commercial market in the USA and several other countries.

Non-pharmacologic approaches

Dietary modifications and implementation of stress-reducing lifestyle changes can be an important component of IBS management. Incorporating a regular exercise routine and improved sleep habits may reduce anxiety and thereby help relieve bowel symptoms. Consuming more frequent smaller meals slowly, as opposed to large meals or eating too quickly, may be helpful. At times, avoidance of caffeinated beverages, and reductions in the amount of nuts, raisins, and bananas consumed may help attenuate symptoms. However, patients need to be cautioned against obsessive preoccupations with, and overly zealous, dietary restrictions, which may inadvertently lead to unbalanced diets and nutritional deficiencies. The use of bulking agents and fiber-enriched diets has been advocated to mitigate constipation, but these can potentially exacerbate bloating and fullness sensations due to enhanced bacterial fermentation within the digestive tract, which leads to gas production.

Depression and anxiety disorders often accompany IBS and should prompt psychiatric referral and treatment. A number of psychotherapeutic interventions, including cognitive behavioral therapy (CBT), interpersonal psychotherapy, and relaxation training/stress management have demonstrated modest benefits in alleviating the symptoms of IBS and the distress associated with it. The research supporting the efficacy of psychotherapeutic interventions in the treatment of pain and related symptoms of IBS has yielded mixed results. These interventions have been shown to be slightly superior to inactive (e.g., wait-listed, controls, and usual care), but the clinical significance of the observed improvements and the sustainability of benefits over time remain uncertain.

Interventional procedures

Acupuncture has sometimes been advocated for use in IBS management. A recent meta-analysis revealed that definitive conclusions regarding efficacy were impossible due to the limited number of high-quality studies and the heterogeneity of interventions employed. Although active acupuncture was more effective in producing improvements in abdominal symptoms and global ratings of well-being as compared with control conditions, active acupuncture did not fare better than sham acupuncture in terms of alleviating abdominal symptoms and defecation difficulties.

Follow-up

Regular visits with the patient in which the clinician imparts empathetic understanding and guidance are of overriding importance. Attentive listening to the patient's perceptions of changes in bowel habits and related abdominal symptoms as well as efficacy of treatment is paramount to establishing a trusting clinician–patient relationship upon which to base a shared treatment alliance to forge further treatment progress. For example, unveiling relationships between symptom exacerbations and types of food ingested and medication use can illuminate what modifications can be made to mitigate future symptoms. Educating patients about the link between psychological and physiological effects can be pivotal to enlisting the patient's participation in psychotherapy and stress management techniques. Ultimately, the goal is to provide sufficient symptom relief and to restore, or enhance, adaptive functioning.

Prognosis

Irritable bowel syndrome may be a lifelong condition. The course of IBS can be variable; for some, there may be periods of months during which symptoms remit and then return, while for others there may be enduring, or worsening, symptoms over time. Symptomatic relief can generally be achieved through diet, stress management, and the use of prescribed medications. A multidisciplinary approach encompassing medical, psychotherapeutic/stress management, and nutritional approaches can be effective in addressing the patient's symptoms, and can achieve improvements in the functional adaptation and quality of life of afflicted patients.

REFERENCES AND FURTHER READING

Chang JY, Talley NJ. An update on irritable bowel syndrome: from diagnosis to emerging therapies. *Curr Opin Gastroenterol* 2011; **27**: 72–8.

Lesbros-Pantoflickova D, Michetti P, Fried M, Beglinger C, Blum AL. Meta-analysis: the treatment of irritable bowel syndrome. *Aliment Pharmacol Ther* 2004; **20**: 1253–69.

Longstreth GF, Thompson WG, Chey WD, *et al.* Functional bowel disorders. *Gastroenterology* 2006; **130**: 1480–91.

Malone MA. Irritable bowel syndrome. *Prim Care Clin Office Pract* 2011; **38**: 433–47.

Zijdenbos IL, de Wit NJ, van der Heijden GJ, Rubin G, Quartero AO. Psychological treatments for the management of irritable bowel syndrome. *Cochrane Database Syst Rev* 2009; (1): CD006442.

29

Groin pain, ilioinguinal, iliohypogastric, and genitofemoral neuralgia

Clinical presentation

Entrapment neuropathies of the ilioinguinal, iliohypogastric, and genitofemoral nerves can be a source of regional abdominal wall and groin pain. Failure to recognize these conditions can lead to extensive and futile efforts to explore and treat presumed intra-abdominal and pelvic sources of discomfort. These neuropathies are generally caused by direct injury, usually in the form of compression or irritation, as the nerves descend from the lumbar plexus through the trunk and iliac region to their terminations in the superficial abdominal wall, upper thigh, and groin. Commonly, nerve irritation arises from trauma or injury sustained during, or fibrous adhesions and scar tissue resulting from, lower abdominal surgery, e.g., appendectomy, herniorrhaphy, and Pfannenstiel incision for hysterectomy or cesarean section. These neuralgias may also arise during pregnancy. Idiopathic causes of all three conditions are rare. However, other causes for the neuropathic symptoms, e.g., at the level of the lumbar plexus, must be considered in the differential of the patient's presentation (see *Differential diagnosis*, below).

The genitofemoral nerve arises from the L1 and L2 nerve roots. It courses in an oblique path through the psoas muscle, emerging from the medial aspect of the psoas muscle approximately at the level of the third or fourth lumbar vertebrae. The nerve divides into a femoral branch, which descends with the external iliac artery (supplying the medial aspect of the thigh), and a genital branch, which then enters the internal inguinal ring, accompanying the spermatic cord or round ligament to supply the scrotum or labia. The genitofemoral nerve also supplies motor innervation for the cremasteric muscle.

Although anatomic variations are possible, the ilioinguinal and iliohypogastric nerves arise from the same femoral nerve root origins, have a similar trajectory in the trunk and along the iliac crests, and then have similar locations for entrapment, but then diverge somewhat to produce slightly different distributions of pain and radiation patterns (Table 29.1).

Table 29.1 Features of ilioinguinal, iliohypogastric, and genitofemoral neuralgia

	Ilioinguinal nerve	Iliohypogastric nerve	Genitofemoral nerve
Nerve root sources	L1 ± T12	L1 ± T12	L2 ± L1
Site of entrapment	Medial to ASIS	Medial to ASIS	Internal inguinal ring
Pain locations	Groin along the inguinal line, pubic symphysis, root of penis, proximal (upper) scrotum, labia majora, anterior and inner aspects of the thigh	Groin, posterolateral aspects of gluteal region	Medial thigh overlying the femoral triangle, bottom of scrotum, labia majora
Tenderness elicited on physical exam	Medial to ASIS	Medial to ASIS	Inguinal ring
Motor weakness	Weakness of lower anterior abdominal wall musculature	Weakness of lower anterior abdominal wall musculature	Possible weakness of lower anterior abdominal wall
Nerve block site	5 cm medial and inferior to ASIS	2.5 cm medial and inferior to ASIS	Lateral to the pubic tubercle (genital branch); middle third of inguinal ligament (femoral branch)

ASIS, anterior superior iliac spine.

Both the ilioinguinal and iliohypogastric nerves arise from the L1 nerve root, with some potential contribution from the T12 nerve root. The ilioinguinal nerve emerges from the lateral aspect of the psoas muscle and courses along the quadratus lumborum muscle before it traverses the inner aspect of the ilium. The ilioinguinal nerve is entrapped medial to the anterior superior iliac spine (ASIS), usually at the midpoint between the iliac crest and the twelfth rib, where the nerve penetrates the transverse abdominis and internal oblique muscles. The nerve is said to penetrate these two muscles consecutively in a stepwise or zig-zag fashion, and therefore is subject to mechanical irritation when strained by muscle or fibrous strands. The entrapment of the ilioinguinal nerve is referred to the groin; there may be an associated weakness of the lower abdominal wall.

Like the ilioinguinal nerve, the iliohypogastric nerve courses along the quadratus lumborum muscle and then caudally along the ilium. It bifurcates into a lateral branch (supplying the skin overlying the posterolateral aspects of the gluteal region) and an anterior branch (supplying cutaneous sensation of the skin of the abdomen above the pelvis).

Signs and symptoms

For each of the three neuropathic conditions, patients typically present with an initial onset of burning pain and paresthesia in the lower abdomen and inguinal region. In the case of both ilioinguinal and genitofemoral neuralgia, the pain often radiates into the upper medial aspect of the thigh and genitals. For iliohypogastric neuralgia, the pain is largely confined to the inguinal region with a band that may extend back along the lateral and posterior gluteal region. Patients may report that the skin over that area is exquisitely sensitive; pain can be aggravated by walking, running, climbing stairs, squatting, prolonged sitting, Valsalva, and hyperextension of the hip. Eventually, in the same distributions, the patient may experience numbness and dysesthesia, i.e., perceived unpleasant sensations in response to normal stimulation such as the touch of one's clothing (allodynia). The neuropathic pain can be alleviated by flexing the hip. For example, because the pain can be exacerbated by leaning backwards or hyperextension of the lumbar spine, patients will often assume a stooped posture, with flexion of the hips and forward inclination of the trunk.

Physical examination will reveal sensory deficits in the skin overlying the inner thigh, the scrotum or labia, e.g., hypoesthesia along the anterior and medial thigh. Diagnosis of iliohypogastric or ilioinguinal neuralgia can be supported by Tinel's sign, i.e., pain is reproduced by palpation/tapping over a circumscribed area over the transverse abdominis muscle 2–3 cm medial to and below the ASIS (approximately below the imaginary line extending between the umbilicus and the ASIS). Hip hyperextension and/or forced flexion of the hip against manual resistance are maneuvers that likewise can reproduce pain. For genitofemoral neuralgia, a Tinel's sign may be elicited by tapping over the nerve at the point it passes beneath the inguinal ligament.

With ilioinguinal and iliohypogastric entrapment, weakness of the lower abdominal musculature may be notable. The presence of motor weakness extending beyond the lower abdomen on neurological examination, or gastrointestinal or urogenital symptoms, would be inconsistent with these neuropathic conditions, suggesting other conditions in the differential diagnosis – an intraabdominal process affecting the lumbar plexus, spinal lesions, a pelvic mass, or myofascial pain syndrome, among other possibilities.

Laboratory tests and diagnostic investigations

Although there are no laboratory tests for ilioinguinal, iliohypogastric, and genitofemoral neuralgia per se, several assessments may be warranted to establish that other conditions are not better accounting for symptoms. These can include complete blood count, erythrocyte sedimentation rate, and a thyroid profile. Although systemic conditions producing symptoms mimicking these conditions would likely have accompanying clinical signs to assist in diagnosis, such laboratory investigations can serve to unveil, or rule out, hypothyroidism, intra-abdominal infection, diabetes mellitus (and related diabetic neuropathy), or other worrisome clinical conditions.

Diagnostic uncertainties arising from the history and/or physical examination can be clarified utilizing electrodiagnostic investigations. Sensory nerve conduction studies (NCS) can confirm the diagnosis of ilioinguinal, iliohypogastric, and genitofemoral impingement. In addition, electromyography (EMG) may assist in distinguishing entrapment neuropathies of these nerves from diabetic polyneuropathy, lumbar radiculopathy, or plexopathy.

Imaging studies

Radiographs are necessary to eliminate the possibility that pathology of the back, pelvis, or hip is not accounting for nerve irritation. Abdominal and/or pelvic CT scanning may unveil a lower abdominal or pelvic process impinging on the lumbar plexus, e.g., retroperitoneal tumor, enlarged abdominal lymph nodes, lipoma, or leiomyomata. MRI may be necessary to assess spinal pathology that may be accounting for the disturbances, e.g., spinal stenosis, intervertebral disc herniation, or mass/space-occupying lesions affecting the nerve roots exiting the intervertebral foramen or infiltrating the lumbar plexus.

Differential diagnosis

The diagnosis of ilioinguinal, iliohypogastric, or genitofemoral neuralgia is usually based on obtaining a supporting history and physical examination. However, the clinician must consider other conditions within the differential diagnosis that can potentially masquerade as symptoms of these conditions. Among the possible etiologies, consideration must be given to:

- ankylosing spondylitis
- endometriosis
- epididymitis, orchitis, testicular torsion, testicular cancer
- hip dysplasia, hip avulsion fracture
- inguinal hernia
- kidney stones
- lumbar diabetic neuropathy
- myofascial pain syndromes affecting the pectineus muscle or the adductor muscles of the hip, among others
- obturator neuropathy

- osteoarthritis or rheumatoid arthritis with hip joint involvement
- scrotal masses, e.g., hydrocele and varicocele
- spinal lesions, e.g., spinal stenosis, mass/tumor, or intervertebral disc herniation at the T12–L1–L2 vertebral levels
- vulvodynia

The clinician ought to bear in mind that some of these conditions can coexist with ilioinguinal, iliohypogastric, or genitofemoral neuralgia. For example, it is possible that neuralgic symptoms may coexist with myofascial pain syndromes.

Pharmacotherapy

Patients may be initially treated with anticonvulsants, trials of alpha-2-delta ligands (e.g., gabapentin or pregabalin) or another class (e.g., carbamazepine). Systematic investigation of their use in patients with ilioinguinal, iliohypogastric, or genitofemoral neuralgia has been lacking, with publications often based on anecdotal reports and small case series. Although not described in the literature specifically with regard to the above-mentioned neuralgias, antidepressant trials may also be useful adjuncts in the treatment of neuropathic pain. Caution would naturally be required with the use of any of these agents; for instance, side effects may limit tolerability and resultant utility, and in some cases may be prohibitive (e.g., during pregnancy). Inadequate responses to these agents may necessitate low-dose opioid analgesics, but the benefits may need to be balanced against potential risks/adverse effects. Topical lidocaine may be helpful to mitigate related neuropathic pains as well. Failure to respond to these agents, along with concurrent non-pharmacologic approaches, may necessitate interventional approaches.

Non-pharmacologic approaches

Non-pharmacologic approaches will include behavior modification, i.e., avoidance of activities that are likely to exacerbate pain, including squatting or sitting for prolonged periods.

Interventional procedures

When pharmacologic modalities produce unsatisfactory relief, treatment may proceed to non-operative interventions including nerve blockade employing local anesthetics (anatomic, ultrasound-guided, or EMG-guided). Ultimately, temporary relief produced by direct ilioinguinal, iliohypogastric, or genitofemoral nerve blockade with local anesthetics can confirm a diagnosis of neuralgia affecting these nerves. Bear in mind that nerve blockade can serve as a therapeutic intervention as well. Failure of peripheral nerve blockade to alleviate symptoms may suggest that the source of the pain may be more proximal, e.g., intra-abdominal, at the lumbar plexus, or at the spine.

Surgical intervention, i.e., neurectomy, is reserved for patients who fail to respond favorably to conservative treatment measures. However, surgical resection of the ilioinguinal or genitofemoral nerves may precipitate a resultant hypoesthesia of the labia/scrotum and potentially a postoperative dysesthesia.

Follow-up

Monitoring of the efficacy of, and potential adverse side effects associated with, medication use and nerve blocks is warranted. Reassessment will be necessary to assess the efficacy of treatment approaches and to determine whether more aggressive interventional approaches (e.g., surgical approaches) warrant consideration.

Prognosis

Generally, groin pain related to ilioinguinal, iliohypogastric, or genitofemoral neuralgia responds favorably to treatment. Patients with mild complaints can achieve sustained relief with nerve blocks. Patients may require repeated nerve blockade when relief is transient, or surgical exploration and neurectomy in severe, refractory cases.

REFERENCES AND FURTHER READING

Harms BA, DeHaas DR, Starling JR. Diagnosis and management of genitofemoral neuralgia. *Arch Surg* 1984; **119**: 339–41.

Melville K, Schultz EA, Dougherty JM. Ilioinguinal-iliohypogastric nerve entrapment. *Ann Emerg Med* 1990; **19**: 925–9.

Murovic JA, Kim DH, Tiel RL, Kline DG. Surgical management of 10 genitofemoral neuralgias at the Louisiana State University Health Sciences Center. *Neurosurgery* 2005; **56**: 298–303.

Starling JR, Harms BA, Schroeder ME, Eichman PL. Diagnosis and treatment of genitofemoral and ilioinguinal entrapment neuralgia. *Surgery* 1987; **102**: 581–6.

30

Coccydynia

Clinical presentation

Coccydynia, also called coccygalgia, coccygeal pain, or coccygodynia, refers to pain that is localized to the area around the coccyx. The coccyx ("tailbone") is the terminal portion of the spine formed from 3–5 small bones, vestigial in humans, the first of which articulates with the sacrum and forms the sacrococcygeal joint. In some individuals there may be a rudimentary disc between the first and second coccygeal segments, but the rest are fused, or synarthroses.

There are a number of nerves and muscles closely related to the sacrum and coccyx which are potential pain generators: spinal nerve roots S4 and S5, inferior rectal nerve, perineal branch of the pudendal nerve, coccygeal nerve, ganglion impar or ganglion of Walther (formed by merging of the distal paravertebral chains), sacrococcygeal ligaments, levator ani (pubococcygeal and iliococcygeal fascicles), coccygeal and gluteal muscles.

Coccydynia may be idiopathic or related to injury to the sacrum, coccyx, or sacrococcygeal joint, such as a direct fall onto the tailbone in the seated position, repetitive minor trauma such as occurs during cycling, or during parturition. These injuries can result in tissue inflammation and contraction of the levator ani and coccygeus muscles, precipitating the characteristic pain of coccydynia.

Non-traumatic causes include frequent or prolonged sitting on a hard surface, referred lumbosacral pain, referred anorectal pain, infection (tuberculosis, osteomyelitis), avascular necrosis of coccyx, meningeal or peridural cyst, or pain referred from pelvic organs.

The unpredictability of the pain in this region of the spine has also been linked to psychological factors, especially in cases of idiopathic or non-traumatic coccydynia in which no clear pathologic etiology is identified.

Signs and symptoms

Patients with coccydynia present with tenderness, pain, or persistent ache in the region of the lower spine, coccyx or in the adjacent muscles and soft tissues; the discomfort is typically exacerbated by pressure from sitting or cycling, or with bowel movements. It may present as sudden, episodic, painful rectal spasms (proctalgia fugax), a persistent sensation of needing to have a bowel movement (tenesmus), or painful intercourse (dyspareunia). Coccydynia may also manifest as backache or accompanying headache.

Coccydynia is more common in women than in men (5 : 1), probably due to the more posterior location of the os sacrum/coccyx and relatively longer coccyx in women, which predisposes it to injury during a fall or difficult childbirth. It may be precipitated by tight-fitting clothing, so-called "jean-seam" coccydynia. There is also evidence of increased incidence of coccydynia in overweight or obese individuals of both genders (BMI > 27.4 in females and > 29.4 in males).

In addition to standard history, physical, and neurological exam, evaluation of coccydynia should include manual examination of the coccyx. Palpation with mobilization of the coccyx may differentiate between nociceptive pain related to ligamentous/muscular support structures and referred pain due to other pathology. The Valsalva maneuver should be positive for coccydynia due to disorders of the sacrococcygeal joint or the attendant muscles but negative for referred causes of pain.

Laboratory tests and diagnostic investigations

There is no specific laboratory test for coccydynia. Laboratory work is generally considered unnecessary in the initial evaluation unless there is suspicion of occult malignancy or infection. Complete blood count with differential (CBC with diff), erythrocyte sedimentation rate (ESR), or C-reactive protein (CRP) should be obtained for these patients.

Imaging studies

Standard lateral spine plain films are always recommended to rule out fractures or dislocations. CT may be helpful, although it has been suggested that since coccydynia is a dynamic disorder (occurring with movement) it may be best appreciated utilizing dynamic films. If there is suspicion of occult pathology, MRI should be obtained.

Differential diagnosis

The approach to the differential diagnosis of coccydynia includes consideration of three potential etiologies for the pain: nociceptive (from the coccyx or sacrococcygeal joint, ligamentous or muscular structures), neuropathic (fourth or fifth sacral nerve, sympathetic ganglia, other proximal nerves), or referred visceral pain (pelvic organs, colon).

Sacral fractures, most likely to occur from a direct axial fall, may result in nociceptive pain localized to the coccygeal region, and they are more common than coccygeal fractures. Referred pain from a herniated lumbar disc may masquerade as coccydynia.

Perirectal abscess, pre-coccygeal inclusion cyst, pilonidal cyst, and neoplasm must be ruled out. Urogenital and gynecologic (uterus, fallopian tubes, ovaries, bladder) or retroperitoneal structures (kidneys, ureters) may also cause pain that is referred to the coccygeal region.

Pharmacotherapy

Conservative treatment is successful in approximately 90% of cases and can include simple non-pharmacologic measures, medications, or a combination of both. As in most inflammatory musculoskeletal conditions, non-steroidal anti-inflammatory drugs (NSAIDs) are the first line of treatment. Stool softeners and laxatives are useful for minimizing pain during defecation. Antidepressant medications may be useful as treatment or adjunctive to other modes of therapy.

Non-pharmacologic approaches

In order to effect an altered sitting position, ring-shaped cushions or specially designed padded seats, and ergonomic adaptations to physical therapy, are useful for initial treatment of coccydynia. Hot or sitz baths may be helpful. If a luxation (anterior or posterior displacement) of the coccyx is identified, intrarectal massage and manipulation may be employed. Studies show some improvement with osteopathic manipulative techniques, including direct correction of the coccygeal displacement based on bimanual assessment, myofascial release of pelvic diaphragm, and direct sacrococcygeal release.

Psychotherapy is useful for patients in whom no clear etiology for coccygeal pain is identified, and cognitive behavioral therapy (CBT) may assist patients with behavioral and lifestyle modifications that may prove beneficial in relieving symptoms as well as preventing future episodes.

Interventional procedures

Sacrococcygeal injections have shown a wide variation in results. The ganglion impar (ganglion of Walther) at the terminal end of the sympathetic chain may be localized via CT scan and injected with anesthetic–steroid agents, a technique that has had success for patients who fail conservative treatment. Radiofrequency ablation is another technique that has shown variable results.

Coccygeoplasty and coccygectomy (partial or complete) have been performed for recalcitrant cases of coccydynia. However, there is insufficient evidence to support the efficacy of these invasive procedures.

Follow-up

Depending on the cause of the coccydynia, patients may require frequent follow-up for manipulative treatments, massage, or interventional procedures. Multi-modal therapy may have the greatest impact on pain reduction for these patients.

Prognosis

The prognosis for coccydynia depends upon the etiology. The majority of cases that are due to trauma will respond to conservative treatment and lifestyle modifications such as weight loss and postural and ergonometric adaptation.

REFERENCES AND FURTHER READING

De Andrés J, Chaves S. Coccygodynia: a proposal for an algorithm for treatment. *J Pain* 2003; **4**: 257–66.

Nathan ST, Fisher BE, Roberts CS. Coccydynia: a review of pathoanatomy, aetiology, treatment and outcome. *J Bone Joint Surg Br* 2010 **92**: 1622–7.

Patijn J, Janssen M, Hayed S, *et al.* Evidence-based interventional pain medicine according to clinical diagnoses, 14. Coccygodynia. *Pain Pract* 2010; **10**: 554–9.

31

Interstitial cystitis

Clinical presentation

Interstitial cystitis (IC) is a chronic bladder inflammatory or non-inflammatory condition of unknown etiology. IC is often considered as a neurogenic cystitis. IC presents with urgency, frequency, and pain with bladder filling that is sometimes relieved with voiding. IC is a diagnosis of exclusion in patients with a history of urinary tract infections but negative studies of urine culture and cytology. Women are more likely than men to be diagnosed with IC. The mean age is 40 at onset. Some patients may experience remission of IC, with a mean duration of several months, without regular treatment. The etiology of IC is still unclear, and it could be mutual symptoms related to multiple underlying disease or inflammations. The hypothetical causes of IC may include increased epithelial permeability, neurogenic abnormalities, and autoimmune disorder.

Signs and symptoms

The urinary frequency, urgency, and pelvic pain correlate with bladder filling, and are sometimes relieved by emptying. There may be a history of bladder problems dating back to childhood, and a possible history of exposure to radiation or cyclophosphamide. There may be coexistent symptoms such as dyspareunia. Hunner's ulcers or glomerulations may be reported in cystoscopy but are not pathognomonic of IC. The terms bladder pain syndrome (BPS) or painful bladder syndrome have been designated for symptoms similar to IC with normal cystoscopic finding without inflammation.

Laboratory tests and diagnostic investigations

Infectious etiologies should be ruled out by urinalysis and culture. Urinary cytology is indicated to exclude malignancy. Urodynamic studies can measure bladder sensation and compliance. Cystoscopy and biopsy may detect glomerulations, carcinoma, and eosinophilic or tuberculosis cystitis.

Imaging studies

Ultrasonography studies may offer preliminary screening without radiation exposure. Radiography of the pelvis may detect any bony pathology. MRI or CT scans of the pelvis are indicated to rule out infection, other abnormality, and neoplasm.

Differential diagnosis

Chemical or radiation cystitis reveals a previous history of exposure. Infectious etiologies of cystitis (e.g., bacterial, genital herpes, or vaginitis) can be excluded by history and physical examination in addition to urinalysis and urine culture. Urethral diverticulum or carcinoma should be suspected from palpation of a mass, and then advanced to further work-up.

The urethral syndrome is characterized by suprapubic and low back pain in addition to urinary frequency, urgency, and dysuria. Dysfunction of the pelvic floor was proposed as the etiology of urethral syndrome, based on the clinical efficacy of skeletal muscle relaxants, electrostimulation, and biofeedback. Chronic low-grade infection of the paraurethral glands has been suspected as a likely cause of urethral syndrome in women, given its similar presentation to prostatitis in men.

There may be coexisting medical conditions associated with IC, such as endometriosis or irritable bowel syndrome, which also contribute to chronic pelvic and abdominal pain. Chronic pelvic pain (CPP) describes non-menstrual pelvic pain of over 6 months' duration that is severe enough to cause functional disability and require medical or surgical intervention. Although adhesions or endometriosis are common laparoscopic findings, some CPP cases still have no specific intrapelvic pathology.

Endometriosis describes the presence of endometrial-like tissue outside the uterus and a chronic inflammatory reaction. Endometriosis may present with dysmenorrhea, dyspareunia, infertility, hematuria, chronic fatigue, and pelvic pain. Endometriosis is confirmed by biopsy and histology of ectopic endometrial implants. Endometriosis may be a common incidental finding in otherwise asymptomatic women being worked up for IC.

In an animal model of neurogenic cystitis, bladder-induced pelvic pain was also exacerbated by colonic administration of a sub-threshold dose of capsaicin. These data propose "organ cross-talk" in pelvic pain and modulation of pain responses by visceral inputs distinct from the experimentally inflamed site. Differential diagnosis is aided by knowledge of the innervation of the lower abdominal and pelvic organs. The spinal innervation of the ureter and bladder is from S2–S4 via the ilioinguinal and genitofemoral nerves, with sympathetic supply from the inferior hypogastric plexus. The innervation of the ureter and bladder overlaps with that of pelvic organs such as the inferior portion of uterine segment, the superior vagina, the distal colon, the rectum, and the uterosacral ligaments. The spinal innervation of the lower vagina, vulva, and perineum are from S2–S4 via the pudendal, ilioinguinal, and genitofemoral nerves, with sympathetic supply from the ganglion impar (ganglion of Walther).

Pharmacotherapy

Tricyclic antidepressants (TCAs) such as amitriptyline have been studied, and are frequently recommended as first-line therapy for IC.

Antihistamines such as hydroxyzine, alpha-adrenergic agents such as phentolamine, tizanidine, and clonidine, and calcium channel blockers such as nifedine could also be beneficial options in the treatment of IC.

Systemic immunosuppressants such as methotrexate and cyclosporine, or intravesical instillation of bacilli Calmette–Guérin (BCG), have been studied in IC based on the hypothesis of autoimmune disease.

The oral heparin-like drug pentosan polysulfate (Elmiron) provides synthetic sulfated polysaccharide and has helped some IC cases to restore the integrity of bladder epithelium. Intravesical instillation of dimethyl sulfoxide (DMSO), heparin, corticosteroids, and bicarbonates has been reported to offer some efficacy in clinical trials on IC.

Acetaminophen, non-steroidal anti-inflammatory drugs (NSAIDs), cyclooxygenase-2 (COX-2) inhibitors and skeletal muscle relaxants are commonly used to alleviate mild to moderate bladder/pelvic pain and spasm related to IC, but without evidence-based studies.

Although opioids are commonly prescribed in the management of moderate to severe acute pain, their efficacy in the case of chronic pain from IC has not been well supported by evidence-based studies.

Non-pharmacologic approaches

Bladder hydrodistension has been used as both a diagnostic and a therapeutic process. It may provide short-term reduction in frequency and pain associated with IC.

Current data suggest that citrus fruits, tomatoes, vitamin C, artificial sweeteners, coffee, tea, carbonated and alcoholic beverages, and spicy foods tend to exacerbate symptoms, while calcium glycerophosphate and sodium bicarbonate tend to improve symptoms of IC. Dietary modification may be beneficial in IC.

A significantly higher proportion of women with IC or BPS responded to treatment with myofascial physical therapy than to the more global therapeutic massage. Myofascial physical therapy and pelvic floor muscle exercise programs have also been studied and advocated in the multidisciplinary treatment of IC.

Cognitive behavioral therapy (CBT), counseling, relaxation techniques, biofeedback, and neurofeedback could be beneficial in selected candidates with IC. The physical agents and modalities such as heat, cold, ultrasound, electricity, as well as complementary and alternative treatments such as acupuncture, offer a non-invasive approach and minimize the potential adverse effects of multimodal pharmacotherapy.

Interventional procedures

Epidural blockade with local anesthetic provided short-term efficacy in a case study of IC. However, there is no definite neural blockade that can be used as either a diagnostic or a therapeutic approach for IC. Sympathetic block does not contribute to either confirmation or symptomatic management of IC.

Transcutaneous electrical nerve stimulation (TENS) presented improvement and remission in some case studies of IC. The mechanism of action in neurostimulation in IC is still unknown. The proposed theories may include the gate control theory of Melzack and Wall, release of neurotransmitters, and suppression of excitatory amino acids. Both sacral nerve stimulation (SNS) and spinal cord stimulation (SCS) have been studied in IC for clinical efficacy. SNS offers symptomatic improvement in frequency and urgency. If a percutaneous trial lead of SNS works well in IC, then proceeding to a permanent internalized implant is recommended. However, mixed results were reported in terms of pain control when neurostimulation was used as the only modality in the clinical treatment of IC.

Injection of botulinum toxin A (Botox) appears to have a positive therapeutic effect in multiple urological conditions, such as refractory idiopathic detrusor overactivity, neurogenic detrusor overactivity, IC/BPS, and benign prostatic hyperplasia. However, the US Food and Drug Administration (FDA) has approved botulinum toxin injection only for the treatment of urinary incontinence as a result of neurogenic detrusor overactivity (e.g., spinal cord injury, multiple sclerosis) in adults who have an inadequate response to or are intolerant of an anticholinergic medication. The treatment of IC needs further evidence-based studies of botulinum toxin injection.

Laser obliteration of the bilateral vesicoureteric plexus provided symptomatic relief in a case study. Surgical interventions such as supravesical diversions or cystectomy have been reported, with mixed outcomes. There was a case report of unrelenting bladder pain despite the cystectomy.

Follow-up

There is still some controversy surrounding the disease model and definitive diagnostic criteria of IC. Attentive follow-up of a working diagnosis of IC, and timely management, should always be the standard of care.

Prognosis

The prognosis of IC depends on whether there is any comorbidity such as irritable bowel syndrome, endometriosis, chronic pelvic pain, fibromyalgia, or migraine headache. All these chronic pain syndromes may interfere with the clinical presentation of IC. Whether multimodal approaches are available and synchronized would affect the treatment course and outcome of IC.

REFERENCES AND FURTHER READING

Cheng C, Rosamilia A, Healey M. Diagnosis of interstitial cystitis/bladder pain syndrome in women with chronic pelvic pain: a prospective observational study. *Int Urogynecol J* 2012; **23**: 1361–6.

Fariello JY, Whitmore K. Sacral neuromodulation stimulation for IC/PBS, chronic pelvic pain, and sexual dysfunction. *Int Urogynecol J* 2010; **21**: 1553–8.

Fitzgerald MP, Payne CK, Lukacz ES, *et al.*; Interstitial Cystitis Collaborative Research Network. Randomized multicenter clinical trial of myofascial physical therapy in women with interstitial cystitis/painful bladder syndrome and pelvic floor tenderness. *J Urol* 2012; **12**: 2113–18.

Friedlander JI, Shorter B, Moldwin RM. Diet and its role in interstitial cystitis/bladder pain syndrome (IC/BPS) and comorbid conditions. *BJU Int* 2012; **109**: 1584–91.

Giannantoni A, Bini V, Dmochowski R, *et al.* Contemporary management of the painful bladder: a systematic review. *Eur Urol* 2012; **61**: 29–53.

Hanno PM, Burks DA, Clemens JQ, *et al.*; Interstitial Cystitis Guidelines Panel of the American Urological Association Education and Research, Inc. AUA guideline for the diagnosis and treatment of interstitial cystitis/bladder pain syndrome. *J Urol* 2011; **185**: 2162–70.

Rudick CN, Chen MC, Mongiu AK, Klumpp DJ. Organ cross talk modulates pelvic pain. *Am J Physiol Regul Integr Comp Physiol* 2007; **293**: R1191–8.

Yokoyama T, Chancellor MB, Oguma K, *et al.* Botulinum toxin type A for the treatment of lower urinary tract disorders. *Int J Urol* 2012; **19**: 202–15.

32

Pelvic pain and endometriosis

Clinical presentation

A common complaint in women of childbearing age, but relatively unusual in men, pelvic pain is a clinically complex problem. Pelvic pain may present as acute, episodic, intermittent, and/or chronic. Acute pelvic pain in menstruating women requires immediate evaluation to rule out gynecologic emergencies such as ovarian torsion or ectopic pregnancy. Chronic pelvic pain is defined as pain in the lower abdomen (below the umbilicus), pelvis, perineum, or buttocks which is intermittent or persistent for at least 6 months, and that does not occur exclusively with the menstrual cycle, pregnancy, or sexual intercourse.

Affecting 4–15% of women of reproductive age seen in primary care settings, and up to 40% of those seen by gynecologists, the diagnosis and treatment of pelvic pain is complicated by its relationship to gynecologic, non-gynecologic organic, functional, and neuropsychological causes. Due to the many potential etiologies for pelvic pain, it is possible that more than one painful pelvic condition may coexist, causing significant physical discomfort and emotional distress and having negative effects on functional status and quality of life. Thus, pelvic pain presents a challenging, often multifactorial problem.

Endometriosis, a common cause of pelvic pain, is tissue with the histologic appearance of endometrium (the lining of the inside of the uterus) that is located outside of the uterus. Endometrial tissue can implant in fallopian tubes, ovaries, or intrapelvic organs and peritoneum. Since hormonal changes with the menstrual cycle also affect ectopic endometrial tissue, this tissue undergoes cyclical bleeding that is unable to drain, resulting in scar formation, pain, and infertility. The release of chemical pain mediators (prostaglandin E_2 and F) from endometrial tissue is postulated as one potential pain generator.

Endometriosis pain can occur cyclically or chronically; it is typically associated with dysmenorrhea or dyspareunia. There is evidence that many individuals with endometriosis are completely asymptomatic, and little correlation has been found between the amount of endometriosis in a given individual and the severity of reported pain. Hence, the precise mechanisms by which endometriosis causes pain are not completely understood.

The presentation of pelvic pain may be acute and episodic, cyclically intermittent, or chronic. Cyclical pelvic pain is likely due to a gynecologic source, while pain not related to the menstrual cycle may have either a gynecologic or a non-gynecologic source. Helpful questions for elucidating the cause of pelvic pain include whether the pain is related to the menstrual cycle or to bowel movements, whether it occurs during urination or sexual activity, and whether the patient has had a recent infection or undergone pelvic surgery.

Acute unilateral lower abdominal pain that occurs around the time of ovulation is most likely ovulatory pain, "mittelschmerz"; the pain may occur on the same side every month or may alternate sides. Suprapubic or low abdominal pain, cramping, bloating, or fullness that occurs immediately prior to and/or during menstruation, referred to as dysmenorrhea, is thought to be due to prostaglandin release during endometrial sloughing.

Signs and symptoms

Endometriosis most commonly presents as dysmenorrhea, dyspareunia, and/or chronic pelvic pain. Although asymptomatic in some individuals, endometriosis can cause chronic cyclical discomfort variably described as sharp, crampy, dull, aching, moderate, or severe. The pain of endometriosis may be worse at the beginning of menses or during intercourse, and it may manifest as rectal or low back pain.

Pelvic pain not related to the menstrual cycle may be due to fibroids or adenomyosis, which is the condition of glandular tissue growing in the uterine muscular wall. Endometriosis may also manifest as non-cyclical pain. Interstitial cystitis, urethritis, and cervicitis present with suprapubic tenderness and associated dyspareunia. Both gastrointestinal and urologic etiologies for pain may exhibit presentations similar to gynecologic pain; the clinical challenge is to delineate the most likely cause of the pain and to determine which diagnostic tests are most useful for confirmation.

Women of reproductive age who present with pelvic pain and non-specific symptoms such as nausea, vomiting, fever, and leukocytosis require prompt, thorough obstetric and gynecologic assessment to exclude emergent medical concerns such as ectopic pregnancy, hemorrhagic or ruptured ovarian cyst, ovarian torsion, or pelvic inflammatory disease. Physical signs include tenderness to light touch or deep palpation, as well as abdominal guarding, rebound, or rigidity; the latter are considered peritoneal signs, and as such they warrant prompt diagnostic work-up including imaging procedures and surgical evaluation to rule out intrapelvic emergency. Patients with severe, acute infection or surgical emergencies such as ectopic pregnancy may attempt to limit motion by curling up with flexed knees in a "fetal position." The physical exam should include bimanual pelvic and rectal exams; exquisite tenderness upon uterocervi-cal palpation and mobilization (the so-called "chandelier sign") is indicative of uterine, tubal, or ovarian pathology.

Symptoms of chronic pelvic pain include painful defecation, urination, and sexual intercourse, all of which are non-specific and may indicate gynecologic, urologic, or colonic pathology. Physical examination may reveal tenderness to light touch or deep palpation, antalgic gait, or limitations to mobility and range of motion (ROM) testing. Patients with chronic pain may also exhibit a depressed affect with marked psychomotor retardation.

Laboratory tests and diagnostic investigations

The first step for evaluating pelvic pain in women of reproductive age is the β-hCG to rule out pregnancy. A positive pregnancy test, in addition to raising concern for ectopic pregnancy, carries accompanying concerns for exposure to ionizing radiation diagnostic procedures (see ACR Appropriateness Criteria, below).

Further testing includes a complete blood count with differential (CBC with diff); urinalysis with culture; cervical culture for sexually transmitted infections, e.g., *Chlamydia trachomatis*, *Neisseria gonorrhoeae*; and VDRL for patients in whom infection is suspected.

A comprehensive metabolic profile may give clues to occult disease processes such as malignancy (liver function test [LFT] or protein/globulin abnormalities, elevated serum Ca) or bone disease. Erythrocyte sedimentation rate (ESR) or C-reactive protein (CRP) are non-specific tests which are of limited use in the evaluation of pelvic pain unless a rheumatologic etiology is suspected.

Imaging studies

Transabdominal and transvaginal pelvic sonography are the imaging studies of choice for evaluating gynecologic causes of pelvic pain, especially since it avoids maternal and fetal exposure to ionizing radiation.

Hysteroscopy with hysterosalpingogram can assess fallopian tube patency and presence of ectopic endometrial tissue. However, laparoscopic visualization with biopsy is the definitive test for endometriosis.

Barium enema and/or colonoscopy may be useful to rule out colorectal path-ology such as malignancy or inflammatory bowel disease. Cystoscopy is indicated to evaluate painful bladder syndrome in both males and females.

CT or MRI scanning provides the best diagnostic evaluation for gastrointest-inal and urologic causes of pelvic pain and may also be useful in assessing gynecologic pain under certain circumstances.

ACR Appropriateness Criteria for acute pelvic pain in the reproductive age group list four "variants" to assist with decision making regarding radiographic procedures in women of reproductive age: gynecologic etiology suspected with (1) serum β-hCG positive or (2) β-hCG negative; and non-gynecologic etiology suspected with (3) serum β-hCG positive or (4) β-hCG negative.

Simply stated, the guidelines recommend that for patients with suspicion of either gynecologic or non-gynecologic pelvic pain who also have a positive pregnancy test, x-ray imaging and CT abdomen with or without contrast are strongly discouraged, unless MRI is unavailable and the imaging is essential for urgent diagnosis.

Differential diagnosis

As already noted, the differential diagnosis of pelvic pain must take into account several potential etiologies for pain generators, including gynecologic, gastro-intestinal, urological, musculoskeletal, and neurologic structures.

Gynecologic pelvic pain related to ovulation and/or the menstrual cycle is usually due to mittelschmerz, dysmenorrhea, or endometriosis; non-cyclical pain may be due to adenomyosis, adnexal cysts, cervicitis, leiomyomata, malignancy, pelvic inflammatory disease, pelvic congestion syndrome, or uterine fibroids. It may also result from post-surgical complications such as adhesions or post-hysterectomy ovarian remnant.

Non-gynecologic causes of pelvic pain include referred pain from gastrointestinal sources such as appendicitis, chronic constipation, Crohn's disease, colon cancer, diverticular disease, irritable bowel syndrome, or ulcerative colitis. Acute appendicitis often presents as mid-epigastric pain that migrates to the right lower abdomen/pelvis; it is also associated with anorexia or nausea and vomiting and leukocytosis plus or minus fever. Heel strike and rectal exam may elicit a severely painful response. Signs associated with diverticular disease, Crohn's disease, or other inflammatory bowel conditions are non-specific, but may mimic appendicitis.

Non-gynecologic causes of pelvic pain may result from urologic conditions such as urethritis, interstitial cystitis, urinary tract infection; nervous system disorders such as pudendal neuralgia or trigger points; musculoskeletal issues including disc herniation, tumors, and osteoporotic fragility fractures; and psychological concerns, due to sexual abuse or other personal issues. It may also result from occult malignancy (e.g., lymphoma) or fibromyalgia.

Pharmacotherapy

Non-steroidal anti-inflammatory drugs (NSAIDs) are the drugs of choice for dysmenorrhea and mittelschmerz. Other analgesic agents such as aspirin or acetaminophen may be helpful, either alone or in combination with NSAIDs as co-analgesics.

Birth control pills are useful for hormonal regulation; women with chronic cyclical pelvic pain should receive a 3–6-month therapeutic trial of combined oral contraceptive pill or a gonadotropin-releasing hormone. Ovarian suppression may be effective treatment for pain associated with endometriosis.

Antibiotic therapy directed at causative pathogens (*Chlamydia*, gonorrhea) is indicated for cases of pelvic inflammatory disease. Opioids are generally discouraged for use in chronic pelvic pain.

Non-pharmacologic approaches

In cases of ovulatory pain or dysmenorrhea, reassurance and anti-inflammatory medications are usually sufficient. Patients report relief from warm baths or heating pads to the lower abdomen as well as lumbosacral massage/efflurage. There are a number of herbs or nutriceuticals (e.g., turmeric) that have been touted for relieving menstrual pain; while probably harmless and possibly able to provide a placebo response, there is no medical evidence to recommend their use.

Patients with chronic pelvic pain of unknown or multifactorial cause(s) may require multimodal therapy utilizing an interdisciplinary team approach including relaxation and physical exercises, biofeedback, and psychological counseling. Pelvic pain may also respond to manual medicine techniques (osteopathic or chiropractic) directed at mobilizing lymphatic fluid, including lymphatic pump and craniosacral release techniques.

Interventional procedures

Abdominal trigger-point injections have been used with success for specific painful areas.

If an acute intrapelvic emergency is discovered, surgery is the treatment of choice.

Non-emergent surgical removal of endometriotic lesions has been the cornerstone of management of pelvic pain due to endometriosis for decades; however, there is little correlation between the findings at laparoscopy and prognosis in terms of pain reduction or fertility. Laparoscopy with adhesiolysis may be beneficial for patients with extensive scarring.

Follow-up

Hormonally mediated and/or menstrual pain, including endometriosis, usually diminishes or disappears with menopause. Follow-up for patients with chronic pelvic pain is helpful in assessing response to therapy and making necessary modifications; in most cases, follow-up is supportive in nature.

Prognosis

The prognosis for pelvic pain is contingent upon the etiology of the pain. A particularly troublesome aspect of endometriosis is the risk of infertility with its attendant effects on a woman's sense of identity. The pain may become the symbol of a larger problem, which requires clinical attention to both its physical and psychological aspects.

REFERENCES AND FURTHER READING

ACR Appropriateness Criteria: acute pelvic pain in the reproductive age group. National Guideline Clearinghouse, 2011.

Bruckenthal P. Chronic pelvic pain: approaches to diagnosis and treatment. *Pain Manag Nurs* 2011; **12**: S4–10.

Ghosh M, Ojha K. Medical and surgical management of pelvic pain. *Obstet Gynecol Reprod Med* 2011; **21**: 249–53.

Howard FM. Endometriosis and mechanisms of pelvic pain. *J Minim Invasive Gynecol* 2009; **16**: 540–50.

Learman LA. Chronic pelvic pain. Part 1: prevalence, evaluation, etiology and comorbidities. *Women's Health* 2005; **5** : 306–15.

Spine

33

Acute and chronic back pain, back strain and sprain

Clinical presentation

Back pain is among the most common debilitating conditions for which patients seek medical care. The term *back strain and sprain* describes pain for which no clear pathologic etiology is identified. More than two-thirds of individuals will experience at least one episode of back pain during their lifetime, accounting for an estimated $38–50 billion in annual healthcare costs in the USA; it is the most common cause of work-related disability in those under 45 years of age. The term *strain and sprain* refers to a musculoskeletal origin for pain, and thus represents a diagnosis of exclusion of other pathologies. Some recommend the diagnosis *idiopathic back pain* in lieu of *strain and sprain*.

Strains, sprains, and muscle spasms usually result from activity or injury; most episodes are self-limited with progressive symptomatic improvement and complete resolution over time. An estimated 90% of cases of back pain are due to mechanical musculoskeletal causes and will resolve spontaneously within 6 weeks to 6 months. However, one in three sufferers have continuous, moderate pain 1 year after the acute episode. Acute back pain is defined as lasting less than 4 weeks, sub-acute as 4–12 weeks, and chronic back pain persists for more than 12 weeks. Some patients experience recurrent episodes of back pain, which is similar to exacerbation of a chronic problem for which there is treatment but no definitive cure.

Back pain presents a diagnostic challenge. Due to the small cortical region in the sensory homunculus dedicated to the back, precise localization of the pain is difficult; i.e., the ability to discriminate between two point stimuli on the skin of the back is much less sensitive than on other parts of the body (hands, feet, face). This explains why the complaint of back pain suggests a potentially large number of problems, musculoskeletal and otherwise. Pain may originate from spinal structures (ligaments, facet joints, joint capsules, vertebral periosteum, annulus fibrosis, etc.) as well as from paravertebral muscles, fascia, and vascular supply. Afferent spinal nerve roots carry impulses from abdominal and pelvic organs that refer pain to the back. The ubiquitous presence of nociceptive fibers in the back makes identification of the precise pain-generating structure problematic.

Many sufferers are able to pinpoint a precipitating event (typically a work- or sports-related activity or injury) that suggests a musculoskeletal etiology for the pain. For those reporting no inciting event, or only minor trauma, clinical evaluation must take into account the possibility of referred pain. Mid- to low-thoracic nerve roots refer pain from pulmonary parietal pleura, gastrointestinal viscera (stomach, gallbladder, and pancreas) adrenals, or kidneys. Lumbar and sacral nerves transmit pain from pelvic organs as well as the hip, sacroiliac, and lumbar spine regions. The brain may be unable to distinguish the source of pain impulses traveling through the same nerves or sharing the same somatosensory neurons. Thus back pain may herald disease of the pulmonary pleura, abdominal viscera, abdominal aortic aneurysm, upper and lower urinary tract, adrenals and kidneys, uterus and ovaries, prostate, vertebral, sacral, hip, or other pathology. An example of viscerosomatic referred pain is right subscapular pain from gallbladder pathology.

In order to understand back strain and sprain it is helpful to review the musculoskeletal anatomy of the back. The spine and supporting musculature is an elegant structure that provides protection for the delicate central nervous system (CNS) and internal organs as well as allowing movement in several planes. The spinal column consists of 24 vertebral segments that constitute the cervical (C1 through C7), thoracic (T1 through T12), and lumbar (L1 through L5) spine. The stacked vertebrae surround and protect the spinal cord and provide egress for the spinal nerve roots. Between each rounded or oval-shaped bony vertebral body is an intervertebral disc that acts as a cushion for vertebral motion. Vertebral bodies comprise an outer shell of hard cortical bone housing a center of spongy cancellous bone; intervertebral discs consist of a fibrous outer ring, the annulus fibrosis, encasing a gelatinous central core, the nucleus pulposus. The thoracic spine provides posterior (dorsal) articular surfaces for the ribs; the anterior (ventral) articulatory surface for the ribs is the sternum. The seven cervical segments and 12 thoracic vertebral bodies rest atop five larger lumbar vertebral segments (some individuals have a sixth lumbar vertebra), which in turn rest on five sacral segments that in adults have fused to form the sacrum. The coccyx is the small curved terminal appendage of the sacrum. Lateral margins of the sacrum provide the articulatory interface with the ilium, known as the sacroiliac joint.

The round vertebral body lies anterior to the articular surfaces of the spinous processes, including the superior and transverse processes as well as the pars interarticularis, which is contiguous with the posterior spinous process. This articular arch forms the spinal foramen, which houses the spinal cord, posterior to which is the ligamentam flavum, which connects the laminae of adjacent vertebrae. Ligamenta flava are thinnest in the cervical, thicker in the thoracic, and thickest in the lumbar region. The pars interarticularis articulates with the superior spinous process of the vertebral segment immediately below; anterior and proximal to these articulations are the intervertebral foramina, largest in the thoracic region, where spinal nerve roots exit. A defect in the pars articularis, known as spondylosis, is essentially a break in the articular chain that may allow the anterior articulate displacement of the affected vertebral body on the segment below, known as spondylolisthesis. Spondylosis may be either congenital or acquired.

In addition to bearing the weight of the body, the spine undergoes flexion, extension, and rotatory movements, enabling the normal range of motion seen in healthy individuals. Since the bulk of these forces center on the lower thoracic and lumbosacral vertebral segments, it is not surprising that the preponderance of cases of back strain and sprain occur in the lower back. With increasing age or repetitive trauma, degenerative changes occur in the intervertebral discs, vertebral bodies, spinous and transverse processes, facet joints, and articular surfaces, which may present as back strain or sprain.

Anatomic landmarks useful for identifying the level of spinal segments include the tip of the scapula, which is located at T7; the umbilicus, located at T12; and the iliac crest, which corresponds with the level of L4. Palpation of these structures gives the examiner an idea of which vertebral segments are affected, which can in turn provide clues to the source of the pain.

Signs and symptoms

The focus of evaluation of back pain is to identify those needing urgent attention by seeking symptoms suggesting an underlying condition that may be more serious, and to determine who may need urgent surgical evaluation. To aid in evaluation of patients presenting with back pain, a 2007 Joint Clinical Practice Guideline from the American College of Physicians and the American Pain Society gives specific recommendations regarding the diagnosis and management of low back pain (Chou *et al.* 2007). The first of these recommendations is to conduct a focused history and physical examination, with the goal of placing patients into one of three categories: (1) non-specific low back pain, (2) back pain potentially associated with radiculopathy or spinal stenosis, or (3) back pain associated with another specific spinal cause. A fourth implied category is back pain referred from a non-spinal source. The guidelines recommend assessment of psychosocial risk factors and emotional distress, since they have been shown to be stronger predictors of low back pain outcomes than either physical examination findings or severity of pain.

Acute low back pain typically presents with a sudden onset related to an activity or injury; patients complain of pain and/or spasm exacerbated by movement. Symptoms of radiculopathy include the complaint of radiation of pain along a dermatomal pattern into the lower leg, which necessitates a neurological evaluation of reflexes, heel and toe walking, Patrick's (FABER) test, and seated and straight leg raising tests. Younger male patients who report symptoms for more than 3 months such as alternating buttock pain, awakening with back pain in the latter part of the night, and morning stiffness that improves with exercise have signs and symptoms suggestive of ankylosing spondylitis. Older individuals with non-specific back pain may have degenerative joint disease, facet joint arthritis, and bulging or herniated discs. Neurologic involvement is suggested by the presence of sciatica (radiation of pain into the leg) or neurogenic claudication (leg pain initiated by movement that resolves with rest, usually lying down). Older individuals complaining of neurogenic claudication may have spinal stenosis; they typically report that the pain is improved by forward bending, such as by leaning on a shopping cart while ambulating. Pain with forward flexion may indicate disc disease, and localized paralumbar pain with extension is suggestive of facet disease. Pain in the buttock or leg is often disc or facet disease, but clinicians must also rule out hip pathology in these patients.

"Red flags" alerting the clinician to a potentially serious cause of back pain include thoracic pain, widespread neurological deficit, lower limb weakness or atrophy, drug abuse and/or human immunodeficiency virus, age less than 20 or greater than 50 years, unexplained weight loss, persistent severe restriction of lumbar flexion, night pain, constant progressive non-mechanical pain, upper respiratory symptoms, previous history of cancer, or recent history of trauma. The classic triad of cauda equina symptoms is altered bowel and/or bladder control, saddle anesthesia, and neurologic deficit. While back pain in someone over age 50, unexplained weight loss, and history of cancer are individually concerning factors, the presence of all three is predictive for a malignant cause of back pain.

The US Agency on Health Care Policy and Research (AHCPR) *Clinical Practice Guideline* for low back pain lists several open-ended questions to gauge the need for more detailed inquiry into the source of pain: What are your symptoms? Pain, numbness, weakness, stiffness? Located primarily in back, leg, or both? Constant or intermittent? How do these symptoms limit you? How long can you sit, stand, walk? How much weight can you lift? When did the current limitations begin? How long have your activities been limited? More than 4 weeks? Have you had similar episodes previously? Previous testing or treatment? What do you hope we can accomplish during this visit? The AHCPR "red flags" indicating the possibility of a serious underlying condition include those shown in Table 33.1.

Psychosocial history should focus on risk factors such as overweight or obesity, cigarette smoking, inactivity, history of intravenous drug or alcohol abuse or addiction, and psychological conditions such as anxiety, depression, or frank psychiatric illness. There is evidence that patients with psychological or social stressors are at risk for prolonged recovery from back strain and sprain. The above factors have been called "yellow flags" alerting clinicians to the potential for protracted pain and debility in these patients.

The physical examination should begin with close observation of the patient walking into the room, noting antalgic, paretic, spastic, or otherwise abnormal gait, followed by measurement of vital signs including the use of a validated pain

Table 33.1 AHCPR "red flags" for low back pain

Sign/symptom	Possible etiology
Recent significant trauma, or milder trauma in those age < 50	Fracture
Osteoporosis	Fracture
Unexplained weight loss	Cancer
Immunosuppressive therapy	Cancer
Unexplained fever or recent urinary tract infection	Infection
Intravenous drug use	Infection
Prolonged use of glucocorticoids	Fracture, infection
Age > 70	Fracture, cancer
Pain lasting longer than 6 weeks	Cancer, infection
History of cancer	Cancer
Progressive motor or sensory deficit	Cauda equina syndrome
Saddle anesthesia, bowel/bladder incontinence or retention	Cauda equina syndrome

scale. Assessment should consider whether the pulse and blood pressure correlate with the amount of pain the patient is reporting, bearing in mind that patients with chronic pain typically exhibit no elevation in these readings. Inspection of the back should seek any deviation from the normal thoracolumbar curves (thoracic kyphosis [convexity] and lumbar lordosis [concavity]), and note the presence of scoliosis or other obvious deformities.

Neurological exam should evaluate patellar and ankle reflexes, motor strength, sensation, and rectal exam if bowel or bladder complaints are present. Motor testing can be easily accomplished by having a seated patient push one leg at a time against the examiner's resisting hand, anteriorly/posteriorly (quadriceps strength), and cephalad by having the patient lift his/her thigh against the downward pressure of the examining hand (hip flexors) and flexing/extending the feet against resistance (plantar and dorsiflexion strength). Motor strength in the supine position can be evaluated by asking the patient to lift each leg, one at a time, off the table, either with or without passive resistance by the examiner; to flex, rotate, and extend the ankle; and to bend the leg and bring it toward the chest in a chair position. Discrepancies in reflex or motor function should be scored using a standardized protocol, usually a 1–5-point scale, with 5 being strongest and 1 being weakest. Knee strength and reflexes test the L4 nerve root, while diminished great toe strength and difficulty heel walking (dorsiflexing the feet) suggests L5 radiculopathy. Difficulty walking on toes or plantar flexing may be indicative of S1 radiculopathy. The sensory examination of patients with back pain may be accomplished with monofilament testing, two-point discrimination, and hot/cold sensation testing.

A complete musculoskeletal structural examination that seeks abnormality in structure or function (somatic dysfunction) is the next step in evaluation of back pain. Inspection of the musculoskeletal structures of the back may be guided by the mnemonic TART: *tenderness, asymmetry, range of motion modified,* and *tissue texture change.* Tenderness is assessed by light to deep palpation of the paravertebral musculature, moving systematically from vertebral segment to each adjacent segment, repeating this evaluation on both sides of the spine. The paravertebrals are easily located by finding the posterior spinous process, which is the most prominently palpable portion of the spine, and dropping the pads of the fingers into the sulci immediately lateral to it on both sides. The transverse processes are inferior to the fingers here; light pressure exerted anteriorly and laterally will allow for evaluation of the paravertebral muscle mass. Asymmetries of the position of the posterior and transverse spinous processes should be noted. Careful palpation and percussion of the entire spine may discover pain, misalignment, or step-off between vertebrae, which are clues to the presence of an underlying anatomic abnormality such as spondylolisthesis or bony pathology such as compression fractures or metastases. Asymmetry is also assessed through visual observation, noting the presence of erythema, rash, bruising, or scars, and by evaluating discrepancies in muscle bulk and manual strength in lower extremities.

Gross range of motion (ROM) testing should evaluate for asymmetry or loss of functional capacity. ROM testing includes evaluation of forward bending (flexion), backward bending (extension), side bending (side flexion), and rotation. While there is a great deal of inter-individual variation, normal range of motion for lumbar flexion is approximately 40 degrees; lumbar extension (backward bending) is approximately 15 degrees; and side bending is approximately 30 degrees (i.e., the ipsilateral side-bent hand should reach close to the knee in a fully side-bent position). Rotation is approximately 45 degrees. A complete osteopathic evaluation of the spine includes assessment of the motion of individual spinal segments, especially those associated with asymmetry or other abnormality noted in the exam. Vertebral segments are palpated to test for restrictions in flexion, extension, side bending (translation), and rotation.

Tissue texture changes that may be found include heat or redness, induration, edema or bogginess, ropiness, tumors, or skin lesions. In addition, trophic changes such as pigmentation, hair loss, or obvious atrophy are signs of underlying pathology.

The ROM exam gives several important clues to the cause of pain. As noted, patients who exhibit more pain with extension may have spinal stenosis, increased pain with forward flexion suggests the possibility of disc disorder, localized paralumbar pain with extension is suggestive of facet syndrome, and pain in the buttock or leg is often disc- or facet-related. In these cases the examiner must rule out hip pathology, since not all pain that radiates to the lower leg is discogenic. In order to evaluate for pain related to disc disease and to rule out hip pathology, clinicians should evaluate the patient with ROM testing of the hip and Patrick's test.

Patrick's test is a detailed range of motion (ROM) evaluation in which the hip joint is stressed to determine the presence of sacroiliac disease. It involves the "sign of four" (from the position in which the affected leg is placed, resembling the number 4) or FABER sign (from the acronym of the maneuvers involved, which are flexion, abduction, and external rotation). With the patient lying supine, the examiner places the lateral malleolus of the suspected limb over the patella of the opposite side. Downward pressure on the thigh is then exerted by the hand of the examiner, testing for hip joint disease by antagonizing hip flexor spasm brought on by an inflammatory lesion. A positive test is revealed when hip pain, especially in the area of the hip flexors, is elicited. The test may also provoke pain in the sacroiliac joint.

In order to evaluate patients for nerve root compression, the straight leg raising (SLR) test is employed. A positive test, indicating possible nerve root compression, occurs when the patient feels back pain that radiates down the leg (usually the lateral or posterior aspect) at $\leq$ 70 degrees of hip flexion. Aggravation of the pain with ankle dorsiflexion and relief with knee flexion support the positive finding. To perform the test, the examiner should ask patient to localize the pain by pointing; at the point the patient feels pain, lower the leg and dorsiflex the foot to reproduce sciatic nerve pain. Herniated disc correlates with a positive SLR test, usually at a lower degree of elevation, aggravated by ankle dorsiflexion and relieved with knee flexion. A "crossover SLR test" elicits pain in the affected leg when the unaffected side is raised; it is less sensitive (29%) but more specific (88%). Performance of the SLR test with the patient seated may create fewer false positives than when the patient is supine. Patients with no pain while sitting with the leg(s) extended, but who describe pain on supine examination, may be suspected of having a psychogenic origin for their pain, such as malingering. An alternative is the "slump test," in which the seated patient is asked to lean forward or "slump over" his/her thighs while the examiner elevates the lower legs, one at a time. Patients who complain of pain radiating down the leg (as in the SLR test) have positive evidence of a radicular etiology for the pain.

Laboratory tests and diagnostic investigations

There is no specific laboratory test for back strain and sprain, and it is generally considered unnecessary in the initial evaluation of non-specific back pain. However, specific laboratory testing is indicated to differentiate non-specific, musculoskeletal pain from pain from another source. Complete blood count with differential (CBC with diff), erythrocyte sedimentation rate (ESR), or C-reactive protein (CRP) should be obtained for patients in whom vertebral infection or cancer is suspected. A comprehensive metabolic panel may reveal abnormalities indicative of disease processes. For example, elevation of serum alkaline phosphatase is found in patients with Paget's disease of bone, which can cause vertebral compression fractures and spinal stenosis; and calcium levels may be elevated in cases of hyperparathyroidism, which can also cause compression fractures. Prostate-specific antigen (PSA) level elevation may indicate the presence of prostate malignancy, and abnormal proteins in blood and urine may indicate cancer of the plasma cells or multiple myeloma. A rheumatologic evaluation is indicated for those with suspected rheumatoid arthritis (rheumatoid factor, ESR, CBC with diff) or ankylosing spondylitis (HLA-B27).

Imaging studies

Imaging studies should not be routinely obtained for the evaluation of patients with non-specific back pain without the presence of "red flags." Several clinical practice guidelines recommend that imaging be reserved for patients who present with progressive or severe neurologic deficits or for suspected serious underlying conditions, based on focused history and physical examination. For these patients, the imaging study of choice is MRI. CT may also be obtained; however, these studies should be reserved for patients who are potential candidates for surgical or interventional therapies.

Imaging can be misleading, because many abnormalities (e.g., spondylolysis or internal disc disruption) are as common in pain-free individuals as in those with back pain. Studies such as discography may cause pain in previously asymptomatic individuals. For those under age 60, radiographic studies have a low yield: there are unexpected x-ray findings in only 1 of 2500 patients with back pain. Furthermore, radiographic imaging may identify incidental abnormalities that are not the actual cause of pain. For example, bulging discs are found in one in three pain-free individuals, and herniated discs in one in five. Individuals over age 60 who are pain-free all have age-related disc degeneration; imaging may identify herniated disc in approximately 30% and bulging disc in 80%. Spinal stenosis may be found in one in five older patient cases.

A recent review (Deyo *et al.* 2009) notes that "lumbar magnetic resonance imaging (MRI) increased in the Medicare population by 307% during a recent 12-year interval. Others have described rapid increases in spine imaging and for imaging procedures in general. Spine imaging rates vary dramatically across geographic regions, and surgery rates are highest where imaging rates are highest. When judged against guidelines, one-third to two-thirds of spinal computed tomography imaging and MRI may be inappropriate."

For patients with back pain who have severe or progressive neurological deficits or who are suspected of vertebral infection, cauda equina syndrome, or cancer, the imaging study of choice is MRI. Suspected vertebral compression fractures or spondyloarthropathy may be evaluated by plain film radiographs of the spine, and anteroposterior radiographs of the pelvis may be helpful in diagnosing ankylosing spondylitis. It is important to consider the dose of ionizing radiation as well as the age and child-bearing potential of the patient when determining whether or not to order radiologic studies, since the amount of radiation from a single CT scan of the pelvis is significant.

Differential diagnosis

As previously noted, in cases of back pain when there is no specific disease or spinal abnormality identified, a diagnosis of *strain and sprain* is given. *Idiopathic* or *mechanical* back pain are terms that may also be used. Eighty-five percent of cases of low back pain are due to strain (overstretched muscle) or sprain (partly torn/injured ligament). The differential diagnosis includes degenerative disc or facets, herniated disc, osteoporotic compression fracture, spinal stenosis, spondylolisthesis, visceral disease, neoplasia (multiple myeloma, spinal cord tumor), congenital disease (kyphosis, scoliosis), traumatic fracture, and inflammatory arthritis (ankylosing spondylitis).

Detailed discussions of several causes of back pain may be found in the folllowing chapters, including compression fracture, lumbar radiculopathy, sciatica and piriformis syndrome, spinal stenosis, lumbar facet syndrome, sacroiliac pain, coccydynia, and post-laminectomy pain, as well as pain referred from abdominal and pelvic organs. Once satisfied that back pain is due to a musculoskeletal or mechanical cause and not another etiology, the diagnosis of back strain and sprain is given. The differential diagnosis of back strain and sprain may reasonably be presumed to be due to a structural musculoskeletal cause.

A review by Greenman published in 1996 identified six somatic dysfunctions ("the dirty half-dozen") that were present in a cohort of patients presenting with disabling back pain many times more commonly than problems identified by orthopedic or neurologic testing. They are: (1) pelvic tilt and short leg syndrome, (2) non-neutral lumbar mechanics, (3) pubic dysfunction, (4) innominate shear dysfunction, (5) restricted sacral nutation, and (6) muscular imbalance. If one of these dysfunctions is identified by a structural diagnostic process, manual medicine or manipulative therapy may be helpful to correct the underlying process.

Pharmacotherapy

There are a number of medications that may be helpful in the pharmacologic management of non-specific back pain. As with any condition, the choice of medication depends on a number of factors including the severity and duration of symptoms, prior response to treatment, expected outcomes, presence of comorbidities, age and physiologic state of the patient, costs of therapy, and degree of supporting evidence. Further considerations include the goals of treatment and whether treatment is directed at acute symptom management or persistent, chronic pain. In general, response to pharmacologic treatment for acute back pain is favorable, with improvement in function and reduction of pain expected over a 1–2-month course. On the other hand, if back pain has been present for more than 12 weeks, defined as chronic back pain, the likelihood of significant improvement from pharmacotherapy is much lower.

The initial choice of treatment for acute back strain and sprain is the analgesic acetaminophen or non-steroidal anti-inflammatory drugs (NSAIDs) such as aspirin, ibuprofen, or naproxen. Many patients initiate self-treatment with these medications, which are available over the counter. Prescription-strength NSAIDs or the cyclooxygenase-2 (COX-2) inhibitor celecoxib decrease pain and relieve pain by inhibition of prostaglandins. NSAIDs are available in multiple formulations including tablets or capsules, topical patches, and gels. However, their use is limited by the risk for gastrointestinal bleeding or adverse renal effects. All NSAIDs, including topical preparations (which have a lower serum concentration), have a Food and Drug Administration (FDA) black box warning against the risk for heart attack or stroke.

Skeletal muscle relaxants have been shown to be helpful in the acute phase of back strain and sprain to reduce muscular spasm but are not recommended as first-line therapy; their use is limited by the presence of sedation and other CNS adverse effects. The addition of a skeletal muscle relaxant to acetaminophen or an NSAID may be more effective than the use of either medication alone. Benzodiazepines have sedative, anxiolytic, and antiepileptic effects and have been used as skeletal muscle relaxants, but they lack FDA approval for this indication. Muscle relaxants are not indicated for chronic back pain, and most guidelines recommend their use for no more than 1–2 weeks, if needed.

Opioid analgesics may be effective in the treatment of acute back strain and sprain, but they are not considered first-line therapy and should be used at the lowest effective dose for the shortest time possible. A potential use of opioid analgesics for back pain is for patients with known gastrointestinal bleeding, renal impairment, or advanced age, since NSAIDs and skeletal muscle relaxants have limited safety profiles for such individuals. Systemic corticosteroids and antiepileptic medications are not recommended in the treatment of back strain and sprain.

Non-pharmacologic approaches

There are a number of non-pharmacological treatment options for back strain and sprain, including complementary and alternative medicine (CAM) modalities. The AHCPR has issued guidelines for the non-pharmacological treatment of back strain and sprain. Recommendations included in the *Clinical Practice Guideline* define a paradigm shift away from focusing care exclusively on the pain and toward helping patients improve activity tolerance. Spinal manipulation (by chiropractors, osteopaths, or physical therapists) and massage have evidence of effectiveness.

However, there is no evidence to support the use of prolonged bed rest, immobilization, traction, or bracing for back strain and sprain. Bed rest should be recommended for no more than 48 hours for individuals who are unable to tolerate routine activity. Hot and cold packs have been successfully used as self-care options, and the current evidence suggests that there is some benefit to heat applied to the painful area but little evidence for the use of cold beyond the acute phase of spasm/inflammation. Clinicians may advise the use of cold or heat as tolerated, and provide recommendations for gentle stretching.

Spinal manipulative techniques, such as offered by osteopaths (osteopathic manipulative medicine, OMM), or chiropractic treatment have been shown to have efficacy, but there is little evidence to support the use of acupuncture for back strain and sprain. Massage is a commonly utilized self-care modality which has been shown, anecdotally, to be helpful, and there is some evidence for its use.

Patients should be advised to remain as active as possible but to avoid heavy lifting, twisting, or bodily vibration for several weeks until the pain has resolved. It is important to remember that up to 80% of the population experience back pain at some time, and it is usually a self-limited condition with estimates showing that 50% are better in 1 week and 90% of cases of low back pain are resolved in 6 weeks. Clinicians should offer reassurance that low back pain typically resolves without permanent sequelae, but that recurrence is common, so education about careful lifting methods, seated and standing posture, and simple preventive exercise modalities should be offered.

Prevention of back strain and sprain includes proper postural alignment while standing, sitting, and lying down. Standing posture can be assessed by observing the patient from the side; ideally, one can visualize a vertical line running from the top of the head just anterior to the earlobe and shoulder, down the center of the hip, behind the kneecap and just in front of the ankle. Standing posture can also be assessed by standing against a wall: the back of the head, shoulders, and buttocks should touch the wall and there should be enough room to slide a hand between the wall and the lumbar area. When standing, the head should be held level with the chin parallel to the floor, not thrust forward, while the shoulders are relaxed and the abdominal muscles are pulled in. Good seated posture can be achieved by sitting in a straight-backed chair with shoulders against the chair, chest lifted and arms on the armrests with the upper back straight, not stooped.

Exercise is an important component of self-care for back strain and sprain. The Williams flexion exercises are useful, as is yoga or pilates. The focus of an exercise program is to strengthen the muscles in the back and abdomen while stretching the muscles in the back. Proper lifting technique requires bending at the knees and carrying the object close to the body. Holding objects at arm's length increases the load significantly and can put undue strain on back muscles. Patients with back strain/sprain should be encouraged to lose extra weight and to maintain a healthy body mass index; they should also be advised to quit smoking, since this is a major risk factor for osteoporosis and also decreases circulation to the intervertebral discs, speeding their degeneration.

Interventional procedures

Interventions aimed at reducing the pain and disability associated with back pain are based upon the presence of an identifiable musculoskeletal abnormality such as a herniated nucleus pulposis. Patients diagnosed with idiopathic, mechanical back pain or back strain and sprain by definition lack a specific anatomic problem that might be amenable to surgical or radiologic intervention.

Discussion of specific interventions such as diagnostic neural blockade, therapeutic lumbar epidural steroid injections, lumbar discectomy, total disc replacement, laminectory, and other spinal surgical options for treatment of radiculopathies caused by herniated discs, spinal stenosis, or vertebral compression fractures may be found in the following chapters.

Follow-up

Patients with recurrent or chronic (persisting longer than 3 months) back strain and sprain warrant evaluation by an interdisciplinary team of providers to develop a plan of care that will reduce pain and disability, improve and maintain functional capacity, and assist the patient in finding methods to ameliorate or cope with the problem of pain. Some patients benefit by attending "back school," a program designed to modify or eliminate factors that may be contributing to the pain and disability.

Prognosis

The prognosis for patients with back strain and sprain is generally very good. Patients should understand that the goal of therapy is to maintain function and manage psychosocial distress, even if complete resolution of pain is not possible. Functional outcome depends more on individual patient behavior than on medical treatments.

Spontaneous recovery rate is approximately 50–75% at 4 weeks and over 90% at 6 weeks. Most people will not require surgery to achieve pain control even with herniated discs. However, subacute or chronic low back pain can be difficult to treat, and exacerbations can recur over time. Patients with ongoing back strain and sprain should be referred for interdisciplinary pain management.

REFERENCES AND FURTHER READING

Chou R. Therapy in practice: pharmacological management of low back pain. *Drugs* 2010; **70**: 387–402.
Chou R, Qaseem A, Snow V, *et al.* Diagnosis and treatment of low back pain: a joint clinical practice guideline from the American College of Physicians and the American Pain Society. *Ann Intern Med* 2007; **147**: 478–91.
Clinical Guideline Subcommittee on Low Back Pain; American Osteopathic Association. American Osteopathic Association guidelines for osteopathic manipulative treatment (OMT) for patients with low back pain. *J Am Osteopath Assoc* 2010; **110**: 653–66.
Deyo RA, Weinstein JN. Low back pain. *N Engl J Med* 2001; **344**: 363–70.

Deyo RA, Mirza SK, Turner JA, Martin BI. Overtreating chronic back pain: time to back off? *J Am Board Fam Med* 2009; **22**: 62–8.

Ferguson F, Holdsworth L, Rafferty D. Low back pain and physiotherapy use of red flags: the evidence from Scotland. *Physiotherapy* 2010; **96**: 282–8.

Greenman PE. Syndromes of the lumbar spine, pelvis, and sacrum. *Phys Med Rehabil Clin N Am* 1996; **7**: 773–85.

Last AR, Hulbert K. Chronic low back pain: evaluation and management. *Am Fam Physician* 2009; **79**: 1067–74.

Ong CK, Doll H, Boedeker G, Stewart-Brown S. Use of osteopathic or chiropractic services among people with back pain: a UK population survey. *Health Soc Care Community* 2004; **12**: 265–73.

Pelz DM, Haddad RG. Radiologic investigation of low back pain. *CMAJ* 1989; **140**: 289–95.

34

Compression fracture

Clinical presentation

Vertebral compression fractures do not typically occur in the absence of forceful injury or direct trauma such as a fall from height or an automobile accident. However, in the presence of disease states (osteoporosis, Paget's disease, primary or metastatic malignancy, or hyperparathyroidism) something as minor as a sudden movement or cough can cause compression fracture. Also referred to as fragility fractures, they can cause significant pain and disability, limitations in activities of daily living, social isolation, depression, and decreased quality of life. Vertebral compression fractures are the most common type of compression fracture. One out of six in a survey of 500 individuals over age 60 who presented to an emergency department had an incidental finding of vertebral fracture on chest x-ray.

Despite widely available screening procedures and increased awareness of the consequences of osteoporosis, many older persons have low bone mineral density, which places them at risk for compression fractures. Most common in middle-aged and older Caucasian or Asian women, osteoporosis may also occur in frail nursing home residents of both genders due to impaired mobility and vitamin D deficiency (inadequate nutrition and exposure to sunlight), and in cardiac and liver transplant patients. Other risk factors for osteoporosis include cigarette smoking, low body weight, low estrogen or testosterone levels, lack of weight-bearing exercise, chronic steroid or antihormonal drug use, and excessive alcohol consumption. There is also an association between osteoporosis and prolonged use of proton pump inhibitors (PPIs), gastrectomy, and Crohn's disease.

Noting that up to 65% of compression fractures go unrecognized until a radiographic image reveals them, the presentation is variable. Some patients may complain only of loss of axial height, while others may report the sudden onset of excruciating, immobilizing pain, usually during a specific movement such as twisting, turning, or bending forward. The fracture may result from a fall or from placing a load on outstretched arms, such as raising a window or lifting a bag of groceries. Such fractures usually occur in the anterior portion of the vertebral body.

It is estimated that 25% of women over the age of 50 will experience one or more compression fractures during their lifetime; in contrast, men account for only one-seventh of vertebral compression fractures associated with osteoporosis.

Signs and symptoms

When assessing acute back pain, one diagnostic screen for compression fracture utilizes three "red flags" plus gender: age 70 or older, prolonged use of corticosteroids, significant trauma, and female gender. As already noted, however, many vertebral compression fractures are asymptomatic and are discovered incidentally on x-rays obtained for other reasons. Loss of 6–8 cm in height has been associated with vertebral compression fracture.

A simple procedure that may pinpoint an occult fracture is spinal percussion: the examiner lightly taps each spinal segment in the same way that a Lloyd's test is performed over the lateral lumbar area to test for kidney pain. An area of pain or tenderness may indicate fracture or other spinal pathology.

Pain may be immediate upon fracture or may occur 1–2 days later, and it generally worsens during activities that involve twisting or bending; it frequently will not be relieved by bed rest. Fractures in the lower lumbar region may result in transient neurologic symptoms such as difficulty urinating or defecating. If such symptoms persist, neurosurgical evaluation is indicated for urgent spinal cord decompression.

The anatomic compromise that occurs from compression fractures can result in long-term structural changes. Thoracic or lumbar pain causes postural and ambulatory changes that lead to muscle fatigue (with resultant asthenia, decreased appetite, depression, disordered sleep, and social isolation); increased kyphosis and loss of height ("dowager's hump") lead to consequences such as the loss of intrathoracic and intra-abdominal space for vital organs, thus compromising respiration, digestion, and ambulatory function. These changes may be associated with failure to thrive and increased mortality.

Laboratory tests and diagnostic investigations

Serum alkaline phosphatase (enzyme released by osteoblasts) level is elevated in patients with Paget's disease. Calcium levels are increased in cases of hyperparathyroidism. Prostate-specific antigen (PSA) elevations may be indicative of prostate cancer (although the antigen is also elevated in benign prostatic hypertrophy). Abnormal urine and serum proteins (UPEP and SPEP) may reveal plasma cell cancer, multiple myeloma.

Imaging studies

Lateral plain film radiographs, CT, or MRI scan may be utilized for imaging compression fractures. Positron emission tomography (PET)-CT diffusion and perfusion MRI are helpful for differentiating osteoporotic or traumatic compression fractures from those due to a malignancy-related diagnosis. Increased fluorodeoxyglucose (FDG) uptake indicates a potential neoplastic cause for fracture. Bone single photon emission computed tomography (SPECT) is another modality that may help to differentiate between malignant and non-malignant causes of compression fracture.

Differential diagnosis

The differential diagnosis of compression fracture includes most of the diagnostic possibilities associated with back pain. Clinicians must be alert to "red flags" indicating medical emergencies such as spinal cord compression, dissecting thoracic or abdominal aortic aneurysm, and tumors.

Pharmacotherapy

Salmon calcitonin is the pharmacologic treatment of choice, especially if initiated in the first few days after fracture. It may be administered intranasally, intrarectally, or subcutaneously. Side effects include dizziness and epistaxis (for intranasal calcitonin); allergy to salmon is a contraindication.

Bisphosphonates, ibandronate, and strontium ranelate may be useful for prevention of additional symptomatic fractures in patients with osteoporosis. They help to preserve bone mass by slowing bone resorption. Side effects of bisphophonates are predominantly gastrointestinal, including indigestion, diarrhea, stomach pain, heartburn, and peptic ulcers, as well as muscle cramps.

Since the etiology of pain in metastatic pathologic fractures is prostaglandin release, non-steroidal anti-inflammatory drugs (NSAIDs) may be helpful. Analgesics such as acetaminophen, aspirin, tramadol, and other opioid analgesics may be useful, and for intractable pain hospitalization may be required to establish an appropriate oral regimen based on parenteral requirements for pain control.

Estrogen in women and testosterone in men help to maintain bone mineral density, which declines with age due to loss of sex hormones; women may lose up to 20–30% of their bone mass in the first decade following menopause. Hormonal preparations such as estrogen and calcitonin are useful for maintaining bone mineral density. Selective estrogen receptor modulators (SERMs) mimic some, but not all, of the actions of estrogen with the goal of providing the bone-stabilizing effects of estrogen without some of its negative consequences. The recently approved RANK ligand inhibitor denosumab is a monoclonal antibody for treatment of osteoporosis in women only.

Non-pharmacologic approaches

Treatment of spinal compression fractures includes minimal bed rest, guided exercise, and fall prevention. In patients with only mild to moderate pain, bracing and supportive care may be all that is required. Physical therapy is essential for maintaining proper posture and ambulatory function.

Interventional procedures

In patients with neurologic compromise or in those with persistent severe pain, surgical intervention may be indicated. Kyphoplasty is a percutaneous procedure in which a balloon is inserted into the vertebral body, inflated to restore the original height of the compressed bone, and then filled with bone cement.

Although kyphoplasty is still considered somewhat controversial for osteoporotic compression fractures, the American Academy of Orthopedic Surgeons recently made a strong recommendation against the use of vertebroplasty for treatment of vertebral compression fractures, since studies have shown it to be no more effective than placebo. An adverse effect of vertebroplasty is leakage of cement into the spinal foramen or proximal to facet joints and nerve roots, which can result in neurologic compromise and/or pain.

Injection of anesthetic agents in the posterior segments (facet joints, pedicles) of vertebrae has been shown to eliminate pain as well, suggesting that these structures may be pain generators in compression fractures.

Follow-up

Compression fractures occurring from frank trauma, primary bone disease, or metastasis will require ongoing follow-up with orthopedic, endocrine, or oncologic specialists as indicated. Osteoporotic compression fractures may be best managed by primary care providers utilizing a multidisciplinary approach that includes physical therapy, nutrition, and psychological support as needed.

Prognosis

The prognosis for patients with traumatic or metastatic compression fractures depends on the extent to which the pain is controlled and return to function is achieved. For patients with osteoporotic compression fractures, it is vital that preventive measures be instituted to correct the anatomic deformity and return the individual to function, as well as to prevent future compression fractures.

REFERENCES AND FURTHER READING

Esses SI, McGuire R, Jenkins J, *et al.* The treatment of symptomatic osteoporotic spinal compression fractures. *J Am Acad Orthop Surg* 2011; **19**: 176–82.

Mukherjee S, Lee YP. Current concepts in the management of vertebral compression fractures. *Oper Tech Orthop* 2011; **21**: 251–60.

35

Lumbosacral radicular pain and lumbar radiculopathy

With contributions from Jeffrey Loh

Clinical presentation

Lumbosacral radicular pain and radiculopathy are two pain disorders commonly encountered within the field of pain management. Their combined annual prevalence varies between 9.9% and 25% in the general population, with a point prevalence of 4.6–13.4% and a lifetime prevalence of 1.2–43.0%. Based on these numbers, lumbosacral radicular pain and radiculopathy clearly represent one of the most commonly occurring forms of neuropathic pain.

While these two disorders share many similar attributes, their diagnoses are based on clearly differentiated neurologic criteria. Lumbosacral radicular pain is characterized by a radiating pain in one or more of the lumbar or sacral dermatomes, while lumbar radiculopathy is characterized by a motor or sensory abnormality on neurologic examination, in addition to radicular pain. Although the two diagnoses consist of different definitions, the clinical presentation for these two disorders often appears similar.

Signs and symptoms

The typical presentation of a patient complaining of radicular pain or radiculopathy consists of a pain that may affect an extremity, with involvement of the feet or toes. Pain commonly ranges from sharp and shooting in nature, to dull, piercing, throbbing, or burning. The common levels involved in a lumbar radiculopathy are typically related to disc herniations involving the L4 and L5 levels. Depending on whether the radicular pain or radiculopathy is due to a disc herniation, patients may state that their pain is increased with forward bending. On physical examination, patients with radicular pain will typically demonstrate normal motor strength and intact sensation. However, patients with a radiculopathy will commonly demonstrate decreased strength in the extremity with the radiculopathy, compared to the non-affected extremity. Sensory changes are also evident in a radiculopathy, with patients often noting decreased sensation to touch and temperature following a dermatomal distribution, and not a peripheral nerve distribution. Deep tendon reflexes at the patella and Achilles tendons may also show hyper- or hyporeactivity. Patients suffering from radicular pain or radiculopathy will often demonstrate a positive straight leg raising (SLR) test at less than 60 degrees elevation, but absence of this sign does not exclude a diagnosis of radicular pain or radiculopathy.

Laboratory tests and diagnostic investigations

To better assess the multiple different etiologies associated with radicular pain and radiculopathy, electrodiagnostic tests consisting of electromyography (EMG) and nerve conduction studies (NCS) have proven to be useful adjuncts. These studies should be obtained if there is difficulty in determining whether a patient's radicular pain or radiculopathy originates from within the spine or from a peripheral nerve distribution.

While the sensitivity and specificity for these tests are suboptimal, a meta-analysis of electrodiagnostic studies indicates the utility of these diagnostic tests for aiding in the evaluation of lumbar radiculopathy. Current evidence indicates that peripheral limb EMG, paraspinal EMG for lumbar radiculopathy, and H-reflex testing all provide a beneficial utility in determining the diagnosis of lumbar radiculopathy. In electrodiagnostic studies evaluating somatosensory evoked potential of the L5 or S1 dermatomes, paraspinal EMG of sacral radiculopathy, or motor evoked potentials, evidence is inadequate to reach a definitive conclusion on the utility of these studies for aiding in the diagnosis of radiculopathy.

Imaging studies

Besides electrodiagnostic studies, imaging studies often play a significant role in the work-up of a radicular pain or radiculopathy. In acute-onset lumbosacral radicular pain, radiographic imaging provides minimal benefit, as 60–80% of patients have improvement of their pain within 6–12 weeks. In those patients that continue to have radicular pain or radiculopathy after 12 weeks' duration, imaging studies have proven useful. X-rays prove beneficial as an initial diagnostic study, as they allow for evaluation of fractures, facet hypertrophy, or degenerative disc disease as potential causes for a patient's radicular pain and radiculopathy. In cases where patients demonstrate a spondylolisthesis, x-rays of the lumbar spine with flexion and extension views help to evaluate for underlying spinal instability, which could be causing nerve root compression and associated radicular pain and radiculopathy. If a patient's radicular pain is thought to be due to a bony etiology, CT scans prove useful as an adjunctive imaging modality to x-rays, as CT scans provide enhanced evaluation of the spine. Common conditions associated with radicular pain or radiculopathy that benefit from CT-based evaluation include facet arthropathy, pars fractures, and sacroiliitis.

MRI studies also aid in evaluating the underlying cause of a patient's lumbo-sacral radicular pain, as this imaging modality helps to assess the correlation with findings ascertained on physical examination. MRI allows for better evaluation of a patient's soft tissue structures, helping to determine whether the cause of a patient's pain is from a herniated disc, annular tears, central spinal stenosis, or foraminal narrowing. While MRI findings may indicate the cause of a patient's radicular pain, the clinician should not rely solely on an MRI for guidance. The specificity for an MRI to determine the underlying cause of radicular pain is low, given that 20–36% of asymptomatic patients demonstrate a disc herniation on MRI. The correlation between the severity of radicular pain and the magnitude of disc herniation is also unpredictable, and in many cases patients with radiculo-pathy may not demonstrate any observable findings on MRI.

Differential diagnosis

While physical examination is helpful in the initial diagnosis of radicular pain and radiculopathy, many different clinical states can mimic the presentation. Because pain radiating down an affected extremity can occur from varying points, from the level of the spine to the peripheral nerves innervating the affected extremity, the clinician should be aware of the multiple different causes that may mimic radicular pain and radiculopathy. Spinal stenosis is often associated with radicular pain and radiculopathy, with patients complaining of low back pain that worsens when standing upright, and pain that improves when sitting or bending forward. Patients with spinal stenosis will often complain of increased weakness in their lower extremities following prolonged periods of standing upright, due to the increased pressure placed on the spinal cord, with the pain and weakness typically resolving quickly when at rest.

Facet arthropathy, sacroiliitis, and piriformis syndrome are common disorders associated with low back pain, and can mimic the symptoms of radicular pain and radiculopathy, although the radiating pain associated with these disorders does not typically radiate to the foot of the affected extremity. The typical exam finding that correlates with facet arthropathy is pain that localizes to the para-median regions of the lumbar spine, with this pain becoming worsened by posterior extension of the lumbar spine when combined with lateral rotation. In contrast, sacroiliac pain localizes specifically over the sacroiliac joint itself, and is typically worsened by direct pressure to the sacroiliac joint, either through palpation or through loading of the joint using maneuvers such as the Patrick's, Gaenslen's, or Yeoman's tests. Piriformis pain commonly localizes to the mid-lateral aspect of the gluteal region, and is reproducible with direct palpation of the piriformis muscle or with stretching of the piriformis muscle by flexing and internally rotating the ipsilateral hip.

Metabolic disorders that can affect peripheral nerve function, such as diabetes complicated by peripheral neuropathy, should also be considered as part of the differential for radiating leg pain. Although post-herpetic neuralgia does not typically affect the lumbosacral region, this condition often mimics radicular pain, given the dermatomal distribution on presentation of this disease. Conditions such as ankylosing spondylitis and arachnoiditis are less common causes of radiating pain that also need to be excluded in the diagnosis of radicular pain.

Pharmacotherapy

Studies of non-steroidal anti-inflammatory drugs (NSAIDs) and cyclooxygenase-2 (COX-2) inhibitors have shown them to be efficacious in improving lumbar radicular pain. In situations where a patient's radicular pain or radiculopathy is unresponsive to these medications, the use of an oral steroid regimen or methylprednisolone (Medrol) dose pack can be considered, but only after careful consideration of a patient's medical situation.

The use of tricyclic antidepressants (TCAs) such as amitriptyline and nortriptyline has been found to be beneficial for the treatment of chronic pain and neuropathic pain. TCAs have been studied predominantly in diabetic neuropathy and post-herpetic neuralgia, however, and there is less evidence-based research on their use in lumbar radicular pain and radiculopathy.

Anticonvulsant agents such as gabapentin and pregabalin are an additional class of medications useful in the treatment of radicular pain and radiculopathy. Though post-herpetic neuralgia is the current Food and Drug Administration (FDA) indication for gabapentin and pregabalin, with pregabalin having an additional indication for diabetic neuropathy, extensive literature published on off-label use of gabapentin has shown benefit in radicular pain and radiculopathy. While many clinical studies support the use of gabapentin for the treatment of chronic radicular pain, these studies also note that gabapentin's efficacy is often hindered by side effects and difficulty with dosage optimization.

Opioids are prescribed in acute and chronic pain management, but the use of opioids for radicular pain and radiculopathy has not been supported by evidence-based studies.

Non-pharmacologic approaches

A randomized study of physical therapy and conservative treatments compared to conservative treatments alone showed a statistically significant improvement in perceived benefit in those patients who received physical therapy in conjunction with conservative care. However, the cost-effectiveness in patients receiving physical therapy and conservative management was the same as in patients randomized to receive conservative management only.

Physical therapy provides many modalities with which to improve a patient's radicular pain, with many exercises focused on stabilizing the spine by strengthening the core abdominal and back muscles. Transcutaneous electrical nerve stimulation (TENS), massage, postural alignment, and myofascial treatments are additional modalities.

Interventional procedures

In situations where lumbar radicular pain and radiculopathy persist after 12 weeks of conservative management, guidelines and studies indicate the use of interventional treatments for the management of a patient's pain. Multiple studies have shown that intervertebral discs are composed of inflammatory mediators. Herniation of the intervertebral disc allows these inflammatory mediators to contact the spinal column and cause nerve irritation. Epidural steroid injections allow the anti-inflammatory effects of corticosteroids to be deposited near the inflamed nerve root.

Three different approaches for the administration of epidural corticosteroids are often utilized under fluoroscopic guidance: interlaminar, transforaminal, and caudal. To perform an interlaminar injection, the interlaminar space between two vertebrae is identified. A needle is then advanced in the midline of a patient's back through this space, until the epidural space is entered. The evidence for the use of interlaminar injections for short-term relief is strong, but studies on long-term relief are lacking. Studies also show that the number needed to treat (NNT) for 50% pain reduction for short-term (1 day to 3 months) and long-term pain relief (3 months to 1 year) are relatively small. The decision to utilize an interlaminar approach is usually based on a patient's MRI showing multiple levels of disc bulges/herniations at the upper levels of the lumbar spine, or on the patient having extensive degenerative disease that precludes a transforaminal approach.

In contrast to interlaminar injections, transforaminal injections are utilized when patients show localized levels of disease on MRI or physical exam. To appropriately perform a transforaminal injection, the entrance of the neural foramen at the inferior aspect of the transverse process is visualized from an oblique view. A needle is then placed ventral to the exiting nerve root at the neural foramen. Recent meta-analyses indicate strong support for short-term relief and moderate strength for long-term improvement with the use of transforaminal epidural steroid injections.

Caudal epidural steroid injections have also been shown to have a strong level of evidence for short-term relief of radicular pain and radiculopathy, and evidence of moderate strength for long-term relief of pain. The use of this injection is typically considered in patients with extensive degenerative disease, resulting from disc herniations/bulges, spinal stenosis, or prior lumbar laminectomy, as caudal epidural steroids injection provide diffuse coverage in the lumbar spine. Under fluoroscopy, the entrance of the sacral hiatus is visualized from a lateral aspect, with a needle advanced through the sacral hiatus until the epidural space is entered. A catheter is then guided as close as possible to the targeted level for administration of medications. Studies have shown that up to 71–80% of patients report a benefit with caudal epidural administration of steroids, and that caudal epidural steroid injections have the potential to provide significant healthcare cost savings.

In situations where conservative treatments and interventional procedures fail to provide significant benefit for lumbar radicular pain or radiculopathy, surgical options provide an additional treatment modality. For lumbar radiculopathy due to a herniated disc, a microdiscectomy to remove the herniation often proves beneficial. In patients where foraminal stenosis impinges an exiting nerve root, a foraminotomy to decompress the nerve root can be beneficial. For patients where spinal canal stenosis is the underlying cause of a radiculopathy, a decompressive surgery may be indicated. Studies overall indicate positive short-term benefits with surgical treatments, although the long-term benefit of these surgeries remains to be established.

Follow-up

To assess the efficacy of a patient's treatment, the patient should typically be evaluated on a monthly basis during the initial management phase. Monthly visits allow for review of a patient's diagnostic studies and evaluation of the efficacy of a treatment modality in regards to pain modulation. Follow-up visits also allow for assessment of a patient's functional capacity in both the work environment and activities of daily living. However, once a patient's lumbar radicular pain or radiculopathy has become stabilized, that patient can be followed every 3 months or on an as-needed basis.

Prognosis

If the condition is managed appropriately, the prognosis for patients with lumbar radicular pain and radiculopathy can be promising. In the acute phase, most patients typically show a resolution of symptoms with conservative management. For those patients experiencing an acute flare of pain beyond their pain of a chronic duration, the numerous conservative and interventional treatments available may improve both symptoms and functionality, especially when utilized in a multidisciplinary approach.

REFERENCES AND FURTHER READING

Abdi S, Datta S, Trescot AM, *et al.* Epidural steroids in the management of chronic spinal pain: a systematic review. *Pain Physician* 2007; **10**: 185–212.

Carragee E, Alamin T, Cheng I, *et al.* Are first-time episodes of serious LBP associated with new MRI findings? *Spine J* 2006; **6**: 624–35.

Cho SC, Ferrante MA, Levin KH, Harmon RL, So YT. Utility of electrodiagnostic testing in evaluating patients with lumbosacral radiculopathy: an evidence-based review. *Muscle Nerve* 2010; **42**: 276–82.

Chou R, Baisden J, Carragee EJ, *et al.* Surgery for low back pain: a review of the evidence for an American Pain Society clinical practice guideline. *Spine (Phila Pa 1976)* 2009; **34**: 1094–109.

Luijsterburg PA, Lamers LM, Verhagen AP, *et al.* Cost-effectiveness of physical therapy and general practitioner care for sciatica. *Spine (Phila Pa 1976).* 2007; **32**: 1942–8.

Van Boxem K, Cheng J, Patijn J, *et al.* Evidence-based interventional pain medicine according to clinical diagnoses, 11. Lumbosacral radicular pain. *Pain Pract* 2010; **10**: 339–58.

36

Sciatica and piriformis syndrome

Clinical presentation

Sciatica (sciatic neuralgia) is a radiculopathy characterized by pain and/or paresthesia that follows the path of the sciatic nerve as it exits the lumbar spine, traverses the buttocks and posterior thigh, and extends down the back of the leg into the foot. Spinal nerve roots that supply the sciatic nerve are the L4, L5, S1, and S2. The most common cause of sciatica is herniated disc. There are an estimated five cases per 1000 adults in Western countries.

Piriformis syndrome, also a peripheral sciatic neuritis, is a neuromuscular condition characterized by hip and buttock pain. The etiology of piriformis syndrome pain is due to trauma, inflammation, or injury of the piriformis muscle, or anatomic variations in the muscle as it relates to the sciatic nerve. The piriformis is a pear-shaped muscle that originates at the anterior surface of the sacrum and attaches to the superior medial aspect of the greater trochanter. Piriformis syndrome most commonly presents during the fourth or fifth decades of life, and it affects individuals of all occupations and levels of activity.

Sciatica frequently presents with incident pain while walking or driving a vehicle. The onset of the pain is usually sudden, due to an identifiable injury while bending, twisting, or lifting. Males and females are equally affected.

Piriformis syndrome tends to have a more insidious onset, for example due to prolonged sitting on a hard surface ("wallet neuritis"), but it may also present suddenly following physical injury. Females are more frequently affected, with a reported female-to-male ratio of 6 : 1. Pelvic biomechanics associated with the angle of the quadriceps femoris muscle ("Q angle") in females may predispose to piriformis syndrome.

Signs and symptoms

The symptoms of sciatica are those of an L4–S1 radiculopathy: pain and/or paresthesia in the distribution of the sciatic nerve. Evaluation of both sciatica and piriformis syndrome should begin with a focused history and physical to assess the onset and duration of the pain, precipitating, aggravating, and alleviating factors, and level of disability. Range of motion (ROM) testing may be useful in pinpointing the site of pain.

Signs of sciatica that might alert the clinician to a ruptured or herniated disc include weakness of plantar flexion, inability to push off, toe walk or heel walk with the affected foot, diminished or absent patellar and ankle reflexes, and decreased sensation to pinprick on the dorsum or sole of the affected foot. Palpation of the lumbar paraspinal muscles may reveal segmental tenderness in the region of L4–S1. Patients with sciatica due to herniated disc may exhibit apprehension to flexion and extension during ROM testing. The straight leg raising (SLR) and crossover SLR tests are useful for evaluating for disc herniation.

Typical symptoms of piriformis syndrome include pain that improves with ambulation and worsens with no movement or with sitting, standing, or lying for longer than 15–20 minutes; pain/paresthesia radiating from the sacrum through the gluteal area and down the posterior aspect of the leg, usually stopping above the knee; weakness and/or numbness in the ipsilateral lower leg and foot; dyspareunia in women; pain with bowel movements; and occasionally headache and neck pain.

Patients may exhibit a "piriformis sign." In the recumbent supine position, the leg on the affected side is actively externally rotated, and subsequent passive internal rotation of the leg precipitates pain. Palpatory examination reveals tenderness in the region of the sacroiliac joint, greater sciatic notch, and piriformis muscle. The contracted piriformis muscle, in the form of a sausage-shaped mass lateral to the sacrum on the affected side, may also be palpable.

Laboratory tests and diagnostic investigations

No laboratory studies are indicated in the evaluation of sciatica or piriformis syndrome.

Imaging studies

Patients with pain present for more than 6 weeks or with signs suggestive of a ruptured or herniated disc may be evaluated by CT or MRI. MRI may be helpful in elucidating the presence of muscle injury in piriformis syndrome, but this is rarely indicated. Both diagnoses can typically be made on clinical findings alone.

Differential diagnosis

Sciatica and piriformis syndrome must be distinguished from each other, since they share the same pain generator: the sciatic nerve. Each entity may also be confused with intervertebral discitis, lumbar radiculopathy, sacroilitis, primary sacral dysfunction, or trochanteric bursitis.

Pharmacotherapy

Non-steroidal anti-inflammatory drugs (NSAIDs) and acetaminophen, as in many conditions affecting the lower back, have been considered initial choices. Muscle relaxants are also frequently prescribed, and in the case of piriformis syndrome have shown efficacy as compared to placebo. Opioid analgesics may be useful on a short-term basis for patients obtaining inadequate relief from first-line medications. Topical analgesic patches may be tried, and local steroid injections may have an anti-inflammatory effect for some patients.

Non-pharmacologic treatment

As with mechanical or idiopathic back pain, bed rest for sciatica or piriformis syndrome is strongly discouraged. Treatment options include topical applications of heat or ice, gentle stretching, and progressive exercise. Multimodal therapies include psychological therapy, invasive/physical rehabilitation modalities (e.g., osteopathic manipulative medicine, chiropractic treatment, acupuncture), complementary medicine, or interventional therapy.

Interventional procedures

Piriformis muscle injection with local anesthetics under fluoroscopic or ultrasound guidance may be considered for diagnostic and therapeutic purposes. Botulinum toxin injection has been studied for pain management and functional restoration in piriformis syndrome.

Epidural steroid injections may be considered when sciatica is caused by a herniated disc. Please see Chapter 35 for further discussion of interventional procedures.

Prolotherapy (also known as sclerotherapy or ligament reconstructive therapy), which consists of injecting an irritating solution at the origin or insertion of ligaments to strengthen weakened or damaged connective tissue, has been utilized in the treatment of piriformis syndrome, but there is little published research to support its use.

Lumbar disc surgery is frequently performed in patients with severe, debilitating sciatica that does not resolve in 6 weeks. It has been observed in clinical trials that patients assigned to early surgery and those who received conservative treatment and eventual surgery, if needed, had similar 1-year outcomes.

Therefore, patient selection should focus on the goals for surgery, such as the need for faster recovery, or should be based on other quality-of-life measures.

Follow-up

Subsequent care for sciatica and piriformis syndrome includes assessment of pain, function, and quality-of-life measures. Patients should expect to remain active and to experience progressive improvement of symptoms with selected therapy.

Prognosis

The natural history of sciatica is favorable, with resolution of leg pain occurring within 6–8 weeks in the majority of patients.

REFERENCES AND FURTHER READING

Boyajian-O'Neill L, McClain R, Colerman MK, Thomas PP. Diagnosis and management of piriformis syndrome: an osteopathic approach. *J Am Osteopath Assoc* 2008; **108**: 657–64.

Cramp F, Bottrell O, Campbell H, *et al.* Non-surgical management of piriformis syndrome: a systematic review. *Phys Ther Rev* 2007; **12**: 66–72.

Peul WC, van Houwelingen HC, van den Hout WB, *et al.* Surgery versus prolonged conservative treatment for sciatica. *N Engl J Med* 2007; **356**: 2245–56.

37

Lumbar spinal stenosis

Clinical presentation

An increasingly common cause of radicular pain in the aging population, lumbar spinal stenosis causes leg pain and/or neurogenic claudication, defined as pain in the buttocks or legs with walking or standing that resolves with lumbar flexion or rest. Lumbar spinal stenosis is caused by narrowing of the vertebral canal, lateral recess, or intervertebral foramina due to degenerative changes of the lumbar spine such as hypertrophy of the ligamentum flavum, osteoarthritic facet joints, or herniated disc. A congenitally narrow spinal canal may contribute to the problem by limiting the ability to tolerate encroachment by these structures on the spinal cord and nerve roots.

Patients with lumbar spinal stenosis are typically older than 50; men are affected nearly twice as often as women. Patients may complain of heaviness in the buttocks and/or legs and difficulty with ambulation. The pain is aggravated by walking or standing and relieved by sitting or assuming a flexed (bending forward) posture. Less commonly, lower extremity weakness may be present. A classic presentation of lumbar spinal stenosis is the patient who finds that leaning forward, such as on a shopping cart, helps with the pain and ability to tolerate ambulation.

Signs and symptoms

The onset of lumbar spinal stenosis is usually insidious and progressive, reflecting the progressive nature of degenerative osteoarthritic changes in the spine. In addition to the slow development of pain over time, it is episodic or incident pain, as opposed to continuous pain, which occurs with activity (walking) and is exacerbated by certain positions, such as standing upright. The pain is relieved by rest, sitting or lying down, with side lying generally better tolerated than supine or prone. Lumbar spinal stenosis sufferers may assume a slight compensatory forward flexed position.

There are no specific physical tests for lumbar spinal stenosis. However, a thorough examination of the lower back and legs, including assessment of muscle mass, asymmetry, range of motion, reflexes, and focused neurologic testing for sensory and motor abnormalities, may be useful in delineating the level of nerve impingement.

Laboratory tests and diagnostic investigations

No laboratory studies are indicated in the evaluation of lumbar spinal stenosis unless there is suspicion of infection or malignancy. Signs of infection include fever or sudden onset of pain following trauma. Age over 60, unexplained weight loss, and symptoms of cauda equina syndrome (saddle anesthesia, bowel and/or bladder incontinence) should prompt investigation for occult malignancy. Electrodiagnostic testing can help in the evaluation of lumbar stenosis, as it can rule out a concomitant peripheral neuropathy that can mimic some of the complaints seen in lumbar stenosis. It may also help stratify patients according to their potential to respond to epidural steroids or possible surgical decompression.

Imaging studies

Radiographic studies may help to identify arthritic changes that are causative. However, it has been noted that a large percentage of persons over the age of 60 have evidence of spinal stenosis on imaging yet remain asymptomatic. MRI and/or CT myelography are the studies of choice for demonstrating areas of impingement on the spinal cord or nerve roots. Electrodiagnostic testing can localize the level of nerve root involvement, as the level of stenosis on imaging studies may not correlate with physical examination or electromyography (EMG) findings.

Differential diagnosis

Critical in establishing the diagnosis, the symptom of neurogenic pain due to walking must be differentiated from claudication from a vascular cause. Vascular claudication is typically expressed as cramping or sharp pain in the calf that extends proximally with walking; this pain is exacerbated by activity in any position and relieved by rest in any position. In contrast, neurogenic claudication is aggravated by backward bending (extension) or activity and relieved by forward bending (flexion) and rest. Patients with neurogenic claudication, unlike those with vascular claudication, are able to tolerate cycling without inducing pain, because of the forward-flexed position on the bike.

Degenerative disc disease that causes lumbar radiculopathy may be mistaken for lumbar spinal stenosis. A potential distinguishing feature of spinal stenosis is the insidious, progressive nature of the pain, in contrast to the usual presentation of degenerative disc disease, which can frequently be linked to an injury or trauma.

Pharmacotherapy

Non-steroidal anti-inflammatory drugs (NSAIDs) and acetaminophen, as in many conditions affecting the lower back, are initial analgesic choices. Topical analgesic patches or gels may also be useful.

Several other medications have been studied including calcitonin, gabapentin, limaprost, and methylcobalamin. A recent evidence-based review suggested that parenteral, but not intranasal, calcitonin gave transient (less than 3 months) analgesic benefits. Evidence for efficacy of the other medications is limited.

Non-pharmacologic approaches

Conservative care for lumbar spinal stenosis focuses on maintenance of function. Patient education is a mainstay of treatment. Physical therapy, core muscle strengthening exercises, and supplemental vitamins have also been utilized as potential treatment modalities. Bed rest is generally discouraged. Physical therapy recommendations, in order of decreasing importance, include flexibility, stabilization, and strengthening exercises, application of heat or ice, acupuncture, and joint mobilization.

Interventional procedures

Epidural steroid injections have been widely studied for their efficacy in spinal stenosis; patients may obtain short-term relief (1–3 months) post-injection. Epidural block and adhesiolysis (prolotherapy or sclerotherapy) have been tried as well as acupuncture for pain relief. The different approaches to epidural steroid injection are described in Chapter 35.

Lumbar spinal stenosis is the leading cause for spinal surgery in the population of older adults. Numerous studies support the usefulness of surgery for reduction of pain, but post-surgical functional improvement has been less impressive and relies heavily on rehabilitation and patient education. Careful patient selection has been shown to improve outcomes of both pain and functional measures.

Follow-up

Lumbar spinal stenosis is a chronic, debilitating condition that requires ongoing patient support and follow-up. Postoperative care may include physical therapy, patient education, self-directed exercise, and pain management; hence, care of patients with lumbar spinal stenosis is ideally multimodal.

Prognosis

Prognosis for lumbar spinal stenosis is generally favorable, especially in patients who tolerate exercise and interventional procedures.

REFERENCES AND FURTHER READING

Tomkins CC, Dimoff KH, Forman HS, *et al.* Physical therapy treatment options for lumbar spinal stenosis. *J Back Musculoskelet Rehabil* 2010; **23**: 31–7.
Tran de QH, Duong S, Finlayson RJ. Lumbar spinal stenosis: a brief review of the nonsurgical management. *Can J Anaesth* 2010; **57**: 694–703.
Weinstein JN, Tosteson TD, Lurie JD, *et al.* Surgical versus nonoperative treatment for lumbar spinal stenosis: four-year results of the Spine Patient Outcomes Research Trial. *Spine (Phila Pa 1976)* 2009; **35**: 1329–38.
Yuan PS, Albert TA. Managing degenerative lumbar spinal stenosis. *J Musculoskelet Med* 2009; **26**: 222–31.

38

Lumbar facet syndrome

Clinical presentation

Lumbar facet syndrome (LFS) is a non-inflammatory degenerative process of progressive joint stiffness and decreased range of motion that results in loss of mobility and pain. Estimates of the prevalence of low back pain due to LFS range from 10–20% in injured workers and 36% in the general population to more than 50% in the elderly.

Facet joints are zygapophyseal: synovial joints between the superior articular process (zygapophysis) of a vertebra and the inferior zygapophysis of the vertebra immediately above it. Facet joints are the only synovial joints in the spine, and their normal biomechanical functioning allows side bending, extension, and flexion, limits axial rotation, and serves to prevent the vertebral body from sliding forward in extreme flexion. They also assist in the distribution of vertebral load in the standing position. Anatomically, facet joints are similar to the sacroiliac joint and so are subject to degenerative or traumatic changes that can impact on neuronal structures (e.g., dorsal root ganglia) and adjacent musculature (erector spinae and multifidus muscles) which can become pain generators. The facet joint is innervated by nociceptive and autonomic neurons, with dual innervation from the medial branch of the dorsal ramus of its vertebral segment and the one immediately above (e.g., innervation to the L4 facet joint is from L4 and L3).

Not limited to articular cartilage, lumbar facet degenerative changes also occur in periarticular bone, synovial lining, and connective tissues. The etiology of these changes is multifactorial, a combination of genetic and biochemical factors, repetitive strain (such as recurrent rotational forces) with low-grade trauma, increasing age, joint instability or malalignment, muscle weakness, and peripheral neuropathy. Lumbar disc herniation or degeneration with subsequent alteration in biomechanics, as well as acute trauma, e.g., from a motor vehicle accident, has been linked to facet joint degeneration. LFS occurs most commonly at the L5–S1, L4–L5, and L3–L4 levels in decreasing order, reflecting the increased load borne by lower lumbar joint segments.

Signs and symptoms

LFS typically presents later in life or related to occupational or traumatic injury and is more common in males than in females. The association with intervertebral disc lesions is due to consequent increased axial loading of the lumbar facets. Patients complain of pain that radiates to the buttock, hip, or groin that is increased in the morning and after periods of inactivity. Stress, exercise, lumbar spine extension (back bending) and rotational movements, standing, and sitting are exacerbating factors, while flexion of the lumbar spine and lying down cause remission of pain.

There is no pathognomonic confirmatory physical test that is diagnostic of LFS. Patients with LFS complain of axial low back pain, sometimes with radiation into the groin or thigh. The pain is typically bilateral, differentiating it from sacroiliac joint pain, which is usually unilateral. Pain in the flank, hip, and lateral thigh may be associated with the upper facet joint, and posterior thigh pain is usually associated with the lower facet. Pain that extends below the knee is usually not due to lumbar facet pathology.

Pain elicited during pressure placed by the examiner on the paravertebral muscles may help to localize the source of pain to the facets.

Laboratory tests and diagnostic investigations

Laboratory testing is indicated for "red flag" conditions such as fever or unexplained weight loss to rule out infection, malignancy, or other autoimmune disease. Inflammatory conditions such as rheumatoid arthritis or ankylosis spondylitis can be evaluated with erythrocyte sedimentation rate (ESR) and rheumatoid profile. Electromyography (EMG) and nerve conduction studies (NCS) can be considered for diagnosis of LFS only to rule out lumbar radiculopathy, peripheral neuropathy, or other pathology.

Imaging studies

Pain suggestive of an urgent medical condition such as abdominal aortic aneurysm or spinal cord compression should prompt immediate evaluation with CT scan or MRI.

Radiographic findings of degenerative change at the lumbar facet joints are ubiquitous in older persons, and thus radiographic evidence of osteoarthrosis is a poor predictor of pain. Oblique views are required for visualization of the facets; standard posteroanterior and lateral films with flexion/extension views may show degenerative changes, spondylosis, or spondylolisthesis which are non-specific, for LFS.

The facet joint space itself is best visualized with CT scan or MRI. However, since there is no definite correlation between imaging findings and the severity of pain, the presence of facet arthropathy does not rule out the diagnosis of LFS.

Differential diagnosis

The differential diagnosis of LFS includes referred pain from kidneys/ureters (e.g., renal calculus), pelvic and gastrointestinal organs. An ominous condition that may mimic the pain of LFS is abdominal aortic aneurysm, suspicion of which should prompt immediate imaging studies.

Muscle strain/sprain (mechanical low back pain), discogenic pain, ligamentous injury, and stress fracture (pars interarticularis) may present with complaints similar to LFS. Inflammatory arthritides may also be confused with LFS.

Please refer to Chapter 33 for further discussion and differential diagnosis regarding LFS.

Pharmacotherapy

Medications that may be useful for the pain of LFS include non-steroidal anti-inflammatory drugs (NSAIDs), cyclooxygenase-2 (COX-2) inhibitors, and skeletal muscle relaxants. Topical analgesics may provide time-limited relief. Because of the chronic nature of LFS, opioid analgesia should be used only in carefully selected and consented patients and for the shortest duration possible to allow pain relief that is sufficient to maintain or restore physical function.

Non-pharmacologic approaches

As with most causes of back pain, emphasis should be placed on maintenance of range of motion, ambulation, and functional status. A multimodal approach utilizing weight loss (if appropriate), progressive exercise including stretching and aqua-therapy, cognitive behavioral therapy (CBT), and/or psychiatric modalities may be helpful.

Osteopathic or chiropractic manual medicine techniques are useful for reducing muscle tension, correcting somatic dysfunctions, and restoring range of motion. Physical therapy and rehabilitation modalities may further augment these interventions.

Interventional procedures

Since LFS pain cannot be diagnosed clinically or radiographically, image-controlled diagnostic medial nerve or intra-articular anesthetic blocks are useful. They may also be utilized for treatment of lumbar facet joint pain. Diagnostic blocks utilize a minimal volume of local anesthetic and are still associated with false positive rates. Therapeutic blocks use larger anesthetic volumes to flood the area around the suspected nerve. Both procedures require correct positioning of the needle, facilitated through the use of electrical stimulation, fluoroscopy, and ultrasound.

Temperature-controlled radiofrequency neuroablation (neurotomy or rhizotomy) is currently considered the gold standard for treatment of diagnostic-block-proven LFS (pain reduction of > 50%). Some investigators have reported good results lasting up to 12 months, although the scientific evidence remains controversial. Complications of this treatment include transient, localized burning pain and self-limiting back pain. Patients who fail to respond to neurotomy may be candidates for a one-time intra-articular anesthetic block.

There is currently no evidence to support surgical intervention for diagnostic-block-proven LFS.

Follow-up

The chronic degenerative changes may be progressive and require ongoing supportive and restorative care utilizing multiple modalities, as described above. The goal of therapy is to achieve analgesia adequate to allow for optimum physical functioning and mobility.

Prognosis

The prognosis for LFS is generally favorable if the emphasis is on maintenance of function and quality of life.

REFERENCES AND FURTHER READING

Beresford ZM, Kendall RW, Willick SE. Lumbar facet syndromes. *Curr Sports Med Rep* 2010; **9**: 50–6.

Cavanaugh JM, Lu Y, Chen C, Kallakuri S. Pain generation in lumbar and cervical facet joints. *J Bone Joint Surg Am* 2006; **88** (Suppl 2): 63–7.

Kalichman L, Dunter DJ. Lumbar facet joint osteoarthritis: a review. *Semin Arthritis Rheum* 2007; **37**: 69–80.

Van Kleef M, Vanelderen P, Cohen SP, *et al.* Evidence-based interventional pain medicine according to clinical diagnoses, 12. Pain originating from the lumbar facet joints. *Pain Pract* 2010; **10**: 459–69.

Varlotta GP, Lefkowitz TR, Schweitzer M, *et al.* The lumbar facet joint: a review of current knowledge. Part II: diagnosis and management. *Skeletal Radiol* 2011; **40**: 149–57.

39

Sacroiliac joint pain

Clinical presentation

Sacroiliac joint pain (SIJP) is a relatively common cause of low back pain that may be overlooked or misdiagnosed. Estimates of prevalence vary, but SIJP accounts for approximately 20% of cases of low back pain. The terms sacroiliitis and sacroiliac joint (SIJ) dysfunction are used to describe acute and chronic pain in the gluteal region, low back, or hip, with or without radiation into the upper lumbar area, groin, abdomen, and lower extremity. The International Association for the Study of Pain (IASP) defines SIJP as pain localized in the region of the SIJ, reproducible by stress and provocation tests, and reliably relieved by selective infiltration of the SIJ with a local anesthetic.

SIJ dysfunction occurs from malposition of the sacrum on the innominate bones due to mechanical forces of pelvic rotation, joint locking, and hypo- or hypermobility with or without attendant muscular imbalance. It typically results from direct or indirect trauma, postural or anatomical abnormalities. Sacroiliitis refers to an inflammatory condition caused by spondylitis. As opposed to using the terms *strain* or *sprain*, many clinicians refer to SIJ dysfunction as sacral *torsion* or *shear*.

The SIJs are mainly innervated by dorsal sacral rami, S1–S4. Encased by strong ligaments, the SIJs provide the interface between the sacrum and paired innominates (flared bones composed of the ilium, ischium, and os pubis). With the sacrum and coccyx, the innominates form the pelvic girdle. The SIJs thus act as shock absorbers, allowing torque and transverse rotations that take place in the lower extremity to be transmitted through the pelvis to the spine. Like most paired spinal joints, the SIJs operate in concert. As in the knee joint, the SIJ has a "self-locking" mechanism: the joint opposite the one undergoing motion achieves a tightly opposed state, called the *close-packed position*, that prohibits further motion and provides joint stability. During load transfer from one leg to the other and through the pelvis, the SIJ becomes close-packed on one side as the weight of the body is transmitted from the sacrum to the hip bone.

The SIJs are unusual in that they do not undergo typical range of motion through extension/flexion, abduction/adduction, but go through subtle rotation and flexion when subjected to the larger movements of the hip, pelvis, and legs. To describe the positional relationship of the sacrum the term *nutation* has been used; it represents the forward-nodding (flexion) motion of the sacral base (the widest, cephalad portion), while *counter-nutation* refers to posterior-nodding (extension) of the sacrum. Motion of the pelvic bones affecting the SIJ include: anterior innominate tilt of both innominate bones on the sacrum (where the left and right move as a unit); posterior innominate tilt of both innominate bones on the sacrum (where the left and right move together as a unit); anterior innominate tilt of one innominate bone while the opposite innominate bone tilts posteriorly on the sacrum (antagonistic innominate tilt), which occurs during gait; and sacral flexion (nutation) or sacral extension (counter-nutation).

Since the sacrum is the pyramidal base or "keystone" of the vertebral column, the SIJs are continually subject to mechanical stress: coupled with gliding pelvic motions, the weight of the spine exerts pressure on the SIJs. The SIJ can indirectly be put into a pattern of strain as a result of postural habits, muscular asymmetries, or trauma; such forces may result in SIJ dysfunction and cause inflammation, or sacroiliitis.

Several ligaments support the stability of the SIJ, including the anterior and posterior sacroiliac ligaments, interosseous, sacrotuberous, and sacrospinous ligaments. Muscles that attach to the sacrum or ilia include the gluteus medius and minimus, piriformis, iliacus, and rectus femoris. When these structures are stretched or injured, the SIJ may undergo excessive motion, causing inflammation and disruption of the joint and adjacent nerve endings. On the other hand, a too rigid SIJ may prevent normal nutation and rotation of the sacral base, also resulting in sacroiliac joint dysfunction.

Sacroiliac pain presents as dull, aching pain in the low back, hip, buttocks, thigh, or in the sciatic distribution, which may become sharp or shooting with certain movements. The pain is frequently localized to one side, but compensatory change at the other SIJ may cause pain over both joints. Patients complain of difficulty sitting in one place for too long or back/hip pain with rolling over in bed, stiffness in the hips and low back upon arising in the morning, and difficulty arising from a seated posture or getting out of bed.

Common causes of SIJP are degenerative disease, especially in older adults; history of a traumatic accident (e.g., fall onto the hip or buttocks) or repetitive trauma (e.g., heavy physical exertion); pregnancy and childbirth; or prior surgery such as lumbar fusion. Anatomical risk factors include leg length discrepancy with compensatory postural change, abnormal patterns of gait, or scoliosis.

Degenerative joint disease, particularly of the lumbosacral spine and hips, may cause alterations in posture and/or ambulatory patterns (e.g., favoring a painful hip joint) that result in shearing or torsional forces on the SIJ. Direct pelvic trauma (e.g., a head-on collision in which the leg on the affected side is locked in extension) may predispose one to SIJP; however, disruption of the SIJ due to repetitive day-to-day trauma should not be discounted as etiologic, since the simple act of sitting places stress on the joints and may cause recurrent micro-trauma resulting in SIJP.

Pregnancy/childbirth has been implicated in SIJP. The mechanics of childbirth require that the pelvic joints loosen to allow the neonate to pass through the pelvic outlet. This is accomplished through release of the hormone relaxin, which causes ligamentous relaxation. Postpartum levels of relaxin decrease, allowing the ligaments to return to their former tightness, yet female patients often identify the onset of chronic gluteal/low back pain with pregnancy or childbirth.

Lumbar fusion surgery results in non-mobile spinal segments and causes increased motion to segments above or below the fusion, which can alter pelvic mechanics and place stress on SIJs.

Signs and symptoms

Somatic dysfunctions that occur at the SIJ can be characterized as innominate rotations or sacral torsions/flexions. Manual medicine techniques (e.g., osteopathic palpatory exam) are useful in assessing and delineating the nature of the lesion at the SIJ. As noted, the diagnostic criteria for SIJP include pain in the region of the SIJ and positive results on provocative testing (maneuvers to reproduce pain in the SIJ), with relief of pain from anesthetic injection (under x-ray guidance) into the SIJ itself.

A focused range of motion and palpatory examination of the lumbar spine and SIJ help the clinician to differentiate between lumbar or spinal structures (e.g., herniated disc or facet disease) and the SIJ as the pain generator. For example, patients with SIJP should have negative straight leg raising (SLR) tests and may not complain of pain on extension or flexion. The affected SIJ sulcus may show tissue texture changes (edema, bogginess), asymmetry, and tenderness; direct palpation may reproduce the pain. Patients may be unable to sit on the affected side.

There are several provocative tests designed to reproduce a patient's pain at the SIJ, but no one test has predictive reliability. One meta-analysis suggests that the presence of three or more positive provocative tests has discriminative power for making the diagnosis of SIJP.

The Fortin finger test refers to the patient's ability to localize the pain with one finger placed over the region of the SIJ within 1 cm of the posterior superior iliac spine, consistent over two or more trials. Other provocative tests include the distraction and compression tests, Gaenslen's and Patrick's tests, thigh thrust (posterior shear) and Gillet tests. A brief descripton of each of these follows:
- The distraction (gapping) test is performed with the patient supine. The examiner's hands grasp each anterior iliac spine and apply pressure in a dorsolateral vector, attempting to "pull them apart" to elicit pain in the affected SIJ.

- The compression (approximation) test is performed with the patient lying on his/her side with the affected side up and hips flexed to 45 degrees; the examiner grasps the anterior iliac crest and exerts downward (medial) pressure, attempting to "force them together" with the objective of eliciting pain.
- Gaenslen's (pelvic torsion) test is performed with the patient lying supine or on the side with the affected leg dropped over the edge while the opposite leg, supported by the examiner, is flexed at both the hip and knee and passively flexed until the knee pushes against the abdomen. The examiner then exerts downward pressure to bring the leg on the affected side into hyperextension and light pressure is applied to the knee, eliciting pain at that SIJ.
- Patrick's test (or FABER, an acronym for the motions involved: flexion, abduction, external rotation) is also known as the "sign of four," since the affected leg is placed in a position that resembles the number 4. With the patient lying supine, the examiner bends the affected leg at the hip and knee, placing the lateral malleolus over the patella of the opposite side. Downward pressure on the thigh is then applied by the hand of the examiner, provoking pain in the sacroiliac joint. (Patrick's test also tests for hip joint disease by antagonizing hip flexor spasm brought on by an inflammatory lesion. A positive test is revealed when hip pain, especially in the area of the hip flexors, is elicited.)
- The thigh thrust test (posterior shear test) is performed with the patient supine and the unaffected leg extended. The examiner flexes the affected leg at the hip to an angle of 90 degrees with slight abduction while applying light pressure to the bent knee to elicit pain at the affected SIJ.
- The Gillet test is performed by having the patient stand on one leg and pull the other leg up to his or her chest, causing pain on the affected side.

Laboratory tests and diagnostic investigations

There is no specific laboratory test for SIJP, and such tests are generally considered unnecessary in the initial evaluation of non-specific back pain. However, as previously noted, specific laboratory testing is indicated to differentiate non-specific, musculoskeletal pain from pain from another source, especially in the case of patients with "red flags" suggesting an underlying serious problem (see Chapter 33).

Complete blood count with differential (CBC with diff), erythrocyte sedimentation rate (ESR), or C-reactive protein (CRP) should be obtained for patients in whom infection or cancer is suspected, and are useful in differentiating ankylosing spondylitis, reactive arthritis, or psoriatic arthritis from sacroiliitis.

Imaging studies

The diagnosis of SIJP rests on clinical evaluation alone, since there is no demonstrable radiographic abnormality; imaging is important only to rule out "red flags." Plain films of the lumbosacral spine and pelvis are frequently obtained, as are CT scans or MRIs. Results of the latter are frequently misleading, perhaps identifying lesions that are not the actual pain generator. In one study, CT scans were negative in 42% of patients with symptomatic SIJP. MRI has not been proven to have a positive correlation with sacroiliitis or SIJ dysfunction.

Differential diagnosis

Clinicians must differentiate SIJ dysfunction from SIJ pathology, since the latter includes infection, traumatic disruption such as fractures, metabolic bone disease, and spondyloarthropathies. SIJP may be confused with facetogenic or discogenic disease, lumbar nerve root compression, endometriosis, myofascial pain, or piriformis syndrome. Ankylosing spondylitis or other rheumatologic disease may also mimic sacroiliitis.

Since several levels of spinal nerve segments that exit the lumbar spine and sacrum cross over the SIJ and into the leg, SIJP may have associated referred leg pain. SIJP may be confused with other conditions that cause hip or buttock pain or pain radiating into the legs, such as sciatic pain. SIJP that mimics discogenic or radicular pain can potentially lead to misdiagnosis, resulting in unnecessary lumbar surgery; the provocative tests described above therefore are very useful.

As in all cases of low back pain, "red flags" such as unexplained weight loss or fever should be aggressively pursued. Also, like low back pain, many cases of SIJP will resolve in 6–8 weeks. Whether the pain at the SIJ is acute or chronic will influence both diagnostic testing and treatment decisions.

Pharmacotherapy

There is no definitive medication to cure SIJP. Non-steroidal anti-inflammatory drugs (NSAIDs) are helpful in the acute phase. Steroid injections directly into the SIJ not only have been used to confirm diagnosis but also may provide short- or long-term resolution of the pain. Topical anti-inflammatory patches or gels may be useful, either alone (especially for patients in whom oral NSAIDs are contra-indicated, such as elderly patients and those with known gastritis/ulcer or renal disease) or in addition to oral medications. Muscle relaxants have not been shown to be useful for SIJP.

Non-pharmacologic approaches

Treatment aimed at restoring anatomic function and normal range of motion is the cornerstone intervention for SIJP, and should be initiated as soon as possible, utilizing a multimodal, interdisciplinary approach. Beneficial osteopathic manipulation and/or chiropractic manual therapies include muscle energy, direct and indirect corrective techniques. These may be coupled with physical therapy or rehabilitative strategies directed at loosening/stretching muscles and ligaments in the case of SIJ hypomobility, or tightening/strengthening in the case of hypermobility. Other modalities include heat, ice, ultrasound, and focused exercise. Cognitive behavioral therapy (CBT) and/or psychiatric evaluation may be of benefit for some patients.

Aquatherapy that moves pelvic structures through gentle, repetitive range of motion may also assist in normalizing SIJ function and reducing pain. A pelvic supporter in the form of a belt wrapped tightly around the hips, designed to limit motion at the SIJ, may be helpful for selected patients.

Complementary and alternative medicine techniques that lack scientific evidence for efficacy may be helpful, including but not limited to prolotherapy, balneotherapy, massage, and acupuncture.

Interventional procedures

Articular injections with local anesthetic and long-acting corticosteroids are the most commonly used interventional procedure for SIJP. Studies suggest that both intra- and extra-articular injections may be beneficial.

Radiofrequency (RF) ablation is an interventional technique that employs a probe to cauterize small nerves that provide sensation to the SIJ, destroying potential pain generators. The technique is not always successful; nerve endings may regenerate over time, causing return of the pain. Since RF treatment is symptomatic and does not address the mechanical problem of SIJ mobility, it should be coupled with the non-pharmacologic strategies outlined above.

Complications of articular injections and RF procedures include infection, hematoma formation, neural damage, trauma to the sciatic nerve, and others. Dysesthesia or hypokinesia and temporary worsening of pain have also been reported. Patient selection and education are crucial for the success of these interventional procedures.

Follow-up

Because of the anatomical and mechanical/functional nature of SIJP, it may become a chronic condition that requires ongoing multimodal follow-up for corrective manipulative treatment, education, exercise prescription, interventional procedures, and judicious use of pain medication.

Prognosis

The prognosis for SIJP is favorable, especially for patients who are willing and able to make modifications in postural or lifestyle factors that may be predisposing to inflammation and somatic dysfunction.

REFERENCES AND FURTHER READING

Clavel AL. Sacroiliac joint dysfunction: from a simple pain in the butt to integrated care for complex low back pain. *Tech Reg Anesth Pain Manag* 2011; **15**: 40–50.

DePalma MJ, Ketchum JM, Saullo T. What is the source of chronic low back pain and does age play a role? *Pain Med* 2011; **12**: 224–33.

DonTigny RL. A detailed and critical biomechanical analysis of the sacroiliac joints and relevant kinesiology: the implications for lumbopelvic function and dysfunction. In Vleeming A, Mooney V, Stoeckart R, eds., *Movement, Stability and Lumbopelvic Pain: Integration of Research and Therapy*, 2nd edn. Philadelphia, PA: Elsevier; 2007; pp. 265–78.

Nicholas AS, Nicholas EA. *Atlas of Osteopathic Techniques*, 2nd edn. Philadelphia, PA: Lippincott Williams & Wilkins; 2012.

Vanelderen P, Szadek K, Cohen S, De Witte J, *et al.* Evidence-based interventional pain medicine according to clinical diagnoses, 13. Sacroiliac joint pain. *Pain Pract* 2010; **10**: 470–8.

40

Lumbar post-laminectomy syndrome

With contributions from Christine Lee and Talin Evazyan

Clinical presentation

Patients with lumbar post-laminectomy syndrome, also known as failed back surgery syndrome, present with persistent or recurrent low back and/or radicular pain after lumbosacral surgery. It is a common condition that affects patients who undergo lumbar spine surgery. Post-laminectomy syndrome can significantly impact a patient's quality of life and functional status. Patients may experience deterioration in physical and psychological health and productivity.

Post-laminectomy syndrome consists of a myriad of surgical and non-surgical etiologies. It includes a heterogeneous group of disorders that have common pain symptoms after lumbar surgery. The etiology of post-laminectomy syndrome can be divided into three groups: preoperative, intraoperative, and postoperative factors.

Preoperative factors include the patient's psychological condition, such as anxiety, depression, poor coping strategies, and hypochondriasis. All these tend to have poor outcomes. The patient's preoperative social situation can also lead to poor outcome, for example in the case of those involved in litigation and worker compensation. Another issue is poor preoperative surgical evaluation, including poor candidate selection (e.g., microdiscectomy for axial pain), type of surgery chosen (e.g., inadequate decompression in multilevel pathology), and revision surgery opted for when there is a higher risk of spinal instability with subsequent revisions.

Intraoperative factors that lead to post-laminectomy syndrome include technique, incorrect level of surgery, and inability to achieve the aim of surgery.

Postoperative factors include progression of the original disease process, epidural fibrosis, surgical complications (e.g., epidural hematoma, infection, nerve injury), and new spinal instability. Early identification and management of the acute complications from surgery is essential, as they can lead to rapid permanent neurologic deficits. Post-surgical pseudomeningocele is a rare complication from spinal surgery that can result from inadvertent meningeal tear or inadequate closure. Nerve root damage during surgery or prolonged injury to nerve root from compression from the original disease process can cause persistent radicular pain. During surgery, dissection and prolonged retraction of the paraspinal muscles can result in denervation and atrophy. Lumbar lordosis can be lost due to pedicle screw fixation, and paraspinal and hamstring muscles may develop spasm and atrophy.

Signs and symptoms

Though non-specific, symptoms may include pain localized to the spine and/or radiating to the extremities described as burning or shooting pain. Pain in the low back may be described as sharp or dull, and the location of pain may be reported as different than the level surgically treated. Accompanying the pain, patients may have neurological symptoms including numbness or tingling in the lower extremities as well as bladder, bowel, and sexual dysfunction. Psychiatric comorbidities such as depression, anxiety, and poor coping mechanisms may contribute to worsening the perception and interpretation of pain associated with post-laminectomy syndrome.

On physical examination there may be areas of tenderness and muscle spasm. One may find sensory dysfunction, changes in deep tendon reflexes, and motor weakness that may or may not follow a nerve distribution or dermatomal pattern.

Laboratory tests and diagnostic investigations

It is important that diagnostic evaluations be performed prior to further intervention. Routine laboratory studies can be ordered to rule out infection or an inflammatory process. Electrodiagnostic studies may be useful to detect the involvement of a particular nerve root when in the case of a radiculopathy or peripheral nerve disease.

Imaging studies

After a thorough history and physical and review of treatment administered, diagnostic imaging studies to further elucidate the etiology of disease include MRI, CT, as well as plain film x-rays. Plain x-rays can show loss of disc height as well as determine instability on extension and flexion views. CT and MRI may help determine the etiology of the pain by looking at the detailed structure of the spine, including evidence for annular disc bulge or herniation, retained disc, central canal stenosis, lateral recess stenosis, compression of nerve roots, or osteophytes. MRI is more helpful to determine soft tissue abnormalities. CT myelography can help in postoperative spine imaging, because on MRI there can be a distortion of images from surgical hardware.

Differential diagnosis

Common clinical conditions that may present similarly to post-laminectomy syndrome include myofascial pain syndrome, lumbar radiculopathy, spondylolisthesis, recurrent disc herniation, epidural hematoma, and arachnoiditis. Some patients who have had lumbar fusion may develop accelerated degeneration at adjacent structures from the level of fusion because of extra stress.

Arachnoiditis is commonly misdiagnosed. It is caused by inflammation of the arachnoid tissue in the central nervous system secondary to an adverse reaction to chemicals, infections, direct injury to the spine, chronic compression of the nerves, or complications from spinal surgery or other invasive spinal procedures. In patients with arachnoiditis, the complaint of pain will be out of proportion to clinical findings.

To differentiate between these differential diagnoses one must look at the overall clinical presentation, signs and symptoms, diagnostic tests, and imaging studies. In general, MRI findings may not correlate to the degree of pain the patient reports.

Pharmacotherapy

Pharmacotherapy in conjunction with other treatment modalities can be used to meet treatment goals of mitigating pain and improving quality of life. The choice of therapeutic agents depends on the type of pain. Often both neuropathic and nociceptive pain is present in post-laminectomy syndrome.

Over-the-counter oral agents that can be used for treatment of pain include non-steroidal anti-inflammatory drugs (NSAIDs) and acetaminophen. Prescribed oral agents can include antidepressants such as tricyclic antidepressants (TCAs), dual serotonin–norepinepherine reuptake inhibitors (SNRIs), anticonvulsants, and muscle relaxants. Topical agents such as lidocaine cream or patches can be used for adjuvant therapy.

The next line of therapy can include tramadol and tapentadol. Although opioids are commonly prescribed in moderate to severe acute pain, their efficacy in chronic pain management of post-laminectomy syndrome has not been supported by evidence-based studies.

Non-pharmacologic approaches

Paramount in the treatment of post-laminectomy syndrome is prevention. Often, this syndrome occurs when the outcome of lumbar spinal surgery does not meet the patient's and surgeon's expectation. Thus, it is important that the surgeon communicates with and educates the patient concerning the objectives and possible outcomes of surgery. Multidisciplinary management has been found to be important in many chronic pain conditions, and it can be useful in the management of post-laminectomy syndrome. Other therapies that may help manage pain include spinal manipulation, massage, psychotherapy, and family therapy.

Patients with post-laminectomy syndrome often are deconditioned, leading to weakness of the abdominal muscles that are responsible for maintaining a stable spine. Physical therapy can decrease pain, improve posture, stabilize the spine, improve fitness, and reduce mechanical stress on the spinal structures. Developing an exercise program that includes core muscle strengthening and stretching has also been shown to improve outcomes.

Psychological therapy, including cognitive behavioral therapy (CBT), has been shown to improve patients' ability to cope with chronic pain. The common components of CBT include teaching and maintenance of relaxation skills; behavioral activation such as goal setting and pacing strategies; interventions to change perception such as visual imagery, desensitization, or hypnosis; and promotion of self-management.

Interventional procedures

Many patients with post-laminectomy syndrome will not obtain sufficient analgesia and functional improvement with conservative management only, and will require more invasive interventions including injections, implantable therapies, and further surgery. Epidural steroid injections can help to control symptoms of pain related to epidural fibrosis, discogenic pain, recurrent disc herniation, and spinal stenosis. Though epidural injections are the most commonly performed non-surgical intervention for treatment of chronic low back pain, only a moderate percentage of patients show improvement in pain and functional status following the procedure.

Spinal cord stimulation is currently indicated for patients with post-laminectomy syndrome who have failed conservative management and have no obvious indication for surgical correction. This modality of pain control is based on neuromodulation, though the exact mechanism of action for spinal cord stimulation is yet to be discovered. The goal of therapy is to deliver electrical stimulation to the level of the spinal cord generating areas of pain and replace this sensation with paresthesias. Psychological assessment is of major importance for a successful outcome with this treatment modality.

The efficacy of intrathecal opioid administration has been studied in cancer-related pain. However, as patients with post-laminectomy syndrome are often refractory to treatment, intrathecal opioid administration may be considered as a therapeutic option. With both spinal cord stimulation and intrathecal opioid therapy, a trial prior to implantation is essential to demonstrate efficacy of the implantable treatment device.

In patients with post-laminectomy syndrome, surgery is indicated only when absolutely necessary, such as in cases of hardware complication, adjacent level disease, epidural abscess, epidural hematoma, and cauda equina syndrome. Surgical intervention should be carefully considered, as it important to keep in mind that it may lead to worsening of low back pain symptoms.

Follow-up

It is important for patients who suffer from post-laminectomy syndrome to have close and frequent follow-up with a primary treating physician to assess both functional status and pain. This should be performed on a regular basis, especially if patients are on medication for which adverse events need to be monitored. Should pain worsen or new neurological dysfunction develop, this may be an indication of worsening disease requiring further diagnostic studies.

To maintain functional status, regular exercise as well as physical therapy should be encouraged. If pharmacotherapy is being used as a treatment modality, drug–drug interactions need to be checked as well as compliance. One may consider referral to pain management consult if a patient does not improve with conservative therapy.

Prognosis

Post-laminectomy syndrome is a complex pain condition requiring a multidisciplinary approach to improve outcome. Failed back surgery syndrome is also a term used to describe this condition, but it is associated with a negative connotation which labels patients inappropriately. It is important to focus on those aspects of post-laminectomy syndrome that can be treated, in order to help improve the quality of life and functional status of patients suffering from this condition.

REFERENCES AND FURTHER READING

Chan C, Peng P. Failed back surgery syndrome. *Pain Med* 2011; **12**: 577–606.
Deyo RA, Nachemson A, Mirza SK. Spinal fusion surgery: the case for restraint. *N Engl J Med* 2004; **350**: 722–6.
Miller B, Gatchel RJ, Lou L, *et al.* Interdisciplinary treatment of failed back surgery syndrome (FBSS): a comparison of FBSS and non-FBSS patients. *Pain Pract* 2005; **5**: 190–202.

Slipman CW, Shin CH, Patel RK, *et al.* Etiologies of failed back surgery syndrome. *Pain Med* 2002; **3**: 200–14.

Turk DC, Wilson HD, Cahana A. Treatment of chronic non-cancer pain. *Lancet* 2011; **377**: 2226–35.

Van Buyten JP, Linderoth B. "The failed back surgery syndrome": definition and therapeutic algorithms. An update. *Eur J Pain Suppl* 2010; **4**: 273–86.

Hip and lower limb

41

Hip arthritis and bursitis pain

Clinical presentation

Hip region pain can result from multiple factors and may represent many possible etiologies. It can significantly impact on mobility and quality of life. Hip arthritis (degenerative joint disease, DJD) refers to degenerative joint changes noted at the femoroacetabular joint. It is typically associated with painful and limited internal rotation of the hip. This may be due to degenerative wear and tear changes over time, or it can be traumatically induced. Impaction-type injuries of the femoral head or neck with or without associated fracture can lead to damage of the articular cartilage or surrounding labrum.

Femoral neck fractures, particularly transcervical level fractures, or fractures associated with significant displacement of the femoral neck and head, can give rise to avascular necrosis (AVN). This in turn can lead to femoral head collapse and fairly rapidly progressive DJD of the hip joint.

Labral pathology can result in hip joint dysfunction, and associated pain in the groin region, but range of motion will typically be maintained.

Femoroacetabular impingement (FAI) occurs as a result of a bony "bump" at the anterolateral quadrant of the femoral head–neck junction. This "bump," while commonly associated with degenerative changes, is also seen in younger patients, and the association of FAI with DJD is therefore controversial. FAI results in impingement of the labrum, which is thought to lead to altered mechanics, which in turn results in degenerative changes.

Hip bursitis, more commonly called trochanteric bursitis, typically manifests with lateral thigh region pain.

Lumbar radiculopathy involving the L5 nerve root can atypically present with complaints of lateral thigh region pain. Since patients will note pain with weight bearing on the affected limb in all of the above scenarios, other specific complaints should be evaluated in order to differentiate the etiology of hip region pain. Other complaints therefore need to be elucidated in an attempt to develop a thoughtful differential diagnosis.

The clinical presentation of hip pain varies, but there are common features. Almost any derangement of the hip joint or trochanteric region will cause pain with weight bearing and associated gait compensation. All derangements of the hip will cause a compensated Trendelenburg gait, which refers to the shifting of the body's center of mass over the painful weight-bearing limb to functionally deactivate the gluteus medius and minimize joint compressive forces.

Signs and symptoms

Patients with DJD of the hip will note pain with weight bearing as well as start-up pain, which manifests as pain when transitioning from sit to stand. However, they will usually not complain of pain at rest. Entering or exiting a car may be painful if the problematic hip has to be placed into internal rotation while entering the cabin of the car. Trochanteric bursitis commonly manifests with pain along the lateral hip and peritrochanteric region. Patients will note significant pain on attempts at lying on the symptomatic side. Palpation of the region will be poorly tolerated.

FAI can manifest with pain on weight bearing. It may also cause complaints of pain during a particular arc of range of motion. FAI and labral pathology can thus mimic one another clinically, as both may present with a focal painful arc of motion, without restricted range.

Peritrochanteric region pain can be an atypical presentation for an L5 level radiculopathy. Pain in this situation is secondary to gluteus medius weakness and resultant chronic muscle strain.

Physical examination is critical to elucidate the etiology of hip pain. Observation of gait pattern to assess for a compensated Trendelenburg gait is critical. A compensated gait pattern with decreased stance time on the involved side is diagnostic of a painful hip syndrome, such as DJD, trochanteric bursitis, or labral pathology. FAI will not typically present with diminished stance time on the affected limb unless it has resulted in secondary labral pathology. A patient who has a compensated Trendelenburg without a shortened stance time may have issues of painless weakness. This can be seen in L5 radiculopathy, old poliomyelitis patients, or patients with underlying primary or secondary muscle disorders, which can include patients with myopathies, adult-onset muscular dystrophies, and statin-induced myopathies.

Range of motion (ROM) assessment is critical. In the seated position with the knee flexed to 90 degrees, the hip should be ranged through its full arc of both internal and external rotation. Pain with internal rotation, particularly if associated with decreased range of motion, is consistent with symptomatic DJD of the hip joint. Pain with internal rotation, but with symmetric and full range of motion, can be seen in early DJD, labral pathology, and sometimes FAI. Many times with labral issues as well as in FAI the painful arc is very discrete and focal.

Manual muscle testing of both lower extremities, including proximal as well as distal muscles, must be performed. Symmetric proximal weakness in the lower extremities that is also noted in the upper extremities should raise the suspicion of an underlying myopathic process. A very high index for suspicion should exist if the patient has a waddling type gait pattern, or bilateral Trendelenburg gait pattern. In the patient with an L5 level radiculopathy, weakness of the extensor hallucis longus (EHL) as well as the foot evertors and invertors may be noted. A positive straight leg raising (SLR) test may also be appreciated. In this case the SLR may reproduce the lateral thigh pain as opposed to classic radicular complaints.

Muscle stretch reflexes should be assessed in the lower extremities to evaluate for a possible radiculopathy. Though not commonly tested, the medial hamstring reflex allows for assessment of L5 level root function. It is performed by pressing the fingers of one hand against the medial hamstring tendon, just proximal to the knee, and then percussing the fingers with a reflex hammer much as in the manner of performing a biceps reflex. The patella reflex can assess L4 root function, and the Achilles reflex can be used to investigate S1 root function.

Palpation of the trochanteric region is critical in the assessment of trochanteric bursitis. Palpation should reproduce the pain if the patient truly has trochanteric bursitis. In contradistinction to iliotibial band syndrome, which can also cause trochanteric region pain, trochanteric bursitis causes focal pain at the level of the greater trochanter. An iliotibial band syndrome will cause more diffuse lateral thigh pain down to the level of the lateral knee.

Imaging studies

Evaluation of the hip must include plain film radiographs of the hip. A basic anteroposterior view of the pelvis will allow for side-to-side comparison of the hip joints.

MRI will be helpful in the patient with pain on internal rotation in the face of an unremarkable x-ray. In this scenario an MRI with contrast will be helpful to evaluate for a labral tear. MRI may also be useful in the evaluation of chondral defects which can cause focal discrete pain in a particular arc of range. In patients with findings suggestive of an atypical presentation for an L5 radiculopathy, plain films of the lumbar spine and possible MRI are appropriate.

Differential diagnosis

As one can see, a myriad of issues can cause hip joint and hip region pain. Common mimics for hip joint DJD include labral pathology and FAI. Both of these entities tend to be seen in younger patients and may result in pain with internal rotation of the hip, but range of motion will be maintained.

An L5 level radiculopathy can mimic trochanteric bursitis, but careful exam may reveal blunting of the medial hamstring reflex on the involved side.

Additionally, a positive SLR may be manifest along with weakness of the EHL and L5 innervated foot invertors (tibialis posterior).

Myopathies can mimic the gait deviation commonly associated with hip dysfunction. This class of disorders should be strongly considered in patients with bilateral Trendelenburg gait pattern, and in those with demonstrable proximal weakness in the upper and lower extremities. Statin-induced myopathies need to be considered in this group, as older patients frequently take cholesterol-lowering agents and also have an increased incidence of hip DJD.

Pharmacotherapy

Treatment is guided by the degree of disability and functional impairment. First-line treatment for hip DJD and peritrochanteric region pain should include a trial of non-steroidal anti-inflammatory drugs (NSAIDs) unless contraindicated.

Non-pharmacologic approaches

Application of ice to the trochanteric region several times a day may be very helpful for symptomatic relief of the pain from trochanteric bursitis. Physical therapy with the use of modalities such as ultrasound may be helpful for chronic trochanteric bursitis.

Use of a cane in the ipsilateral hand will effectively offload the painful hip during stance phase and can give good symptomatic relief in patients with hip DJD as well as trochanteric bursitis, labral tears, or FAI.

Interventional procedures

Patients who fail conservative intervention or are profoundly uncomfortable may benefit from more aggressive interventions. Trochanteric bursitis can be treated with corticosteroid injection. If the patient does not respond to the injection the diagnosis should be questioned.

Repeat injections are not recommended, as they are associated with an increased incidence of gluteus medius tendon rupture. Failure to respond to the injection should give strong consideration for an atypical presentation of an L5 level radiculopathy.

Intra-articular hip joint injection under ultrasound or fluoroscopic guidance has diagnostic and therapeutic utility. In patients with DJD or labral pathology a dramatically positive response to intra-articular corticosteroid injection is common and should be expected. Similarly, a positive response will be noted in FAI. Again, failure to see a significantly positive response, even a transient one, should call the diagnosis of intra-articular hip pathology into question.

Surgical intervention is appropriate for patients who are symptomatic and noting a decreased quality of life as a result of their severe hip DJD. Total hip arthroplasty has a long and well-documented track record of improving pain and quality of life in the appropriate patient population.

The treatment of hip pain and associated peritrochanteric region pain is both challenging and rewarding.

Follow-up

Follow-up is dependent upon the cause of the pain. In most cases, the follow-up will be on an as-needed basis. The exception is the patient who has undergone a total hip arthroplasty. He or she will require surgical follow-up to monitor the wear of the endoprosthesis.

Prognosis

Prognosis for hip arthritis is one of slow progression. In appropriate individuals total hip arthroplasty can dramatically improve pain, mobility, and quality of life. The prognosis for trochanteric bursitis is one of flares and remission.

REFERENCES AND FURTHER READING

Beck M, Kalhor M, Leunig M, Ganz R. Hip morphology influences the pattern of damage to the acetabular cartilage: femoroacetabular impingement as a cause of early osteoarthritis of the hip. *J Bone Joint Surg Br* 2005; **87**: 1012–18.

Fox KM, Hochberg M, Resnik C, *et al.* Severity of radiographic findings in hip osteoarthritis associated with total hip arthroplasty. *J Rheumatol* 1996; **23**: 693–7.

Ganz R, Parvizi J, Beck M, *et al.* Femoroacetabular impingement: a cause for osteoarthritis of the hip. *Clin Orthop Relat Res* 2003; **417**: 112–20.

Nilsdotter AK, Aurell Y, Siösteen AK, Lohmander LS, Roos HP. Radiographic stage of osteoarthritis or sex of the patient does not predict one year outcome after total hip arthroplasty. *Ann Rheum Dis* 2001; **60**: 228–32.

Tubach F, Ravaud P, Baron G, *et al.* Evaluation of clinically relevant changes in patient reported outcomes in knee and hip osteoarthritis: The minimal clinically important improvement. *Ann Rheum Dis* 2005; **64**: 29–33.

42

Meralgia paresthetica

Clinical presentation

Meralgia paresthetica (MP) is a sensory syndrome often associated with injury, usually in the form of compression or irritation, of the lateral femoral cutaneous nerve (LFCN). The reported incidence is estimated to be approximately 1–4 per 10 000 person-years; the condition affects men and women equally. The LFCN is formed from the fusion of the posterior divisions of the spinal roots emerging at the L2 and L3 levels. Often, the compression/irritation is due to entrapment of the nerve by the inguinal ligament as it courses along the anterior superior iliac spine (ASIS) on its way to the thigh. However, other causes for the symptoms, e.g., proximal to the ASIS, must be considered in the differential of the patient's presentation (see *Differential diagnosis*, below).

Signs and symptoms

Patients typically present with an initial onset of burning pain in the anterior and lateral aspect of the thigh. Patients may report that the skin over that area is exquisitely sensitive, with pain that can be aggravated by exercise, squatting, and wearing clothing that constricts the ASIS, e.g., work-belts, tight pants, corsets, or belts. It is likely to be alleviated by sitting. The patient may eventually, in the same distribution, experience numbness and dysesthesia (perceived unpleasant and frankly painful sensations) in response to normally non-painful stimulation such as the touch of one's clothing (allodynia). Factors predisposing one to MP include significant abdominal protuberance, e.g., resulting from pregnancy and obesity. As the LFCN does not have a motor nerve component to it, there is an absence of any muscle weakness in MP. The presence of motor weakness on neurological examination, or gastro-intestinal or urogenital symptoms, would be inconsistent with MP, suggesting other conditions in the differential diagnosis, e.g., an intra-abdominal process affecting the lumbar plexus, spinal lesions, a pelvic mass, or myofascial pain syndrome, among other possibilities.

Physical findings that corroborate the diagnosis of MP include Tinel's sign and lateral compression testing. Reproduction of the all-too-familiar unpleasant sensations and burning in the nerve's distribution by tapping over the LFCN at the level of the ASIS (Tinel's sign) would be supportive of the diagnosis. Additional sensory testing may reveal reduced pinprick sensation (hypoesthesia) along the anterior and lateral thigh. In the compression test, the patient lies in the lateral decubitus position on the asymptomatic side, while compressive forces are applied over the pelvis on the symptomatic side for approximately 45 seconds. This maneuver effectively reduces constriction of the LFCN by the inguinal ligament; a positive test is considered to be present if the patient reports an improvement in symptoms during the procedure.

Laboratory tests and diagnostic investigations

Although there are no laboratory tests for MP per se, several assessments may be warranted to establish that other conditions are not better accounting for symptoms. These can include complete blood count (CBC), erythrocyte sedimentation rate (ESR), antinuclear antibody (ANA) testing, and a thyroid profile. Although systemic conditions producing symptoms mimicking MP would likely have accompanying clinical signs to assist in diagnosis, such laboratory investigations can serve to unveil, or rule out, hypothyroidism, intra-abdominal infection, rheumatoid arthritis, or other worrisome clinical conditions.

Diagnostic uncertainties arising from the history and/or physical examination can be clarified utilizing electrodiagnostic investigations. Sensory nerve conduction studies (NCS) can confirm the diagnosis of LFCN impingement; however, somatosensory evoked potentials may be helpful in clarifying dysfunction arising from lesions proximal to the ASIS, e.g., lumbar radiculopathy or diabetic femoral neuropathy.

Ultimately, temporary relief produced by direct LFCN blockade with 0.25% bupivacaine can confirm a diagnosis of MP. Bear in mind that nerve blockade can be employed as a therapeutic intervention as well. Failure of peripheral nerve blockade at the level of the ASIS to alleviate symptoms suggests that the source of the pain may be proximal to the ASIS, e.g., intra-abdominal, at the lumbar plexus, or at the spine.

Imaging studies

Radiographs are necessary to eliminate the possibility that pathology of the back, pelvis, or hip is not accounting for the LFCN irritation. Abdominal and/or pelvic CT scanning may unveil an intra-abdominal process impinging on the lumbar plexus. MRI may be necessary to assess spinal pathology that may be accounting for the disturbances, e.g., spinal stenosis, intervertebral disc herniation, or mass/space-occupying lesions affecting the nerve roots exiting the intervertebral foramen. MRI of the abdomen/pelvis can clarify whether a mass/tumor is infiltrating the lumbar plexus.

Differential diagnosis

The diagnosis of MP is usually based on obtaining a supporting history and physical examination. However, the clinician must consider other conditions within the differential diagnosis that can potentially masquerade as MP. Among the possible etiologies, consideration must be given to injury of the LFCN produced by the ASIS; lipoma or other masses compressing the inguinal area; spinal lesions, e.g., spinal stenosis, mass/tumor, or intervertebral disc herniation at the L2–L3 level; postoperative irritation such as secondary to hip arthroplasty, cesarean section, or other pelvic surgeries, direct pelvic trauma, accidental or possibly postoperative (such as hip replacement or obstetric/gynecologic), impacting the lateral cutaneous nerve; lumbar radiculopathy; diabetic neuropathy; and myofascial pain syndromes affecting the sartorius muscle or the tensor fasciae latae, among others. The clinician ought to bear in mind that some of these conditions can coexist with MP: for example, it is possible that the symptoms of MP may coexist with lumbar radiculopathy.

Pharmacotherapy

Patients may be initially treated with non-steroidal anti-inflammatory drugs (NSAIDs), acetaminophen, or cyclooxygenase-2 (COX-2) inhibitors. These agents may be sufficient to mitigate physical discomfort. As MP can be associated with neuropathic pain, consideration may be given to treatment with those antidepressants typically used to treat neuropathic pain (tricyclics and certain serotonin–norepinephrine reuptake inhibitors) and/or alpha-2-delta ligands, e.g., gabapentin or pregabalin. Caution would naturally be required with the use of any of these agents, and in some cases may be prohibitive, e.g., during pregnancy. Inadequate responses to these agents may necessitate low-dose opioid analgesics, but the benefits need to be balanced against potential risks/adverse effects. Topical lidocaine may be helpful to mitigate MP-related neuropathic pain; topical capsaicin may relieve itch and skin hypersensitivity in the distribution of the anterolateral thigh. Failure to respond to these agents, along with concurrent non-pharmacologic approaches (delineated below), may necessitate interventional approaches.

Non-pharmacologic approaches

Non-pharmacologic approaches will include weight-loss programs. These should address nutritional consultation (diet) and participation in an exercise regimen. Patients should be apprised of measures to reduce risks of incurring pain during such exercise, and should wear loose-fitting clothing to reduce dysesthesias during exercise. Be mindful that a report by the patient of a recent weight gain might prompt not only inquiry into recent oral intake patterns, but also an assessment of recently initiated medications with the potential for weight gain. Examples would include atypical antipsychotics and antidepressants, which if modified in dose or replaced with alternatives might result in weight reduction, thereby mitigating symptoms of MP.

Interventional procedures

When pharmacologic modalities produce unsatisfactory relief, treatment may proceed to non-operative interventions including nerve blockade (anatomic or ultrasound-guided) employing local anesthetics (either 1% lidocaine or 0.25% bupivacaine) and/or 40 mg methylprednisolone. Recently, ultrasound pulsed radiofrequency neuromodulation of the LFCN has been employed to treat MP; however, further empirical investigation is warranted to assess its utility and efficacy.

Surgical intervention is reserved for patients who fail to respond favorably to conservative treatment measures. Available surgical approaches include neurolysis of the constricting tissue along with transposition of the LFCN or direct transaction along with resection of the nerve. The former approach offers the advantage of preserving sensory functioning of the nerve over the anterolateral thigh.

Follow-up

Patients will need follow-up and encouragement to reinforce efforts directed at weight-loss measures, particularly if obesity is a predisposing factor. Monitoring of the efficacy of, and potential adverse side effects associated with, medication use are warranted, e.g., hypertension and gastric irritation from NSAID use. Reassessment will be necessary to assess the efficacy of treatment approaches and to determine whether more aggressive interventional approaches warrant consideration.

Prognosis

Generally, MP responds favorably to treatment. A majority of patients can achieve sustained relief with non-operative measures. Patients may require repeated nerve blockade when relief is transient.

REFERENCES AND FURTHER READING

Haim A, Pritsch T, Ben-Galim P, Dekel S. Meralgia paresthetica: a retrospective analysis of 79 patients evaluated and treated according to a standard algorithm. *Acta Orthop* 2006; **77**: 482–6.

Harney D, Patijn J. Meralgia paresthetica: diagnosis and management strategies. *Pain Med* 2007; **8**: 669–77.

Reza Nouraei SA, Anand B, Spink G, O'Neill KS. A novel approach to the diagnosis and management of meralgia paresthetica. *Neurosurgery* 2007; **60**: 696–700.

Van Slobbe AM, Bohnen AM, Bernsen RMD, *et al.* Incidence rates and determinants in meralgia paresthetica in general practice. *J Neurol* 2004; **251**: 294–7.

43

Knee arthritis and bursitis pain

Clinical presentation

Knee pain is a common complaint. It can lead to mobility and activities of daily living (ADL) deficits. Patients may complain of pain with activity, a sense of joint instability, or impaired tolerance for stair climbing, kneeling, or squatting activities.

The incidence of knee arthritis increases with aging, either as a result of cumulative "wear and tear" or secondary to antecedent trauma. Arthritis of the knee can involve the true hinge joint of the knee, the femorotibial articulation, or the patellofemoral joint. The femorotibial joint is composed of a medial and lateral joint space. The medial joint space is more commonly involved in degenerative joint disease (DJD) of the knee. The mechanics and weight bearing through the medial joint and the medial meniscus cartilage predispose the medial joint space to preferential involvement.

Prepatellar bursitis commonly results from prolonged kneeling activities. Low-grade repetitive trauma is also a common cause for prepatellar bursitis. Swelling of the prepatellar bursa will result in rather impressive distension of the prepatellar region. Despite the swelling, significant pain is an uncommon complaint. Evaluation of a patient with prepatellar bursitis must always include consideration of an infected bursa, especially if the patient complains of pain.

Anatomically, the pes anserine bursa serves as a mechanical buffer between the bony medial tibial flare and the attachment of the semitendinosus, sartorius, and gracilis muscles. Pes anserine bursitis will present with pain along the medial tibial flare, below the true knee joint. It typically results from direct blunt trauma to the area. A Baker's cyst may also develop in the osteoarthritic knee. It is a collection of fluid located in the popliteal fossa at the origin of the gastrocnemius muscle. It is a non-specific finding, but its presence has been correlated to internal derangements of the knee. Most commonly it is seen in DJD and meniscal cartilage tears.

Signs and symptoms

Patients with knee arthritis will have several common complaints. Pain with weight bearing is a frequent complaint. Additionally, patients will complain of pain when transitioning from sit to stand. Not infrequently they will also note a sensation of knee instability or buckling. If present, swelling is usually mild, unless there is an underlying inflammatory process such as rheumatoid arthritis, infection, or superimposed acute trauma. Structural deformity of the knee may also be seen in long-standing knee DJD. As the medial joint space is typically preferentially involved in DJD, medial joint collapse with varus knee deformity is common.

Rheumatoid arthritis typically involves synovial and ligamentous structures early on, and results in ligamentous laxity. This in turn leads to accentuation of the normal anatomic structural valgus at the knee. Therefore observation of a valgus knee deformity should raise the question of possible underlying rheumatoid arthritis. As the deformity progresses, range of motion will be lost. Patients will lose end-range terminal extension, which will contribute to the sensation of knee instability or weakness. A loss of flexion will impair the patient's ability to come from sit to stand, and patients may note that they avoid soft chairs or chairs without armrests. Crepitus on range of motion is a common feature. Patients will describe the crepitus as clicking, grinding, or popping. They may also describe it as a sensation of sand in the joint.

Prepatellar bursitis will commonly present with marked swelling of the prepatellar bursa. Significant pain is not a common feature, and when noted should raise the question of an infected bursa. In the case of infection the overlying skin may well be red and warm to the touch. Patients with recurrent episodes of prepatellar bursitis may also demonstrate thickened callused skin over the patella.

Pes anserine bursitis is less common than prepatellar bursitis, and typically results from direct trauma to the bursa. Pain is a common feature in this scenario, despite the lack of significant swelling. In the case of pes anserine bursitis pain is a major complaint, whereas in prepatellar bursitis swelling is the dominant complaint.

Physical examination of the knee starts with visual inspection. Inspection should include observation of overall alignment of the knee as well as any obvious swelling. Observation of gait is also critical to assess for dynamic instability, which is commonly seen in DJD of the knee with progressive varus and, less commonly, valgus deformity. Analysis of stance time on the involved limb will give information regarding pain with standing. A symmetric stance time argues against pain even in the face of deformity. Shortened stance time on the involved limb is consistent with pain or instability of the limb, increasing the significance of any structural deformity that might be observed.

Palpation allows for the assessment of swelling. It also allows one to press over the medial and lateral joint lines, as well as over the medial and lateral collateral ligaments, and lastly the pes anserine bursa region. Palpation of the medial and lateral joint lines may be painful, depending on which joint compartment is more involved with DJD. The medial collateral ligament will shorten and the lateral collateral ligament will stretch in the patient with a varus knee deformity. Attempts at stretching the medial collateral ligament by applying a valgus force will elicit pain. The opposite will happen with the patient who has an underlying valgus knee deformity from DJD or rheumatoid arthritis. Gentle downward pressure over the patella compresses the patellofemoral joint and allows for assessment of retropatellar DJD (chondromalacia patellae), a common source of knee pain. Palpation of the pes anserine bursa will be exquisitely painful in an acute traumatic bursitis.

Range of motion should be assessed. The normal range of motion of the knee is full extension to 120 degrees of flexion. Notation of loss of terminal extension or flexion beyond 90 degrees has functional implications. Loss of terminal extension increases the patient's sensation of instability and "buckling" during weight bearing. Loss of flexion beyond 90 degrees makes ascending stairs and transitioning from sit to stand problematic.

Reflexes should always be evaluated. Loss of the patella reflex on the involved side may be secondary to an L4 radiculopathy or an incomplete femoral nerve neuropathy. Both scenarios complicate the rehabilitation of the patient with a painful knee, since weakness and associated instability may persist even after structural deformity issues are addressed.

Laboratory tests and diagnostic investigations

Synovial fluid analysis is needed to establish the diagnosis of gout, and is critical in the work-up of a suspected septic joint.

Electrodiagnostic studies may be indicated in case of suspected L4 radiculopathy or femoral neuropathy.

Imaging studies

Standing plain film x-rays are most appropriate for the evaluation of knee DJD. It allows for side-to-side comparison of the knees while weight bearing. This allows for the accurate assessment of a structural deformity. MRI is rarely needed, and should only be considered if meniscal or ligamentous pathology is suspected.

Differential diagnosis

Gout and calcium pyrophosphate disease (CPPD) can both cause knee pain. Typically the pain is abrupt in onset and severe. Swelling is also a common feature. The diagnosis of CPPD can be established on x-ray, as calcification of the medial and lateral meniscus cartilages will be noted. Under polarizing light microscopy CPPD crystals are weakly birefringent.

The diagnosis of gout can be established on aspiration and analysis of the synovial fluid for gouty crystals, which are strongly birefringent under polarizing light microscopy.

Abrupt onset of a painful, swollen, erythematous knee may be a "red flag" for a septic joint. Prompt aspiration and Gram stain of the fluid is necessary, and referral to orthopedics is appropriate to ensure definitive management, including surgery if needed.

Pharmacotherapy

The pain and episodic swelling associated with DJD of the knee can respond to judicious use of non-steroidal anti-inflammatory drugs (NSAIDs). Periodic monitoring of renal function and liver function is recommended if NSAIDs are to be used on a chronic basis.

Prepatellar and pes anserine bursitis usually respond well to conservative management, including the use of NSAIDs and ice for control of inflammation.

Non-pharmacologic approaches

Physical therapy that focuses on strengthening of lower extremity musculature may have utility in early DJD of the knee. Assistive devices, such as a cane used in the contralateral hand, can be helpful for pain control and an improved sense of stability.

In cases of prepatellar and pes anserine bursitis, the use of knee pads may help prevent recurrence in patients who spend significant amounts of time on their knees as part of their occupation.

Interventional procedures

Injections of local anesthetic with corticosteroid can be both diagnostic and therapeutic in cases of knee pain secondary to DJD, CPPD, and gout. Injections of high-viscosity hyaluronic acids have shown efficacy for management of knee pain from DJD.

While knee arthroscopy has been used in the treatment of knee DJD, there are no studies that conclusively establish its efficacy. For this reason, it is a controversial intervention without clear demonstrable benefit.

Total knee arthroplasty offers the opportunity for dramatic reduction in pain and improved mobility for patients with severe painful DJD of the knee. Unicompartmental joint replacement is a more recent interventional strategy for management of single-compartment DJD of the knee. It can have efficacy for management of isolated medial or lateral compartment DJD. There are strict inclusion and exclusion criteria that should be met before a unicompartmental knee replacement is contemplated.

Follow-up

Knee DJD is a progressive disorder associated with aging. Management and follow-up are dictated by intervention. Not uncommonly, follow-up will be on an episodic basis to treat flares of pain and swelling. Total joint arthroplasty should be considered when pain and debility progress to the point that quality of life is affected.

Prepatellar and pes anserine bursitis are usually self-limiting. Use of knee pads may decrease the risk for recurrence.

Gout and CPPD require periodic follow-up with rheumatology for pharmacologic management.

Prognosis

Prognosis for knee DJD is one of slow progression of symptoms and pain over time. Initial management is exercise, as-needed use of NSAIDs (with the caution for potential renal and gastrointestinal toxicity), and injections as required. Total knee arthroplasty is reserved for those patients with intractable pain, loss of function, or impairment of quality of life.

REFERENCES AND FURTHER READING

Chilappa CS, Aronow WS, Shapiro D, *et al*. Gout and hyperuricemia. *Compr Ther* 2010; **36**: 3–13.

Fransen M, McConnell S, Bell M. Therapeutic exercise for people with osteoarthritis of the hip or knee: a systematic review. *J Rheumatol* 2002; **29**: 1737–45.

Lombardi AV, Berend KR, Walter CA, Aziz-Jacobo J, Cheney NA. Is recovery faster for mobile-bearing unicompartmental than total knee arthroplasty? *Clin Orthop Relat Res* 2009; **467**: 1450–7.

Lyons MC, MacDonald SJ, Somerville LE, Naudie DD, McCalden RW. Unicompartmental versus total knee arthroplasty database analysis: is there a winner? *Clin Orthop Relat Res* 2012; **470**: 84–90.

Valderrabano V, Steiger C. Treatment and prevention of osteoarthritis through exercise and sports. *J Aging Res* 2010; **2011**: 374653.

44

Knee sprains and tendinitis

Clinical presentation

The knee is a complex joint. It allows for flexion and extension as well as tibial rotation during pivoting activities. The stability of the knee depends primarily upon the ligaments that span between the femur and the tibia and fibula. These include the medial and lateral collateral ligaments as well as the anterior and posterior cruciate ligaments. The meniscal cartilages functionally deepen the tibial plateau and disperse weight-bearing forces over a larger surface area. Additionally they serve as secondary stabilizers.

Tendinitis of the knee most commonly involves the patellar tendon, which is the tendinous extension of the quadriceps muscle. Less commonly, knee tendinitis can involve the hamstring group tendons at their distal insertions on the posterior-medial tibia or fibula head regions respectively. Iliotibial band (ITB) tendinitis can result in lateral knee pain, and is more commonly seen in runners. Tendinous injuries are typically classified grades I through III, with grade I strains manifesting with pain, up to catastrophic grade III ruptures of the tendon.

Ligamentous injuries or sprains are also graded I to III. Grade I sprains are usually associated with low-energy type injuries and are stable on examination. Grade II injuries typically are associated with a higher energy or external force application, and demonstrate varying degrees of instability. Grade III ligamentous sprains are most commonly associated with high energy or high force applications, and are unstable on exam.

The clinical presentation for ligamentous or tendinous injuries can range from minimal to profound disability and dysfunction. Mechanisms of injury can include stepping awkwardly into a hole, trying to pivot while the foot is anchored to the ground, jumping from a height and landing awkwardly, as well as the application of various external loading forces common to sporting events.

Signs and symptoms

Injury to the medial collateral ligament (MCL) can occur with the application of a valgus stress or load placed upon the knee when the foot is anchored to the ground. Isolated MCL injuries can occur in isolation with low-energy type injuries, and will present with medial knee pain, mild swelling, and pain on palpation of the medial knee along the MCL.

Application of a valgus stress will also case pain. Patients will rarely complain of a sense of instability. Higher-energy MCL injuries are commonly associated with concomitant medial meniscus cartilage injuries, as these two structures are physically attached to one another. In these injuries, typically the more severe grade II and III injuries, patients will complain of medial knee pain, obvious swelling will be noted, and the patient will have poor tolerance for weight bearing on the affected limb. A sense of instability will also be noted.

Patients may also complain of a tearing or snapping sensation at the time of injury. If the medial meniscus cartilage has been torn, patients will typically complain of a sense of instability, buckling, and locking of the joint. Locking of the joint will be manifested by the patient being unable to fully extend the knee. Patients will complain of feeling as if there is something in the joint that has the durometer of firm rubber.

Similar complaints will be manifested with lateral collateral ligament (LCL) sprains. In LCL sprains the external force is usually a varus loading force driving the knee into a bow legged posture. This injury is less common than an MCL injury. Patients with an isolated LCL injury will complain of lateral knee pain with mild swelling, and tenderness will be noted along the anatomic course of the LCL. Pain with varus stressing will also be noted.

In grade III LCL injuries patients can potentially complain of paresthesias in a peroneal distribution, as the peroneal nerve can be stretched at the level of the fibular head, which is the distal attachment site for the LCL. Concomitant lateral meniscus cartilage injuries are less common than medial meniscus injuries, as the LCL and lateral meniscus cartilage do not share any common points of attachment.

Anterior cruciate ligament (ACL) injuries can present with minimal complaints of pain, and mild swelling, up to significant swelling, hemarthrosis, and gross instability on testing. Patients with grade II and grade III ACL injuries will note instability, poor tolerance for weight bearing, swelling, and marked intolerance for activities that place rotational stress on the tibia, such as attempting to pivot.

Posterior cruciate ligament (PCL) injuries are less common. They are commonly associated with high-energy injuries, such as with a significant high-energy impact on the anterior knee. Concern in this scenario is for neurovascular injury, and therefore complaints of sensory changes in the foot or loss of dorsi and or plantar flexor function constitute an orthopedic emergency.

Injuries that arise from valgus stress while the knee is driven into flexion expose the patient to the potential for the unhappy triad. This is an injury that includes damage to the MCL, ACL, and medial meniscus cartilage. Multidirectional instability, significant joint swelling, locking, buckling, and an inability to weight bear are common findings. Hemarthrosis will also be noted on aspiration of the swollen knee joint.

Patellar tendinitis may present with pain on eccentric loading of the quadriceps mechanism, when the injury is mild grade I, to knee extensor lag if the strain is a grade II, to complete loss of knee extensor function in a grade III patellar tendon rupture.

ITB tendinitis will typically manifest with lateral knee pain that is intensified with palpation of the distal ITB as it crosses the knee joint.

Ligamentous sprains and tendinous injuries can present a challenge on physical examination. Inspection may reveal an obvious deformity such as a markedly high-riding patella with inability to extend the knee in the case of patellar rupture.

In general, inspection will be of limited utility. A major problem that limits the utility of the physical examination in the evaluation of ligamentous injuries is the reactive muscle spasm that may occur as a protective mechanism. Typically, in grade II–III sprains the quadriceps and hamstring muscle spasm is so significant that a range of motion (ROM) examination of the knee is nearly impossible. In the acute setting on the athletic field, a brief examination may be able to be conducted in terms of assessing varus, valgus, as well as anterior and posterior laxity, but within minutes the swelling and pain associated with significant ligamentous trauma will render the knee examination virtually impossible.

Peroneal motor and sensory function should be assessed in all knee injuries. The peroneal nerve is in a vulnerable position and subject to trauma with varus as well as valgus force application to the knee joint.

Deep tendon reflexes should be evaluated, particularly the patella reflex. An absent patella reflex will occur with complete patellar tendon rupture. An absent Achilles reflex can occur with a severe PCL injury secondary to stretch of the tibial nerve as it courses through the popliteal fossa.

Grade I ligamentous sprains will be amenable to examination. The physical will reveal a stable joint, as the ligamentous structures are intact. A firm endpoint, without joint laxity, will be noted on varus, valgus, anterior, and posterior stress testing. Pain will be elicited upon stressing the involved grade I injured ligament. In the case of MCL and LCL grade I sprains, pain will also be noted on palpation of the involved ligament. Swelling, if present, will be mild.

Patients with grade I tendinous injuries, such as patellar tendinitis, will complain of pain on stressing the tendon. Activation of the quadriceps mechanism against an external load will cause pain. Squatting activities will be poorly tolerated. Swelling will typically be mild. Pain complaints can be significant, and not uncommonly out of proportion to the physical examination findings.

Patients who sustain ligamentous injury and have complaints of locking, clicking, or buckling of the knee should be assessed for meniscal injury.

McMurray's click test can be used to determine the presence of a meniscal tear. The test is performed with the patient supine. The involved knee is fully flexed while the examiner's hand is positioned such that the thumb is over one joint line while the index and middle fingers are over the opposite joint line. While the knee is maintained fully flexed the tibia is rotated medially and laterally.

An audible click, if heard, is suggestive of a torn meniscus. To determine if the click is from a medial meniscus cartilage injury, the examiner can laterally rotate the tibia while extending the knee from the fully flexed starting position. A click while performing this maneuver can be elicited with a medial meniscus tear. A lateral meniscus tear can be assessed by medially rotating the tibia while extending the knee from its fully flexed starting point, once again paying attention for an audible click. Medial meniscus tears can be seen with more significant MCL injuries and/or ACL injuries, and must always be considered.

Imaging studies

Radiography to assess for bony injury is appropriate. MRI to evaluate the status of the ligamentous and tendinous structures is critical when injury to these structures is suspected. MRI should be obtained early in the evaluation and treatment phase to optimize patient management. Any significant ligamentous or tendinous injury may result in early surgical management to optimize outcome.

Differential diagnosis

Ligamentous and tendinous injuries to the knee are not likely to be confused with other types of injuries. The history of a fall, twisting type mechanism, or sudden onset of symptoms in the setting of an athletic event, make the diagnosis fairly evident. The critical element in these situations is not so much in diagnosing the ligamentous or severe tendon injury, but in making sure that concomitant injuries to neurovascular structures have not been missed.

Pharmacotherapy

Treatment depends upon the degree of injury. Simple resolution of pain without ensuring that strength, proprioception, and balance are fully restored is a recipe for repeat injury.

Non-pharmacologic approaches

Grade I ligament sprains can be managed conservatively. Initial management will include control of swelling with ice and protected weight bearing. Early mobilization on physical therapy to maintain knee range of motion is critical. Strengthening of the quadriceps and hamstrings can be started once the swelling and pain are under control.

Grade I tendinous injuries, such as patellar and ITB tendinitis, can be managed by using ice for its local analgesic and anti-inflammatory effect.

Eccentric strengthening exercises can be useful in the rehabilitation of patellar tendinitis. This can be done under the direction of physical therapy.

ITB tendinitis, commonly seen in runners, is usually secondary to tightness of the ITB. Stretching of the ITB and cross-friction massage over the distal ITB at the level of the knee joint can be very helpful.

Physical therapy plays a critical role in the rehabilitation of ligamentous injuries and tendinous injuries to the knee. Recovery of muscular strength as well as joint proprioception is key before returning the athlete or "weekend warrior" to activity. Bracing may be needed to protect the injured knee early on in the return to activities.

Interventional procedures

Grade III ligament and tendon injuries will require referral to orthopedic surgery, as surgical repair will invariably be needed. Isolated MCL tears, without associated medial meniscus cartilage tear, can many times be managed conservatively, even if severe.

Follow-up

Follow-up is dictated by the severity of the injury. Severe injuries will almost invariably require surgical intervention and orthopedic follow-up, as well as prolonged physical therapy. Grade I injuries, once resolved, will not typically require any ongoing follow-up.

Prognosis

Care should be taken to ensure that patients have fully recovered strength, proprioception, and balance before releasing them back to unrestricted activity.

REFERENCES AND FURTHER READING

Chen L, Kim PD, Ahmad CS, Levine WN. Medial collateral ligament injuries of the knee: current treatment concepts. *Curr Rev Musculoskelet Med* 2008; **1**: 108–13.

Clayton RA, Court-Brown CM. The epidemiology of musculoskeletal tendinous and ligamentous injuries. *Injury* 2008; **39**: 1338–44.

Pacheco RJ, Ayre CA, Bollen SR. Posterolateral corner injuries of the knee: a serious injury commonly missed. *J Bone Joint Surg Br* 2011; **93**: 194–7.

Visnes H, Bahr R. Evolution of eccentric training as treatment for patellar tendinopathy (jumper's knee): a critical review of exercise programmes. *Br J Sports Med* 2007; **41**: 217–23.

Wijdicks CA, Griffith CJ, Johansen S, Engebretsen L, LaPrade RF. Injuries to the medial collateral ligament and associated medial structures of the knee. *J Bone Joint Surg Am* 2010; **92**: 1266–80.

45

Degenerative joint disease pain of the ankle, foot, and toe

Clinical presentation

In adults, arthritis is a leading cause of disability and limitations in the work and home environment. Arthritis of the ankle, foot, or toe presents a unique set of challenges as the ankles, feet, and toes are major weight-bearing structures. Additionally, each of these structures allows for efficient interaction with a wide variety of surfaces. These structures are critical not only for weight bearing, but also for maintenance of balance.

The etiology of ankle, foot, or toe arthritis may be secondary to repetitive overuse seen in heavy labor occupation, underlying inflammatory arthritis, trauma, congenital or acquired structural deformities, or crystal-induced arthropathies.

The clinical presentation for arthritis involving the ankle, foot, or toe can be variable, and is dependent upon the etiology of the arthritis. However, certain features will be common to all. Invariably, almost all patients will complain of pain that is worsened with weight bearing. Active range of motion with weight bearing will further increase pain. Walking is therefore usually more painful than static standing.

Patients or family members may note that the patient ambulates with a limp. Patients with an underlying inflammatory arthritis, such as rheumatoid arthritis, which can commonly involve the ankle, foot, and toes, may also have other small joint involvement, and they may thus complain of more diffuse pain.

Crystal-induced arthropathies can involve any joint. Classically gout is associated with involvement of the metatarsal phalangeal (MTP) joint of the great toe. This particular clinical entity is referred to as podagra, and is typically extremely painful. It will also be associated with swelling, redness, and warmth. Gout can involve the ankle joint as well as the joints of the mid foot.

Patients with post-traumatic arthritis will have an antecedent history of trauma, followed by a period of time with relative preservation of pain-free function, with subsequent onset of pain, months to years after the accident.

Congenital deformities such as club foot (talipes equinovarus) predispose to later onset of arthritis as a result of altered mechanics of the foot. The risk increases if there are significant structural residua post correction.

Acquired deformities can occur secondary to underlying neuropathies or myopathies that result in muscle imbalances leading to structural deformity. Classic examples of this include diabetes, with the development of a neuropathic Charcot foot, Charcot–Marie–Tooth (CMT) disease, a hereditary sensory motor neuropathy, spastic diplegic cerebral palsy, and Duchenne muscular dystrophy.

Signs and symptoms

The physical examination of the ankle, foot, and toes should start with inspection, followed by palpation. For the ankle, any obvious bony deformities or malalignment issues should be noted. Swelling in the region of the medial and lateral malleoli may be secondary to chronic degenerative changes at the ankle joint and chronic inflammation from wear and tear. It can also be seen in patients with crystal-induced arthropathies, between flares as well as during flares. Acute flares will also be associated with redness and warmth. Synovial hypertrophy at the ankle may be seen in patients with underlying rheumatoid arthritis.

Palpation of the anterior ankle joint, between the medial and lateral malleoli, may reveal crepitus with plantar flexion and dorsiflexion. This would be consistent with true ankle joint degenerative joint disease (DJD), as the range of motion for the true ankle joint is limited to dorsiflexion and plantar flexion. Crepitus with inversion and eversion of the heel region (hind foot) is found in subtalar joint pathology.

The foot is composed of the tarsal bones, metatarsals, and phalanges. The tarsal bones include the calcaneus, talus, navicular, cuboid, and the three cuneiform bones.

Functionally the foot can be divided into the hind foot, mid foot, and fore foot. The hind foot is composed of the calcaneus, talus, and subtalar joint. The mid foot is made up of the navicular, cuboid, and three cuneiform bones. The fore foot is composed of the metatarsals and phalanges. The foot has multiple articulations, but three joints are of particular interest in regards to arthritis pain and associated gait dysfunction. The subtalar joint allows for hind-foot inversion and eversion. Chopart's joint, also referred to as the midtarsal joint, is made up of the talonavicular articulation as well as the calcaneocuboid articulation. By virtue of its articulations it plays a major role in transmitting load to the mid foot and fore foot during ambulation. The Lisfranc joint, or tarsometatarsal articulation, is important in the gait cycle as weight is transferred over the limb and the body continues through the roll-over phase of the gait cycle.

All of these joints should be placed through their ranges of motion and palpated for crepitus during the exam. Pain with range of motion should be noted, as well as restrictions in range compared to the contralateral foot.

Additional observation of the foot should include assessment of the medial longitudinal arch with and without weight bearing. Loss of the arch with weight bearing, but preservation while not weight bearing, can be seen in ligamentous laxity and a flexible flat-foot deformity. Loss of the arch, with and without weight bearing, speaks to a true bony structural deformity requiring additional assessment of the bony foot.

The phalanges should be viewed as well. Obvious hallux valgus or bunion deformities should be made note of. This can be seen in arthritis of the great toe, and will manifest with pain during the push-off phase of the gait cycle. Range of motion of the great toe should be assessed with and without weight bearing. Loss of the ability to passively dorsiflex the great toe while the patient is weight bearing can be due to tightness of the flexor hallucis longus tendon as well as the Achilles tendon complex, and it is a common source of medial arch pain and a functional hallux rigidus.

Evaluation of the ankle and foot is incomplete without assessment of sensation, pulses, and motor strength for dorsiflexion and plantar flexion, as well as great toe extension and flexion. Achilles reflexes should be checked and compared side to side. Abnormal sensation in both feet with absent Achilles reflexes in a patient with a deformed foot raises the specter of an underlying neuropathy, with a neuropathic etiology for the foot deformity.

Absent dorsalis pedis and posterior tibial pulses can be seen with peripheral vascular disease (PVD), which can be part of underlying systemic issues such as PVD from diabetes.

Imaging studies

Plain film radiographs of the ankle and foot are the standard for assessment of the true ankle joint as well as the joints of the foot. Because of the orientation of the ankle to the hind foot as well as the midtarsal joint (Chopart's joint), multiple views may be required to fully appreciate the arthritis in the hind-foot and proximal mid-foot regions. MRI can be useful in ankle injuries where an osteochondral defect is suspected.

Differential diagnosis

The major challenge in diagnosing arthritis of the ankle, foot, or toes is not so much in making the diagnosis but in establishing the possible underlying etiology. Care must be taken to check motor strength of the ankle dorsal and plantar flexors, reflexes, and sensation to avoid missing more global issues such as CMT, or for example a distal myopathy such as myotonic dystrophy. Incomplete cauda equina spinal cord injuries can manifest with foot and ankle deformities second-ary to unbalanced musculature, but a careful examination including sensory, motor function, and reflexes should make the diagnosis obvious.

Pharmacotherapy

Treatment depends on the degree of pain and dysfunction.

Anti-inflammatory analgesic medications such as non-steroidal anti-inflam-matory drugs (NSAIDs) or aspirin can be very helpful in the patient who is experiencing an acute flare of underlying DJD.

Specific pharmacologic treatments are available for the treatment of acute gout flares. Rheumatology referral is appropriate for the management of the patient with gout, as these patients will in many instances require long-term pharmaco-logic intervention to prevent exacerbations.

Non-pharmacologic approaches

Ankle arthritis may respond nicely to bracing, particularly if the patient's main complaint is pain with ankle range of motion. If the pain is reproduced with subtalar range a lace-up ankle gauntlet that restricts inversion and eversion may be very helpful. If pain is reproduced with dorsiflexion and plantar flexion an ankle-foot orthosis that prevents this range may be useful.

For the patient with severe pain on weight bearing, the use of a patellar tendon bearing ankle-foot orthosis may allow for sufficient weight bearing to be trans-mitted proximally to the level of the patellar tendon as to make weight bearing tolerable.

Hallux valgus if mild may do well with shoe modifications. The use of a shoe with a wide toe box will allow for sufficient room to decrease the pain caused by compression of the joint. The addition of a shoe insert to help protect the joint during the roll-over phase of the gait cycle may also be helpful.

Interventional procedures

In refractory cases of ankle pain, in the patient with severe DJD of the ankle joint and subtalar joint, ankle arthrodesis may offer excellent pain relief, as the painful arthritic joints are fused and motion is ablated.

If conservative measures do not give sufficient pain control to allow for ambulation, surgical referral for possible corrective surgery on hallux valgus should be considered.

Follow-up

Follow-up is dependent upon the degree of intervention. Brace management will require periodic assessment to ensure that the brace remains effective and functional. Periodic replacement may be needed.

Pharmacologic management will require routine follow-up to ensure that the medications are being tolerated. In the case of NSAIDs, as well as the medications that are used to control gout, renal and liver function should be periodically monitored.

Surgical intervention will require follow-up with the surgeon, to ensure satisfactory outcome.

Prognosis

The prognosis of arthritis of the ankle, foot, and toe is one of slow progression. Initial management includes as-needed use of NSAIDs, with the caution for potential renal and gastrointestinal toxicity, and injections of corticosteroids as required. These injections should be limited, however, as repeated injections to weight-bearing joints may ultimately accelerate the degenerative changes.

In patients with refractory ankle pain secondary to severe arthritis, ankle fusion may be helpful for controlling the pain. This will alter gait mechanics, however, and may require shoe modifications to accommodate for the loss of ankle range of motion.

REFERENCES AND FURTHER READING

Hunt KJ, Ellington JK, Anderson RB, et al. Locked versus nonlocked plate fixation for hallux MTP arthrodesis. Foot Ankle Int 2011; 32: 704–9.

Kelikian AS. Technical considerations in hallux metatarsalphalangeal arthrodesis. Foot Ankle Clin 2005; 10: 167–90.

Kwon DG, Chung CY, Park MS, et al. Arthroplasty versus arthrodesis for end-stage ankle arthritis: decision analysis using Markov model. Int Orthop 2011; 35: 1647–53.

Lee WC, Moon JS, Lee HS, Lee K. Alignment of ankle and hindfoot in early stage ankle osteoarthritis. Foot Ankle Int 2011; 32: 693

Mosier-LaClair S, Pomeroy G, Manoli A. Operative treatment of the difficult stage 2 adult acquired flatfoot deformity. Foot Ankle Clin 2001; 6: 95–119.

Thomas MJ, Roddy E, Zhang W, et al. The population prevalence of foot and ankle pain in middle and old age: a systematic review. Pain 2011; 152: 2870–80.

46

Myofascial pain syndrome

Clinical presentation

Myofascial pain syndromes are considered to be among the most common conditions for which patients seek medical attention, although estimates of prevalence vary depending on whether samples are gathered from clinical or community samples, and also across different clinical settings. Pain is generally described along a localized region of the body (often localized to muscle and ligaments/tendons) with a non-dermatomal pattern of radiation. The pain can begin suddenly or insidiously. Patients reporting a sudden onset of the pain can often recall an inciting event, e.g., repeated overuse of a muscle or group of muscles as might be accompanied by exercise, muscle overload, etc. An insidious onset may suggest repetitive movements that may produce microtrauma contributing to the discomfort. Ergonomic factors will often need to be considered among the possible perpetuating factors contributing to pain, disability, and perceived dysfunction.

Afflicted patients may experience significant comorbidities accompanying pain, including sleep disturbances with resultant fatigue and concentration deficits; depression and anxiety also complicates the clinical picture. The emotional distress accompanying myofascial pain syndromes may, in turn, reciprocally contribute to and potentially perpetuate muscle pain and discomfort.

Signs and symptoms

Patients with myofascial pain will report localized pain and tenderness in some region of the body. The discomfort is often characterized as steady, deep, and aching in nature. Occasionally, patients can report lightning-like stabs of pain; rarely is burning described. They may also complain of muscle stiffness and muscle fatigue of affected muscle groups. There can be significant impairments noted in customary activities that limit the capacity to sustain work and functional capabilities.

The indispensible pathognomonic feature of myofascial pain syndromes is the identification of trigger points in affected muscle groups. Often, patients are incapable of localizing the specific trigger point(s) that emit the pattern of pain experienced. On the other hand, during physical examination, when the trigger-point-affected muscle is loaded or stretched, the pain experienced may serve to more precisely identify the location of the trigger point.

Trigger points are circumscribed and slightly enlarged regions palpable along taut bands within the muscle. Taut bands are appreciable cords of ropy structures, 1–4 mm in diameter, that are less compliant than, and therefore distinguishable from, the surrounding pliable muscle tissue. These can be detected by superficial (flat) digital palpation, or, for deeper muscle tissue, through the use of the pincer grasp. It is essential to compare the symptomatic side with the corresponding non-affected side, as the asymmetry in the palpated muscles may assist the clinician in detecting the presence of trigger points. Digital examination typically elicits exquisite tenderness and recreates the referred pain pattern that the patient recognizes as all-too-familiar. On palpation, the patient may be noted to jerk and involuntarily withdraw from the examiner's grip, i.e., the "jump sign." Additionally, strumming of the taut muscular band produces a perceptible localized muscle twitch. The amount of pressure required to elicit pain at trigger points can be approximated through the use of an algometer, and comparisons between symptomatic and asymptomatic sites should be systematically conducted. Physical examination may reveal accompanying muscle shortening and restrictions in range of motion of affected joints that may signal limitations in muscular mobility.

There is a lack of consensus regarding the essential diagnostic criteria for establishing myofascial pain syndromes. This has been fueled, in part, by research investigations demonstrating the poor inter-rater reliability with regard to elicitation and identification of trigger points in patients suspected of having myofascial pain syndromes. The most reliable diagnostic findings in assessing trigger points consist of focal tenderness and pain recognition. Without standardized diagnostic criteria, and in the absence of reliability in the elicitation of trigger points clinically, efforts to improve and refine evidence-driven treatment approaches has, unfortunately, lacked sufficient scientific rigor.

Laboratory tests, diagnostic investigations, and imaging studies

There are no specific laboratory investigations upon which the clinician can rely to make a definitive diagnosis of myofascial pain. Recently, spontaneous motor end-plate needle electrical activity in the vicinity of trigger points has been employed in empirical investigations to confirm trigger-point localization; however, the use of this technique lacks practical clinical utility. Instead, a number of laboratory studies ought to be considered in the work-up of patients presenting with pain in muscle and surrounding fascial tissues, so as to ensure that other potentially treatable conditions are appropriately diagnosed. Toward this end, consideration should be given to conducting a complete blood count (CBC), erythrocyte sedimentation rate (ESR), antinuclear antibody (ANA) testing, rheumatoid factor, a thyroid profile, and assessment of serum vitamin D levels.

Physical examination remains the primary mode for the identification of myofascial pain syndrome. It is important that clinicians recognize that there are other conditions that produce symptoms which can resemble myofascial pain syndromes. The clinician must judiciously employ diagnostic investigations to rule out other potentially treatable medical conditions (see *Differential diagnosis*, below), e.g., x-rays to assess for bony pathology, MRI for assessment of spinal processes that may be contributing to neuropathic and radicular pain, etc.

Differential diagnosis

Several conditions may resemble, or otherwise mimic, the referred pain patterns encountered in the variety of myofascial pain syndromes. Because the referred pain patterns of specific myofascial pain syndromes can be varied and elusive, a number of conditions must be considered among the differential diagnosis. As can be appreciated from review of Table 46.1, comprehensive physical examination (including systematic motor and sensory examination), electrodiagnostic testing, and judicious use of pertinent imaging investigations can help to distinguish myofascial pain from other diagnostic possibilities. It should be noted that identification of trigger points reproducing the patient's referred pain symptoms does not necessarily mean that a comorbid condition does not also exist. For example, although the pain of myofascial pain syndromes is not prototypically neuropathic in nature, one should be aware that neuropathic pains can emerge within the context of a myofascial pain syndrome, e.g., when nerve irritation arises as the nerve passes through an affected muscle or when irritation occurs from compression of the nerve between the affected muscle and bone.

By contrast, fibromyalgia is considered a systemic process, perhaps best conceptualized as a manifestation of central sensitization, in which systemic multifocal muscle tenderness is a feature. Characteristics distinguishing fibromyalgia and myofascial pain syndrome are delineated in Table 46.2. However, the clinician should be aware that there can be considerable overlap of the features, and a given patient may have coexisting conditions.

Pharmacotherapy

A number of medications have been advocated for use as conservative measures to address myofascial pain syndromes, including non-steroidal anti-inflammatory drugs (NSAIDs), cyclooxygenase-2 (COX-2) inhibitors, tramadol, alpha-2-adrenergic agonists (e.g., tizanidine), and serotonin–norepinephrine reuptake inhibitor

Table 46.1 Differential diagnosis of common specific myofascial trigger-point pain syndromes

Possible pain sources	Examples
Joint disorders	Articular dysfunction, osteoarthritis
Regional soft tissue disorders	Bursitis, tendinitis
Myopathy	Secondary to hypothyroidism, secondary to metabolic disturbances, alcohol-related myopathy
Neurological disorders	Radiculopathy, entrapment neuropathies, complex regional pain syndrome
Spinal disorders	Degenerative disc disease, disc protrusion or herniation
Mechanical disturbances	Scoliosis, leg length discrepancies
Infectious disease	Lyme disease, herpes zoster, parasitic infections (e.g., *Giardia* and amoebiasis)
Inflammatory disorders	Polymyositis, systemic lupus erythematosus, polymyalgia rheumatica, rheumatoid arthritis
Fibromyalgia	
Nutritional deficiencies	Vitamin D, B_{12}, folate
Referred visceral pain	Gastrointestinal disorders, cardiac, pulmonary
Vascular-occlusive disease	Peripheral vascular disease
Psychological disturbances	Depression, anxiety, sleep disorders, somatization disorder
Medications	Statins

Adapted from Borg-Stein & Simons 2002 and Simons *et al.* 1999.

Table 46.2 Features distinguishing myofascial pain and fibromyalgia

Myofascial pain	Fibromyalgia
Males = females	Females > males
Regional, localized tenderness	Widespread, multiple tenderness
Asymmetric discomfort/pain	Often symmetric pain/discomfort
Palpated muscles feel tense	Palpated muscles feel soft and doughy
Restricted range of motion	Normal or hypermobile range of motion
Presence of trigger points	Presence of tender points
As many as 20% may have comorbid fibromyalgia	70% have active trigger points suggesting myofascial pain

Adapted from Borg-Stein & Simons 2002 and Simons *et al.* 1999.

(SNRI) antidepressants. For many of these agents, empirical support for clinical efficacy has been very limited, and in some cases it is non-existent. There may be utility in ensuring that nutritional deficiencies be addressed, e.g., in the form of vitamin supplements and concerted efforts to improve nutritional intake. Long-term use of opioid analgesics or benzodiazepines has not received empirical support; concerns arise regarding the potential risks of misuse and dependence.

Non-pharmacologic approaches

Non-invasive approaches recommended for use in patients with myofascial pain syndromes have frequently included physical therapy, passive stretch and spray techniques, massage, low-level laser therapy, transcutaneous electrical nerve stimulation (TENS), electrical muscle stimulation, and ultrasonography. The extant literature has demonstrated inconsistent efficacy as compared with placebo, depending upon the outcome variables assessed, for physical therapy, stretch and spray, laser therapy, electrotherapy, and TENS. The comparative effectiveness of these varied modalities has been difficult to determine because of inconsistencies in the diagnostic criteria employed across empirical trials. Patient education may be useful to encourage adherence with stretching exercises, enhance kinesthetic awareness, and improve dietary intake to ensure nutritional needs. Patients may benefit from psychological therapies, e.g., cognitive behavioral therapy (CBT) and electromyographic biofeedback training, to enhance coping and stress modulation. Education regarding the cultivation of sleep hygiene techniques can also be a particularly useful supplement to treatment.

Interventional procedures

Interventional therapies have been employed for purposes of mechanically stimulating the trigger points. Two approaches are typically employed: dry needling, or needle insertion with introduction of an injectable agent. Dry needling involves insertion of a solid filament needle into the tissues overlying the trigger point (generally at a depth of 5–10 mm) for approximately 30 seconds. If pain persists, the needle may be maintained in position for an additional 2–3 minutes. The precise mechanisms of dry needling are as yet unknown, but they are thought to involve disruptions of motor end plates. By contrast, trigger-point injections, using agents to disrupt the pain, frequently employ lidocaine, mepivicaine, steroids, bee venom, NSAIDs, or botulinum toxin. The two modalities of dry needling and injection techniques have demonstrated comparable efficacy. Data supporting the superiority of one injectable agent over another are lacking; however, steroids and bee venom have produced inconsistent results across investigations.

Use of either modality should never be a stand-alone therapy, but instead should be considered part of a comprehensive treatment approach implemented in combination with pharmacological therapies, physical therapy modalities, and educational strategies to enhance posture, movement, and kinesthetic awareness. Because of the common comorbidity with psychological and psychiatric distress, patients may also benefit from psychotherapeutic modalities directed at mitigating emotional responses to stress and enhancing coping. Psychoactive medications (e.g., antidepressants) may be necessary in conditions where there are significant signs and symptoms meeting diagnostic criteria for mood and/or anxiety disorders; carefully selected, these agents may have pain-mitigating effects.

Follow-up

It is advisable for clinicians to make use of full body figures to schematically represent localized trigger points and the associated referral patterns reported by patients at initial diagnosis/assessment. Referral to the figure at subsequent visits can be helpful to track changes in the progression of pain over time and assess the effectiveness of treatment approaches. Failure to achieve relief should prompt consideration of: (1) the accuracy of diagnosis and whether other conditions ought to be worked up; (2) the accuracy of the localization of trigger points; (3) patient adherence with and efficacy of employed treatment approaches (and whether alternative approaches should be undertaken); and (4) whether other factors, e.g., mood and sleep disturbances, ergonomic factors, nutritional deficiencies, and/or comorbid conditions, may be exacerbating or perpetuating pain.

Prognosis

Complete relief of myofascial pain syndromes, along with restoration of muscle strength, is possible with identification and treatment of acute trigger points. The duration of myofascial pain may be the most significant prognostic factor regarding recovery. Generally, myofascial pain present for 6 months or less is most amenable to full recovery; chronic and recurrent myofascial pain syndromes may be less amenable to full recovery, often with a requirement for long-term symptomatic treatment before appreciable gains can be achieved. Delays in diagnosis and treatment can, therefore, predispose to a relapsing clinical course, necessitating recurrent treatment and elimination of perpetuating factors so as to achieve restoration of adaptive functioning.

REFERENCES AND FURTHER READING

Borg-Stein J, Simons DG. Myofascial pain. *Arch Phys Med Rehabil* 2002; **83** (Suppl 1): 40–7.
Cummings M, Baldry P. Regional myofascial pain: diagnosis and management. *Best Pract Res Clin Rheumatol* 2007; **21**: 367–87.
Harden RN. Muscle pain syndromes. *Am J Phys Med Rehabil* 2007; **86** (Suppl): S47–56.
Lucas N, Macaskill P, Irwig L, Moran R, Bogduk N. Reliability of physical examination for diagnosis of myofascial trigger points: a systematic review of the literature. *Clin J Pain* 2009; **25**: 80–9.
Simons DG, Travell JG, Simons LS. *Travell & Simons' Myofascial Pain and Dysfunction: the Trigger Point Manual*, 2nd edn. Philadelphia PA: Lippincott, Williams & Wilkins; 1999.
Tough EA, White AR, Richards S, Campbell J. Variability of criteria used to diagnose myofascial trigger point pain syndrome: evidence from a review of the literature. *Clin J Pain* 2007; **23**: 278–86.

47

Fibromyalgia pain syndrome

Clinical presentation

Fibromyalgia (FM) is a syndrome perhaps best conceptualized as a state of tonic nociception presumed to possess elements of central sensitization, in which systemic multifocal soft tissue tenderness is a significant feature. Affecting as many as 2–5% of adults in the United States, the epidemiology of FM reveals a female preponderance across all age groups. The prevalence of FM increases with age, with the highest rates in individuals between the ages of 60 and 79 years. Pain associated with FM syndrome can lead to reduced physical function, marked deconditioning and disability, and frequent use of healthcare resources.

Because of the lack of objective physical findings and diagnostic testing corroborating its diagnosis, history obtained from the patient remains the primary mode for the identification of FM syndrome (features of the disorder are elaborated in *Signs and symptoms*, below). The protean nature of symptoms with which patients can present can confound clinicians and has stimulated efforts to standardize diagnosis along objective criteria. For many years, clinicians have relied on operational criteria put forth by the American College of Rheumatology (ACR). Although they have not been validated for clinical use, these criteria stipulated that diagnosis depended upon identifying 11 of 18 possible tender points among specifically designated body regions for a minimum of 3 months' duration (Table 47.1). Tender points must be detectable on the right and left sides of the body, as well as above and below the waist, so as to avoid obscuring the distinction between FM and regional pain syndromes. A tender point was considered to be present when application of a force of 4 kg/cm^2 elicited subjectively reported pain and tenderness.

Since the ACR classification criteria were published, findings from research investigations have raised questions regarding their utility and validity (Table 47.2). Notably, reliance on the tender-point paradigm has been criticized for ignoring the other symptoms commonly experienced by FM patients that substantially contribute to the burden of illness. As a result, there have been recent

Table 47.1 Bilateral tender point locations specified by the ACR criteria

Anterior lower cervical musculature, anterior to the C5–C7 interspaces
Second rib intercostal space, lateral to the second costochondral junction
Lateral epicondyle, 2 cm distal to the epicondyle
Pes anserinus muscle, bilateral and proximal to the knee joint, at the medial fat pad
Occiput, bilaterally at the insertions of the suboccipital muscles
Trapezius, at the midpoint of the upper border of the muscle
Supraspinatus, near the medial border of the scapula
Gluteal, at the anterior fold of the muscle in the upper outer quadrant
Greater trochanter, posterior to the trochanteric prominence

Adapted from Wolfe *et al.* 1990.

Table 47.2 Limitations of the ACR criteria for the classification of fibromyalgia

Limitations	Explanation
Over-reliance on the number of tender points	There can be considerable variability in the number of tender points experienced over time, potentially leading to missed cases
Over-reliance on the number of body quadrants	There can be considerable variability in the number of body quadrants affected, potentially leading to missed cases
The designated tender points are restrictive	Patients may experience tenderness in regions other than those delineated as "acceptable" but yet might otherwise possess other characteristics of the disorder
The digital examination of tender points lacks objectivity	The subjective endorsement of discomfort produced by digital examination can vary depending on the amount of force and the rate at which it is applied
The criteria lack discrimination value	Patients with inflammatory conditions, (e.g., systemic lupus erythematosus, rheumatoid arthritis) are likely to possess symptoms that likewise fulfill the criteria
The criteria introduce bias	The requirement of 11-of-18 tender points potentially erroneously inflates the rate at which the diagnosis is made in women and perhaps older persons

efforts to codify commensurate symptoms, e.g., sleep disturbance, fatigue, etc., as part of the diagnostic criteria.

Signs and symptoms

The pain of FM is chronic and widespread, affecting the axial skeleton, joints, and muscles. For some, the pain begins insidiously and cannot be traced to a specific event; for others, the symptoms may arise after an inciting injury or illness.

Table 47.3 Symptoms commonly associated with fibromyalgia

Neurologic	Headache
	Dizziness
	Atypical numbness
	Restless legs
Cognitive	Impaired concentration
	Impaired speed of performance
	Short-term memory loss
Psychiatric	Depression
	Anxiety
	Sleep disturbances
Gastrointestinal	Abdominal pain
	Bloating
	Diarrhea
	Constipation
Genitourinary	Urinary burning
	Urinary frequency
	Pelvic pain
Constitutional	Fatigue
	Generalized weakness
	Night sweats
	Weight fluctuations

Patients will report pain of moderate to severe intensity; the pain is present throughout the day, with the greatest intensity experienced in the morning and evening. A wide range of sensations may be described, from a deep ache to mild tenderness to intermittent dysesthesia. Morning stiffness, swelling, and paresthesias might also be reported. The patient's symptoms can be variable over time, and can have a fluctuating course. Exacerbations of pain can reportedly be triggered by stress, cold weather, illness, and unaccustomed overexertion. There can be significant impairments noted in customary activities that limit the capacity to sustain work and functional capabilities.

In addition to pain, patients may endorse multiple related somatic, cognitive, and psychological complaints (Table 47.3). For example, FM-afflicted patients may experience sleep disturbances, i.e., non-restorative sleep, with resultant fatigue and concentration deficits. Depression and anxiety often complicate the clinical picture. These complaints, like the widespread tenderness, can be variable and fluctuate in severity over time. It is imperative that the clinician recognize that these varied complaints can represent symptoms of comorbid conditions commonly encountered with FM, such as clinical depression and/or anxiety, irritable bowel syndrome, headache, Raynaud's syndrome, and restless legs syndrome. If unrecognized and therefore untreated, or suboptimally treated, these comorbidities can, in turn, reciprocally contribute to and potentially perpetuate discomfort and functional deficits.

Physical examination will reveal the presence of tender points. These are generally deep to the skin in soft tissue, i.e., in muscle, ligaments, and bursae. Although the presence of tender points can be appreciated on clinical examination, there is no compelling evidence that suggests that the painful tissues are histologically abnormal or distinct from non-tender tissues.

On digital examination, pressure applied to tender points elicits a subjectively reported tenderness, akin to that experienced from day to day. The reliability of tender-point digital examination can be variable, e.g., influenced by the amount of pressure and the rate at which it is applied. The pressure applied to the tender points can be standardized using a pressure gauge algometer. An approximation of the correct amount of pressure corresponding to 4 kg/cm^2 is when sufficient pressure is applied using the belly of the examiner's thumb such that the mid to distal portion of the nail bed blanches.

A thorough history and physical examination can be useful to aid the clinician in distinguishing FM from other sources of pain, such as regional pain arising from myofascial pain syndromes, or inflammatory pain arising from rheumatoid arthritis or systemic lupus erythematosus. In contradistinction to trigger points (see Chapter 46), tender points are *not* palpable, ropy areas of circumscribed muscle which when palpated on digital examination produce pain with predictable referral patterns and related signs, e.g., jump sign and muscle twitch. It is imperative likewise to assess for synovial and extrasynovial findings that would distinguish other rheumatologic conditions (e.g., rheumatoid arthritis) from FM.

Laboratory tests and diagnostic investigations

There are no specific laboratory investigations upon which the clinician can rely to make a definitive diagnosis of FM. Instead, a number of laboratory studies are worthy of consideration in the work-up of patients presenting with widespread pain, so as to ensure that other potentially treatable conditions are appropriately diagnosed (see *Differential diagnosis*, below). Toward this end, consideration should be given to conducting a complete blood count (CBC), electrolytes, liver function tests (LFT), erythrocyte sedimentation rate (ESR), creatine kinase, C-reactive protein (CRP), thyroid stimulating hormone (TSH). Other studies might be considered, depending on the clinical index of suspicion including an assessment of vitamin D 25-OH levels, antinuclear antibody (ANA) testing, rheumatoid factor, and iron studies.

Imaging studies

As with laboratory investigations, the clinician must judiciously employ imaging studies to rule out other potentially treatable medical conditions. Informed by clinical history along with physical findings, diagnostic imaging may be

Table 47.4 Differential diagnosis of fibromyalgia syndrome

Conditions	Examples
Infectious disease	Lyme disease, hepatitis C
Inflammatory disorders	Polymyalgia rheumatica, rheumatoid arthritis, scleroderma, systemic lupus erythematosus
Joint disorders	Osteoarthritis, gout, pseudogout
Medications	Statin-induced myopathy, steroid withdrawal-induced myopathy
Myofascial pain syndromes	Myofascial pain syndromes affecting the torso
Myopathy	Secondary to hypothyroidism, secondary to metabolic disturbances, alcohol-related myopathy
Neurological disorders	Complex regional pain syndrome, multiple sclerosis
Nutritional deficiencies	Vitamin D deficiency, vitamin B_{12} deficiency
Psychological disturbances	Depression, anxiety, sleep disorders, somatization disorder
Spondyloarthritis	Ankylosing spondylitis

warranted. For example, it may be prudent to consider radiographs to assess for trauma, bony pathology, or joint deformity, and MRI for assessment of spinal stenosis or cord compression that may be contributing to neuropathic pain producing widespread pain.

Differential diagnosis

Several conditions may produce symptoms which resemble, or otherwise mimic, those encountered in FM syndrome, including primary inflammatory muscle disease and collagen vascular disease. As can be appreciated from review of Table 47.4, comprehensive physical examination (including systematic motor and sensory examination), and judicious use of pertinent laboratory and imaging investigations, can help to distinguish FM from other diagnostic possibilities. However, the clinician should be aware that there can be considerable overlap between the features of several of these conditions and FM, and a given patient may have coexisting conditions.

Pharmacotherapy

In addition to non-steroidal anti-inflammatory drugs (NSAIDs) and/or cyclooxygenase-2 (COX-2) inhibitors, multiple concurrently administered medications are often required to address the multiple domains of FM, i.e., pain, sleep

Table 47.5 Pharmacotherapy treatment options for fibromyalgia

Class (subclass)	Examples	Adverse effects	Comments
Alpha-2-delta ligands	Pregabalin 150–450 mg/d Gabapentin 1200–2400 mg/d	Dizziness, somnolence, headache, weight gain, edema	No known drug interactions (pregabalin), minimal drug interactions (gabapentin); adjust dose in renal impairment
Antidepressants (serotonin–norepinephrine reuptake inhibitors)	Duloxetine 30–60 mg/d Milnacipran 50–100 mg b.i.d. Venlafaxine 150–225 mg/d	Nausea, dry mouth, insomnia, constipation, sweating, elevated blood pressure	Serotonin syndrome may arise with overdose or when co-administered with serotonergic agents, e.g., triptans, tramadol, monoamine oxidase inhibitors (MAOIs), etc.
Antidepressants (tricyclic antidepressants)	Amitriptyline 10–75 mg/hs Nortriptyline 10–50 mg/hs Desipramine 10–75 mg/hs	Anticholinergic side effects, sedation, orthostasis, weight gain, confusion in the elderly	Avoid if patients have significant cardiac disease; lethal if taken in overdose; risk of serotonin syndrome (as above)
Antidepressants (selective serotonin reuptake inhibitors)	Fluoxetine 20–60 mg/d Paroxetine 10–40 mg/d	Nausea, GI distress, tremor, sexual dysfunction	Limited usefulness in managing pain of FM, may be helpful in treating depression/anxiety
Muscle relaxants (TCA-like)	Cyclobenzaprine 10–40 mg/d	Anticholinergic side effects, sedation	Worsened anticholinergic effects if co-administered with TCAs
Muscle relaxants (alpha-2 agonist)	Tizanidine 4–12 mg/d	Dry mouth, hypotension, dizziness	Hypotension can be problematic; liver function tests need to be monitored every 3 months because of risk of hepatic injury
Dopamine agonists	Pramipexole 3–4.5 mg/d	Nausea, sedation, orthostasis, sleep attacks, hallucinations	Gradual dose increases are required to avoid adverse effects; often used to treat restless legs syndrome
Opioids	Tramadol 50–300 mg/d	Nausea, constipation, sedation, itching, sweating, increased seizure risk	Serotonin syndrome may arise with overdose or when co-administered with serotonergic agents (as above)

disturbances, psychological distress (depression and/or anxiety). A number of medications have been advocated for use (Table 47.5). There are very few data assessing the efficacy of combined pharmacological regimens to address these domains. Strategic polypharmacy may be contoured to the symptoms with which patients present. Psychoactive medications, e.g., antidepressants, may be useful for patients with signs and symptoms meeting diagnostic criteria for mood and/or anxiety disorders, and, carefully selected, these agents may have pain-mitigating effects. For example, low doses of tricyclic antidepressants (TCAs) such as amitriptyline have been demonstrated to improve symptoms of FM on a short-term basis, influencing pain, sleep, and fatigue, although they lack any influence on tender-point counts. Vigilance is required to ensure that drug interactions and potential toxicity arising from polypharmacy are avoided.

Medications that have received US Food and Drug Administration (FDA) approval for treatment of FM include the serotonin–norepinephrine reuptake inhibitors (SNRIs) duloxetine and milnacipran, and the alpha-2-delta ligand pregabalin. A meta-analysis suggested that these three medications do not differ with respect to efficacy, when based upon empirical investigations employing the criterion of producing at least 30% pain relief as compared to placebo. However, the analysis suggested that selection of which agent to employ for a given patient might be based upon the prevailing presenting symptoms. For example, duloxetine was superior to milnacipran and pregabalin with regard to improvement of depression, whereas milnacipran and pregabalin were superior to duloxetine with regard to improvement of fatigue. Duloxetine and pregabalin were more effective than milnacipran in managing sleep disturbances and pain. Drop-out rates due to adverse effects do not differ significantly among the three agents, but differences between their side-effect profiles do exist: e.g., headache and nausea were more likely to arise from use of duloxetine or milnacipran than from pregabalin; diarrhea may accompany the use of duloxetine more than either milnacipran or pregabalin.

In addition, there may be utility in ensuring that nutritional deficiencies be addressed, e.g., in the form of vitamin supplements and concerted efforts to improve nutritional intake. Long-term use of opioid analgesics or benzodiazepines has not received empirical support; concerns arise regarding the potential risks of misuse and dependence.

Non-pharmacologic approaches

Non-pharmacologic therapies recommended for use in patients afflicted with FM have frequently included educational programs (including the provision of educational materials and/or formal educational meetings), cognitive behavioral therapy (CBT), exercise, acupuncture, and massage therapy. Aerobic exercise programs reduce pain and improve functioning, e.g., endurance and capacity for activity. Pain exacerbations are possible during exercise, necessitating modifications in the intensity of the regimen; water aerobics may be an alternative treatment consideration. Patient education may be useful to educate patients about the illness, encourage adherence with exercise, enhance kinesthetic awareness, cultivate sleep hygiene techniques, and improve dietary intake to ensure nutritional needs. Because of the common comorbidity with psychological distress, patients may also benefit from psychotherapeutic modalities such as CBT to enhance coping and stress modulation. An extensive literature exists supporting the utility of interdisciplinary programs, e.g., exercise in combination with CBT and formal patient educational programs, in FM management.

Interventional procedures

Interventional approaches that have sometimes been advocated for FM patients include transcranial electrical stimulation, ultrasound, chiropractic treatment, massage therapy, and tender-point injections. There is some evidence to support the utility of transcranial electrical stimulation in alleviating overall pain, improvements of sleep, and overall quality of life, although accessibility to clinical settings in which transcranial electrical stimulation is available may be a limiting factor influencing the use of this modality. The extant literature has demonstrated inconsistent efficacy, as compared with placebo, of chiropractic treatment, massage therapy, and ultrasound therapy for FM.

There is anecdotal support for tender-point injections as a treatment modality for individuals failing to respond favorably to pharmacologic approaches and other conservative therapeutic measures. Although not currently approved for use by the FDA, the injection of minute quantities of botulinum toxin A directly into identifiable tender points, particularly within affected cervical spine muscles, may be effective in producing needed relief. However, further empirical evidence is required to identify the efficacy and adverse effects associated with botulinum toxin A injections in FM.

Follow-up

Periodic re-evaluation is necessary to determine continued efficacy of treatment interventions, to assess for and manage side effects, and to determine whether modifications in treatment approaches are required. In addition to employing a standard visual pain rating scale, use of full body figures which schematically represent tender points can be helpful to track changes in the progression of pain over time and assess the effectiveness of treatment approaches. It should be borne in mind that the number of tender points, and the pain intensity associated with them, is likely to vary over the course of the illness and should not be the sole basis upon which to base treatment efficacy. Consideration must also be given to follow-up of the patient's physical function, fatigue, and emotional well-being.

The Fibromyalgia Impact Questionnaire, a 20-item scale validated for use in FM, can be easily completed by patients at each visit and is a useful adjunct to assessment.

Failure to achieve improvements in pain severity and related domains of FM should prompt consideration of: (1) the accuracy of diagnosis and whether comorbid conditions ought to be worked-up; (2) whether alternative approaches should be undertaken; and (3) whether other factors, e.g., mood and sleep disturbances, ergonomic factors, nutritional deficiencies, and/or comorbid conditions, may be exacerbating or perpetuating pain.

Prognosis

FM is often a chronic condition; cure is elusive, and multimodal therapies are often necessary to address the multiplicity of symptoms with which patients present. The effects of FM can be enduring and particularly disabling if patients remain inadequately treated. Functional restoration may be possible when patients are regularly followed up and interdisciplinary approaches, combining symptom-based pharmacological and non-pharmacological therapies, are employed and tailored to the specific needs of the patient.

REFERENCES AND FURTHER READING

Bennett R. The Fibromyalgia Impact Questionnaire (FIQ): a review of its development, current version, operating characteristics and uses. *Clin Exp Rheumatol* 2005; **23** (5 Suppl 39): S154–62.

Busch A, Schachter CL, Peloso PM, Bombardier C. Exercise for treating fibromyalgia syndrome. [Update in Cochrane Database Syst Rev. 2007; (4): CD003786]. *Cochrane Database Syst Rev* 2002; (3): CD003786.

Crofford LJ, Clauw DJ. Fibromyalgia: where are we a decade after the American College of Rheumatology classification criteria were developed? *Arthritis Rheum* 2002; **46**: 1136–8.

Hauser W, Petzke F, Sommer C. Comparative efficacy and harms of duloxetine, milnacipran, and pregabalin in fibromyalgia syndrome. *J Pain* 2010; **11**: 505–21.

Jain AK, Carruthers BM, van de Sande MI, *et al.* Fibromyalgia syndrome: Canadian clinical working case definition, diagnostic and treatment protocols: a consensus document. *J Musculoskelet Pain* 2003; **11**: 3–107.

Staud R. Are tender point injections beneficial: the role of tonic nociception in fibromyalgia. *Curr Pharm Des* 2006; **12**: 23–7.

van Koulil S, Effting M, Kraaimaat FW, *et al.* Cognitive-behavioural therapies and exercise programmes for patients with fibromyalgia: state of the art and future directions. *Ann Rheum Dis* 2007; **66**: 571–81.

Wolfe F, Smythe HA, Yunus MB, *et al.* The American College of Rheumatology 1990 Criteria for the Classification of Fibromyalgia: report of the Multicenter Criteria Committee. *Arthritis Rheum* 1990; **33**: 160–72.

48

Pain in rheumatism

Clinical presentation

Musculoskeletal disease related to arthritis is a common cause of joint pain and dysfunction, leading to significant deficits in the functional capabilities of afflicted patients. Osteoarthritis (OA) is the most common form of arthritis resulting in disability among the elderly worldwide. Symptoms are most commonly encountered in persons between the ages of 40 and 50 years, and are most prevalent in women. OA can be idiopathic or secondary to other causes including trauma (e.g., meniscus tear), congenital abnormalities (e.g., acromegaly or Ehlers–Danlos syndrome), metabolic defects (e.g., hemochromatosis or Wilson's disease), post-infectious, and neuropathic. Risk factors for OA include advanced age, female gender, and a history of prior joint injury, such as from trauma incurred during athletic activities and accidents.

OA is characterized by pain, stiffness, swelling, and loss of mobility in one or more joints, brought on by inflammation and degeneration in joint structures such as cartilage, bone, and synovium. Although any joint can be affected, typically weight-bearing joints (hips, knees, low back, and ankles) are prone to OA. Unlike systemic inflammatory disorders, e.g., rheumatoid arthritis and systemic lupus erythematosus, OA is not characterized by extra-articular manifestations such as vasculitis or pericarditis, among others.

The pathology of OA follows a gradual progression, starting with the loss of cartilage matrix, which predisposes the affected joint to further injury. In the process of repairing the injury, chondrocyte activity may, in turn, set off a cascade of inflammatory processes which, over time, leads to progressive wear and tear on the cartilage and alterations to underlying bone, e.g., development of bony outgrowths (osteophytes) at the periphery of the affected joint. Often debris, cartilage, and bone degradation products occupy the joint space and synovial inflammation ensues, precipitated by the release of inflammatory mediators, i.e., cytokines and enzymes. Further cartilage damage and reactive bone formation occurs, and eventually, if unchecked, the affected joint may become dysfunctional.

Estimates suggest that approximately 1% of the population of the United States has rheumatoid arthritis (RA), predominantly affecting women. Although it can occur at any time, RA commonly presents in the second through fourth decades. Risk factors for RA include older age, female gender, a positive family history of RA, and cigarette smoking.

Unlike OA, RA is a systemic inflammatory (autoimmune) disease, producing a symmetric polyarthropathy. Commonly affected joints include the metacarpophalangeal (MCP) joints, the proximal interphalangeal (PIP) joints, knees, ankles, and metatarsophalangeal (MTP) joints. Often, the first manifestations of RA are in the lower extremities, among the weight-bearing joints. In contrast to OA, RA rarely affects the axial spine, except for the cervical spine. In addition, there are several potential extra-articular manifestations of the disorder complicating the patient's condition (Table 48.1).

Signs and symptoms

The pain in OA begins gradually in one or few joints. The pain is characterized as a deep ache that is worsened by movement or weight bearing, and alleviated by rest. As the disease progresses, pain can become constant. In addition to pain, there is restriction of movement. OA patients will complain of gelling and stiffness of the joint which typically lasts less than 30 minutes after awakening or a period of inactivity. Often patients experience crepitus, i.e., a grinding, clicking, or crunching sensation when the joint in question is moved. As the disease progresses, proliferation of cartilage, bone ligament, tendons, joint capsules, and synovium can, along with the joint effusion, produce the joint enlargement observable on physical examination. An altered gait may be present if weight-bearing joints are affected. With further progression, atrophy of the surrounding muscles may be apparent, and eventually flexion contractures may develop. On examination, the affected joints feel warm and swollen, and patients will report tenderness and pain with passive motion. Axial skeletal involvement, i.e., affecting the cervical or lumbar spine, may precipitate symptoms related to radiculopathy; however, this is generally uncommon, as the nerve roots and dorsal root ganglia are well protected.

Patients with RA will report an insidious onset of systemic symptoms such as low-grade fever, fatigue, myalgia, and weakness, with progressive joint involvement. The joints are symmetrically affected. In addition to joint pain, RA patients report morning stiffness, gelling, and fatigue. The pain is usually worse upon awakening or after a period of protracted inactivity. Frequently, RA patients will hold the affected joints in a flexed position to minimize pain. On examination, the affected joints appear red, boggy, and swollen. There may be a blue discoloration of the skin overlying the affected smaller joints, for example in the hands or feet, precipitated by venous congestion. The joints are warm on palpation, and tenderness is often experienced with palpation and passive motion. The muscles around the affected joints may be atrophied.

Table 48.1 Features distinguishing OA and RA

	Osteoarthritis	Rheumatoid arthritis
Pattern of joint involvement	One or more joints	Symmetric polyarthritis
Commonly affected joints	Distal interphalangeal (DIP) joints, proximal interphalangeal (PIP) joints, thumb carpometacarpal (CMC) joint, intervertebral discs and zygopophyseal joints, hips, knees, first metatarsophalangeal joint	PIP joints, metacarpophalangeal (MCP) joints, shoulders, elbows, hips, knees, ankles, metatarsophalangeal (MTP) joints
Other joint findings	Heberden's nodes (on DIP joints), Bouchard's nodes (on PIP joints)	Swan neck deformity, Boutonniere deformity, ulnar deviation
Extra-articular features	None	Low-grade fever, malaise, fatigue, weight loss, rheumatoid (subcutaneous) nodules on extensor surfaces or bony prominences, normochromic normocytic anemia
Systemic complications	None	Carpal tunnel syndrome and entrapment neuropathy, cervical spine C1–C2 instability, pericardial effusion, pleuritic chest pain, mononeuritis multiplex, vasculitis
Laboratory findings	Normal or elevated erythrocyte sedimentation rate (ESR)	Elevated ESR, positive rheumatoid factor, positive anticyclic citrullinated peptide antibody, elevated C-reactive protein, elevated alkaline phosphatase, normochromic anemia
Synovial fluid	Straw-colored, normal mucin clotting, < 2000 WBC/mm^3 with $< 25\%$ polymorphonuclear leukocytes, negative cultures, absence of crystals	Yellow, clots at room temperature, WBC 5000–25000/mm^3 with 85% polymorphonuclear leukocytes, negative cultures, absence of crystals
Radiographic findings	Joint space narrowing, subchondral bone sclerosis and cysts, osteophytes	Early: osteopenia; Late: narrowed joint spaces, joint margins display erosions, possible subluxations

Table 48.2 The American College of Rheumatology diagnostic criteria for RA

The presence of at least four of the following
(a) Morning stiffness $\geq$ 1 hour most mornings
(b) Observable soft tissue swelling affecting $\geq$ 3 joints
(c) Arthritis in proximal interphalangeal, metacarpophalangeal, or wrist joints
(d) Symmetric arthropathy
(e) Subcutaneous nodules
(f) Rheumatoid factor at a level > 95th percentile
(g) Radiological changes, e.g., erosions and/or periarticular osteopenia of hand or wrist joints

Note: Criteria a–d must be present for a minimum of 6 weeks
Adapted from Arnett *et al.* 1988.

Ultimately, the diagnosis of RA is a clinical one (Table 48.2). Patients present-ing with symmetrical joint pain, morning stiffness, and synovitis, especially of the proximal joints of the hands and feet, should raise the clinical suspicion of RA, although other arthropathies may be responsible for the above symptoms (see *Differential diagnosis*, below).

Laboratory tests and diagnostic investigations

Although the diagnosis of RA is essentially clinical, laboratory testing can be confirmatory. A high rheumatoid factor (RF) titer strongly suggests the diagnosis. However, approximately 30% of RA patients have a negative RF, and, conversely, RF can be positive in other disorders, as RF is an autoantibody-reflecting immune dysregulation. A serum anticyclic citrullinated peptide antibody test has been developed which demonstrates high sensitivity and speci-ficity for RA; it is often positive in early stages of RA and can herald disease onset. Other informative laboratory investigations for RA are summarized in Table 48.1. Of note, elevated C-reactive protein (CRP) levels and other acute-phase reactants can be a harbinger of cardiovascular disease accompanying RA. The normally clear, yellow, or straw-colored fluid tends to be turbid with reduced viscosity and predominant polymorphonuclear cells compared to that encountered in other arthropathies.

By contrast, laboratory investigations are not particularly useful in the diagnosis of OA, although negative tests effectively rule out other disorders. Thus, the erythrocyte sedimentation rate (ESR), a sensitive test for systemic inflam-mation, will be normal or only slightly elevated in OA. Additionally, other serological investigations tend to be negative or weakly positive. Synovial fluid analysis is helpful in that results tend to show a relatively non-inflammatory pattern (Table 48.1). Pending clinical findings, work-up for conditions giving rise to secondary OA is prudent, e.g., serum iron, total iron binding capacity, transferrin, and ferritin for suspected hemochromatosis, and serum copper and ceruloplasmin levels for possible Wilson's disease.

Imaging studies

Radiographs and MRI scanning can help in the diagnosis of RA, but erosions do not occur until the disease has progressed. RA erosions can be identified on radiography in 30% of patients within the first year of diagnosis, whereas bone erosions and joint space narrowing can be observable in as many as 90% within 3 years. MRI and ultrasonography may detect RA changes earlier than conventional radiographs. In OA, radiography typically reveals marginal osteophytes, joint space narrowing, bony sclerosis, and some cyst formation as well as malalignment.

Differential diagnosis

A number of arthritides must be considered in the differential diagnosis of OA and RA (Table 48.3). Although many of these conditions share some features in common with OA and RA, physical examination and laboratory and diagnostic assessments can clarify diagnosis and delineate whether alternative treatment approaches are warranted. Importantly, other conditions, such as myofascial pain and fibromyalgia, can co-occur and complicate these arthritic conditions.

Pharmacotherapy

Currently, there are no disease-modifying treatments available for OA. Nonsteroidal anti-inflammatory drugs (NSAIDs) and cyclooxygenase-2 (COX-2) inhibitors have been the mainstay of drug therapy for OA. Although these medications decrease pain, stiffness, and swelling, they do not alter the progression of OA. In fact, there is some evidence that certain NSAIDs, indomethacin and diclofenac, may lead to accelerated progression of disease. Acetaminophen is also useful to treat the pain associated with mild OA, but in patients with moderate to severe OA NSAIDs and COX-2 inhibitors appear to be comparatively more effective in improving pain. Tramadol is a centrally acting analgesic exerting weak opioid influences as well as serotonin–norepinephrine reuptake inhibition; however, it lacks anti-inflammatory properties. It is generally well tolerated, but in some patients there is an increased risk of seizures. Patients in whom NSAIDs, acetaminophen, and tramadol have proven ineffective may require opioid analgesia. Supplementation with chondroitin sulfate 800–1200 mg daily or glucosamine sulfate 1500 mg daily may be a consideration. Available over

Table 48.3 Arthropathies in the differential diagnosis of OA and RA

Arthritic condition	Distinguishing features
Gout	Usually monoarticular arthropathy commonly affecting the first metatarsophalangeal joint; synovial fluid analysis reveals monosodium urate crystals
Pseudogout	Polyarthropathy, usually affecting the knee and larger joints; synovial fluid analysis reveals rhomboid and rod-shaped weakly birefringent crystals on microscopy
Ankylosing spondylitis	Asymmetric polyarthritis; affecting axial skeleton and large joints; can result in cauda equina syndrome; radiographic findings suggest bamboo spine and sacroiliitis
Reactive arthritis	Asymmetric polyarthritis primarily affecting larger joints of the lower extremities; accompanied by constitutional symptoms, tendinitis, and mucocutaneous ulcers
Psoriatic arthritis	Asymmetric polyarthritis primarily affecting DIP joints of the fingers and toes; accompanied by psoriasis
Neurogenic arthropathy	Arthropathy related to impaired deep pain and proprioception leading to joint injury; early radiographic findings resemble OA; ligamentous laxity, muscular hypotonia, and small fractures can evolve
Infectious arthritis	Acute arthritis; related to bacterial (e.g., often *Staphylococcus* or *Neisseria gonorrhoeae*) or viral (e.g, parvoviris or hepatitis B) infection; synovial fluid reveals inflammatory signs
Polymyalgia rheumatica	Affects proximal joints of the extremities; associated with weakness and stiffness of pectoral and pelvic girdles; serology reveals markedly elevated erythrocyte sedimentation rate (ESR) and C-reactive protein level
Scleroderma	Joint pain accompanying sclerodactyly of the skin overlying fingers; telangiectasia; tendon calcinosis; esophageal dysfunction; Raynaud's syndrome
Sjögren's syndrome	Polyarthritis similar in features to RA; associated with dry conjunctivae and mucous membranes, lymphadenopathy, Raynaud's syndrome, vasculitis, glomerulonephritis, mononeuritis multiplex
Systemic lupus erythematosus	Polyarthropathy accompanied by constitutional symptoms, cutaneous symptoms; Raynaud's syndrome, pleurisy; nephritis; vasculitis; peri- and myocarditis
Ulcerative colitis and Crohn's disease	Acute, time-limited arthritis affecting one or two joints, usually knees and ankles; usually resolves without residual joint destruction

the counter, these agents are relatively inexpensive and have been shown to be effective in alleviating pain.

Anti-inflammatory medications, i.e., NSAIDs, COX-2 inhibitors and corticosteroids, can be useful in alleviating symptoms of RA but do not halt disease

Table 48.4 FDA-approved biologics employed for RA treatment

Agent	Target	Route	Dosing	Risks
Etanercept	TNF-alpha	SC	Weekly	Increased risk of infection
Infliximab	TNF-alpha	IV	Every 6–9 weeks	Infusion reactions; increased risk of infection and malignancy
Adalimumab	TNF-alpha	SC	Every 2 weeks	Increased risk of infection
Anakinra	IL-1	SC	Daily	Increased risk of infection
Rituximab	CD-20 on B lymphocytes	IV	Every 24 weeks	Infusion reactions; increased risk of infection
Abatacept	T lymphocytes	IV	Every 2–4 weeks	Infusion reactions; increased risk of infection and malignancy

TNF-alpha, tumor necrosis factor alpha; IL-1, interleukin-1; CD-20, cell-surface antigen; SC, subcutaneous; IV, intravenous.
Source: Leo & Romano 2011.

progression. Corticosteroids can be useful to address severe joint and systemic manifestations associated with RA, but must be employed cautiously in persons with hypertension, diabetes mellitus, peptic ulcer disease, or concurrent infections. As RA can progress rapidly, leading to significant joint destruction/deformity as well as extra-articular effects, early and aggressive treatment is warranted. Disease-modifying antirheumatic drugs (DMARDs), including methotrexate, azathioprine, leflunomide, and cyclosporine, as well as injectable and oral gold salts, used in addition to anti-inflammatory medications, have been shown to slow radiographic progression in patients with RA. Combinations of DMARDs have been shown to be more effective in suppressing RA activity than the use of one agent in isolation. Suboptimal response to combinations of anti-inflammatory medications and DMARDs should prompt the use of biologics (Table 48.4). These agents can be associated with an increased risk of serious infections and slightly increased risk of malignancy. The early use of biologics is indicated once a diagnosis of RA is established, but it is important to weigh the risks and benefits of treatment with biologics against the backdrop that undue hesitation may expose the patient to increased morbidity, given the aggressiveness of RA.

Non-pharmacologic approaches

Patient education is an essential component of comprehensive treatment. The provision of literature and/or educational programs can serve to demystify aspects of the disease and inform patients about how to actively participate in their treatment, and about activity modification, stress reduction, the need for physical therapy, assistive devices, counseling, and other healthcare resources. Exercise, land-based or aquatic, and progressive strength resistance training are essential for preserving joint mobility, maintaining flexibility, reducing the likelihood of muscle atrophy, and reducing deconditioning and pain.

Meta-analysis has suggested that other interventions, including therapeutic ultrasound, acupuncture, and electrical stimulation, may be adjunctive approaches to address pain. However, shortcomings in study design (sample sizes, adequacy of blinding, etc.) limit the degree to which definitive recommendations can be made concerning these modalities.

The psychological sequelae of OA and RA are extensive, and patients are therefore likely to derive benefits from psychological interventions such as cognitive behavioral therapy (CBT). Meta-analyses suggest that patients with arthritis treated with CBT, in comparison to no treatment or to standard treatment, demonstrate small, albeit statistically significant, post-treatment improvements in physical (perceived pain intensity, life interference from pain, health-related quality of life) and psychological functioning (depression severity). However, controversy attends the effectiveness of CBT over time, with studies suggesting that treatment effects are often unsustained at long-term follow-up.

Interventional procedures

If pharmacologic and non-pharmacologic treatments for OA are suboptimal, interventional approaches may be necessary. Intra-articular injection with a corticosteroid and local anesthetic mixture can be quite effective in providing temporary pain relief in an affected joint, even though there is no benefit in terms of halting disease progression. In OA, hyaluronic acids that are normally present within the joint space are degraded, and no longer provide the customary shock absorption and lubrication functions that they previously did. Intra-articular hyaluronan supplementation can be used to help replenish and restore normal joint function. Although viscosupplementation with hyaluronans is indicated for knee osteoarthritis, they can, in principle, be employed in any OA-affected joint. The hyaluronans have a good safety profile – for example, they do not raise blood sugar or adversely affect cartilage or surrounding joint structures, as is often encountered with intra-articular corticosteroid injections – and some evidence suggests that hyaluronans can promote normal cartilage growth. For RA, intra-articular injections of depot corticosteroids or triamcinolone hexacetonide may mitigate joint pain.

Surgical interventions are available for patients with OA and RA, intended to relieve pain, improve joint mobility, and improve the patient's functional capabilities. Arthroscopic synovectomy can be employed to produce short-term relief by removing debris and inflamed synovial tissue. The most definitive improvements generally require conventional surgical procedures including osteotomy, hip resurfacing, partial joint replacement, and complete joint replacement for

OA, and joint replacement and possible tendon reconstruction for RA. Post-operatively, participation in an extensive rehabilitation program is essential to increase the likelihood of achieving optimal results.

Follow-up

Regular medical care is necessary to monitor the course of arthritic conditions. Treatment endeavors must be focused on mitigation of pain and maintaining the functional capabilities of afflicted patients. It is necessary to determine the effectiveness and adverse effects of medication and other treatment interventions, such as osteoporosis resulting from long-term corticosteroid use. Patients with RA are especially prone to develop complications with disease progression, such as entrapment neuropathies (e.g., carpal tunnel syndrome), mononeuritis multiplex, cervical spine instability, vasculitic conditions, and cardiac complications. The development of these complications may warrant modifications in treatment and integrated multidisciplinary care.

Prognosis

The clinical course for both OA and RA can be variable. Generally, OA has a progressive course; however, it can stabilize, and in rare cases reverse. The degree of progression will depend on which joints are involved and the presence of comorbidities. Hence, for example, advanced age, high body mass index, and varus deformity may predict worse prognosis for those with knee OA. Although OA is not a systemic inflammatory disorder (i.e., it lacks extra-articular manifestations), it can nonetheless produce significant pain and disability.

Similarly, some patients with RA may go into remission, while at the other extreme some remain refractory to all interventions. However, most patients have a progressive course with remissions and relapses yet can glean some response to treatment. Poor outcomes are likely to be associated with early development of polyarthropathies and subcutaneous nodules, low functional status at disease onset, and high serological levels of ESR, CRP, and RF. Due to its aggressive nature and pernicious systemic effects, RA is associated with significant mortality.

REFERENCES AND FURTHER READING

Altman R, Asch E, Bloch D, *et al.* Development of criteria for the classification and reporting of osteoarthritis. Classification of osteoarthritis of the knee. Diagnostic and Therapeutic Criteria Committee of the American Rheumatism Association. *Arthritis Rheum* 1986; **29**: 1039–49.

American College of Rheumatology Subcommittee on Osteoarthritis Guidelines. Recommendations for the medical management of osteoarthritis of the hip and knee: 2000 update. American College of Rheumatology Subcommittee on Osteoarthritis Guidelines. *Arthritis Rheum* 2000; **43**: 1905–15.

Arnett F, Edwardworthy S, Bloch D, *et al.* The American Rheumatism Association 1987 revised criteria for the classification of rheumatoid arthritis. *Arthritis Rheum* 1988; **31**: 315–24.

Astin JA, Beckner W, Soeken K, Hochberg MC, Berman B. Psychological interventions for rheumatoid arthritis: A meta-analysis of randomized controlled trials. *Arthritis Rheum* 2002; **47**: 291–302.

Carmona L, Cross M, Williams B, Lassere M, March L. Rheumatoid arthritis. *Best Pract Res Clin Rheumatol* 2010; **24**: 733–45.

Leo RJ, Romano TJ. Management of pain in arthritis. In Ebert MH, Kerns RD, eds., *Behavioral and Psychopharmacologic Pain Management*. Cambridge: Cambridge University Press; 2011; pp. 307–27.

49

Herpes zoster and post-herpetic neuralgia

Clinical presentation

Herpes zoster (HZ) affects 15–20% of the US population, and these numbers are projected to increase as the population ages. Since it occurs more commonly in older and immunocompromised persons, it is estimated that 50% of those who reach age 85 will develop HZ, or "shingles." The illness is caused by reactivation of varicella zoster virus (VZV), which remains dormant in dorsal root ganglia or cranial sensory nerves of the host for decades after the initial infection that caused chickenpox (varicella).

Pain and a characteristic vesicular rash in a dermatomal distribution signal nervous system and integumentary tissue involvement by the recrudescent VZV infection that is HZ. Of equal concern, and the primary target of prevention, is post-herpetic neuralgia (PHN).

HZ pain has been variously defined as acute herpetic neuralgia (pain within 30 days of rash onset), subacute herpetic neuralgia (30–120 days after rash onset) and PHN (pain lasting at least 120 days after rash healing). Second only to painful diabetic peripheral neuropathy as causative of neuropathic pain, PHN is a debilitating condition with significant impact on physical function and quality of life.

The patient complaining of sudden onset of inexplicable aching or shooting pain or dysesthesia (burning, tingling, itching, or numbness) presents the clinician with an opportunity for early intervention when this is correctly recognized as the prodrome to HZ. A prodrome of pain or dysesthesia in a specific dermatomal (< 3 dermatomes) or disseminated (≥ 3 dermatomes) distribution usually precedes the rash within 48–72 hours.

Unfortunately, in most cases, by the time the patient seeks care the characteristic rash is evident, making early intervention less likely. The rash consists of maculopapular lesions which develop into fluid-filled vesicles that appear over 5–7 days. Pustules form during days 4–6, followed by scabbing and cutaneous healing, usually within 2–4 weeks of initial presentation.

As noted above, VZV has potential to cause two illnesses: chickenpox and, years or decades later, HZ. Despite the introduction in 1995 of a varicella vaccine, virtually every long-standing adult resident of the USA has had chickenpox exposure or clinical infection. HZ occurs when an individual's cell-mediated immunity to VZV drops below a critical threshold, as noted in 1965 by Hope-Simpson.

Decreased VZV-specific cell-mediated immunity occurs naturally with aging and also may result from stress, steroids, or immunosuppressive drugs. Chickenpox is accompanied by upper respiratory symptoms and a maculopapular, vesicular rash widely disseminated over the body, while the characteristic dermatomal presentation of HZ reflects the neuronal damage caused by reactivated virus in dorsal root ganglia associated with specific spinal segments.

Signs and symptoms

Reactivation of VZV in the sensory ganglia and peripheral nerves causes a cellular immune response which results in neuronal inflammation and destruction; damaged nerve tissue is the precursor for development of PHN. In rare instances, a patient will complain of neuralgia in a dermatomal distribution in the absence of rash, a condition known as *zoster sine exanthema* or *zoster sine herpete*.

Complications and sequelae of HZ are related to the dermatomal location and severity of infection. They include neurologic (PHN, motor neuropathy, cranial nerve palsy, encephalitis, transverse myelitis); cutaneous (bacterial superinfection, scarring or disfigurement); ophthalmic (stromal keratitis, iritis, visual impairment, retinitis, episcleritis, keratopathy); and visceral (pneumonitis, hepatitis) sequelae.

Occurrence of central nervous as well as peripheral nervous system sequelae bespeaks VZV's retrograde and anterograde pathologic reach. The reactivated VZV may migrate proximally into the spinal cord and CNS as well as distally into visceral, muscle, and cutaneous tissue along the path of the affected nerve roots.

Patients who present with cranial nerve involvement and/or ophthalmic zoster must immediately be started on antiviral therapy; the latter must be referred for urgent ophthalmologic evaluation. Ramsay Hunt syndrome is an eponym describing HZ infection that affects the facial nerve near one of the ears. In addition to painful rash, Ramsay Hunt syndrome can cause facial nerve paralysis and hearing loss in the affected ear.

Patients with HZ affecting cranial nerves or who present with CNS symptoms may require hospitalization for intravenous medications. They should receive immediate antiviral therapy and appropriate referrals for urgent specialized care.

PHN is the most common long-term complication of HZ, occurring in approximately 30% of patients, with higher prevalence in older individuals. PHN is pathologically distinct from the acute (inflammatory) pain of HZ, and is thought to be caused by long-term (neuropathic) changes in affected neurons, an observation supported by postmortem studies of affected individuals. As already noted, HZ pathophysiology includes peripheral and/or central nerve damage.

Peripheral sensitization occurs during the acute phase of infection: nociceptors activated during tissue injury cause ongoing neuronal discharge and hyperexcitability. Deafferentation (destruction of nerve fibers due to necrosis and scarring from VZV infection) and peripheral and central demyelination (destruction of the myelin sheath) can occur, both of which result in neuropathic pain.

Central sensitization is the process by which the CNS undergoes reactive organizational changes with subsequent abnormal sensory processing. Alterations in nerve signaling and neurotransmitter activity cause long-term changes in activation thresholds, nervous system organization, and responses to painful stimuli. The aberrant CNS responds with worsening pain, creating the substrate for prolonged post-herpetic neuropathic pain. Risk factors for the development of PHN include advanced age, female gender, the presence of a painful prodrome, and the severity of acute pain and rash.

Evaluation of PHN should include an accurate patient history with attention to the quality and intensity of the pain symptoms, and a physical examination utilizing simple neurologic tests such as applying light touch, cold, or heat to test for allodynia or sensory deficit; pinprick to test for hyperesthesia; and applying pressure to test for mechanical hyperalgesia. Patients with unusual presentations and those in need of more complex neurological exams should be referred to a neurologist.

Laboratory tests and diagnostic investigations

The diagnosis of acute HZ infection is based on the above clinical findings. No laboratory tests or imaging studies are required, although immunoassays (IFA, EIA), serology (enzyme-linked immunosorbent assay, ELISA), viral culture, and polymerase chain reaction (PCR) are available for confirmation of infection.

Differential diagnosis

The differential diagnosis of HZ includes bullous contact dermatitis, bullous pemphigoid, and herpes simplex virus (HSV) 1 or 2. Features that may distinguish HSV from HZ are multiple recurrences around the mouth or genital area and the absence of chronic pain. Less commonly, erythema exudativum multiforme and disseminated molluscum contagiosum may be confused with HZ.

A rare, poorly defined entity is zosteriform metastasis, characterized by cutaneous vesicobullous, popular, and nodular lesions distributed along dermatomes.

Zoster sine exanthema may be mistaken for myocardial ischemia, pulmonary embolism, cholecystits, renal colic, or other diagnoses having a dermatomal pattern of pain distribution.

Pharmacotherapy

The treatment goals for acute HZ are to reduce pain, promote rash healing, prevent secondary infection, and reduce or prevent PHN. Antiviral therapy (aciclovir, famciclovir, or valaciclovir) shortens the acute illness period when administered in the first 72 hours of symptom onset. Prompt treatment of HZ with antivirals and appropriate medications for pain is also believed to reduce the risk for PHN. Corticosteroids in the acute phase of illness may reduce pain and speed resolution of the rash, but their use remains controversial. Topical corticosteroids should be given only on the advice of an ophthalmologist to patients with ophthalmic zoster. Opioid analgesics and anticonvulsants, which are the mainstay of treatment for PHN, also have efficacy in treatment of acute HZ pain.

No single treatment relieves PHN in all affected individuals; it is often difficult to treat, debilitating to patients, and frustrating for clinicians. Treatment for PHN focuses on alleviation or reduction of pain and improvement in quality of life, including pharmacological, non-pharmacological, complementary and alternative medicine (CAM), and interventional modalities. Antiepileptic drugs, antidepressants, and opioid analgesics are initial treatment options. Topical treatments may be of help after complete healing of the rash has occurred, but their use is limited to intact skin. Interventional treatments, such as epidural injections of corticosteroids and local anesthetic drugs, have an effect on acute HZ pain but are of limited use in preventing PHN.

Administration of commonly used analgesics such as acetaminophen and non-steroidal anti-inflammatory drugs (NSAIDs) including salicylates and cyclooxygenase-2 (COX-2) inhibitors has not been shown to be effective for PHN. Antiepileptic drugs have demonstrated efficacy in treating PHN, including the newer drugs gabapentin and pregabalin, as well as carbamazepine, phenytoin, and valproic acid. Gabapentin and pregabalin are approved by the US Food and Drug Administration (FDA) for treatment of PHN; they bind to the alpha-2-delta subunit of voltage-dependent sodium channels to cause reduction in sodium ion flux. Older antiepileptics such as carbamazepine have been used extensively in the treatment of diabetic neuropathy and trigeminal neuralgia; they also modulate CNS activity by inhibiting voltage-gated ion channel activity. The side-effect profile of older antiepileptic medications (e.g., anticholinergic effects, cardiotoxicity) may limit their use in older individuals. All medications in this class can cause dizziness, drowsiness, and fatigue, but tolerance to these side effects develops with continued use.

Tricyclic antidepressants (TCAs) inhibit the reuptake and increase concentration of serotonin, norepinephrine, and dopamine. They have established efficacy against neuropathic pain, but their use is also limited in older persons due to anticholinergic side effects. The newer serotonin–norepinephrine reuptake inhibitors (SNRIs), venlafaxine and duloxetine, have greater selectivity for serotonin and norepinephrine and generally better side-effect profiles. Duloxetine is FDA-approved for management of diabetic peripheral neuropathic pain and fibromyalgia.

Opioids act as ligands at specific opioid receptors in the central and peripheral nervous system and other tissues, and have been shown to be effective in treating PHN. There are a number of effective opioid medications available for treatment of PHN whose use may be limited by side effects such as constipation and sedation. Since PHN is a persistent problem which will require long-term treatment (possibly for months), patients treated with opioids must be assessed for their risk of misuse, abuse, addiction, or diversion.

Please see Chapter 63 for further discussion of opioid tolerance, dependence, and addiction. Clinicians must seek a balance between pain relief and patient safety. The Federation of State Medical Boards and other agencies have developed policies on prescribing controlled substances including risk management plans that respond to adverse outcomes, which clinicians may find useful. FDA-mandated Risk Evaluation and Mitigation Strategies (REMS) may be required for the use of certain opioid analgesics.

Topical treatment options include capsaicin cream, available over-the-counter for treatment of PHN and arthritis pain. Capsaicin inhibits the release of substance P from cutaneous nerve endings. Pain or allergic reaction at the application site may occur. Topical lidocaine is also available, both as gel and patch formulations; the lidocaine 5% patch was the first FDA-approved medication specifically for PHN. Lidocaine is believed to affect PHN through high-affinity binding and local inhibition of abnormal sodium channels that result from neuronal damage. Side effects from the patch are rash or allergic reaction at the application site.

Non-pharmacologic approaches

Physical and occupational therapy have documented utility as part of comprehensive treatment of PHN to prevent loss of physical function. Cognitive behavioral therapy (CBT) may also be useful for patients who have pain that is resistant to treatment. Other options, which currently lack evidence-based recommendations, include transcutaneous electrical nerve stimulation (TENS) and complementary and alternative medicine (CAM) techniques. A TENS unit delivers pulsed electrical current across intact skin to underlying nerves and has been used as an alternative treatment for PHN; some studies show evidence for its use in neuropathic pain.

CAM techniques include acupuncture, ultrasound treatments, therapeutic massage, herbal supplements, magnet therapy, and thermal techniques, many of which are currently undergoing trials to assess their clinical efficacy. There is insufficient evidence to recommend for or against their use in the treatment of PHN.

Prevention

A one-dose live, attenuated vaccine designed to boost cell-mediated immunity to VZV was licensed by the FDA in 2006, based on the results of the Shingles

Prevention Study (SPS). The Advisory Committee on Immunization Practices of the Centers for Disease Control and Prevention (CDC) recently expanded its guidelines to recommend HZ immunization for all individuals aged 50 years or older. The SPS demonstrated reduced morbidity from HZ and PHN in adults $\geq$ 60 years of age with significant reductions (61%) in the burden of illness (reduced severity of pain and rash) and incidence of infection (51%). It also showed significantly lower (67%) incidence of PHN in the vaccine treatment group compared with placebo, with continuing efficacy in an SPS subgroup followed for 7 years.

Interventional procedures

Invasive procedures are not first-line treatment for PHN but may be useful for blocking autonomic nerve pathways and temporarily "turning off" sympathetic innervation to a region. Options include sympathetic nerve block, stellate ganglion block, peripheral nerve, epidural, or plexus block, neurolysis, and ablation.

Follow-up

Treatment of PHN requires an ongoing physician–patient interaction that includes pain assessment, evaluation of treatment options, and adjustment of treatment modalities as indicated. Assessment of pain is a mainstay for treatment of PHN, enabling the clinician to gauge the effect of various therapies and the patient to note progress toward return of function and improved quality of life. The Short-Form McGill Pain Questionnaire is a well-validated self-report questionnaire that uses selected questions from the longer McGill Pain Questionnaire in addition to the Present Pain Intensity (PPI) index and Visual Analog Scale (VAS). The Neuropathic Pain Scale specifically assesses features of neuropathic pain. The Zoster Brief Pain Inventory, which assesses health-related quality-of-life measures such as general activity, mood, walking, work, relations with others, sleep, and enjoyment of life, was specifically developed to assess the pain associated with acute HZ and PHN. Clinicians may utilize one or more of these assessment tools as part of the diagnostic and treatment process for patients with HZ.

Prognosis

The natural course of HZ infection is generally favorable, with symptoms subsiding within several weeks to months. The prognosis is worse for individuals with CNS or visceral involvement and for those who develop PHN. Development of PHN is related to the location and extent of the rash, the number and severity of the lesions, and the amount of prodromal pain and acute herpetic neuralgia during the course of the rash. With the advent of HZ immunization, it is hoped that the incidence of this debilitating disease will be lessened.

REFERENCES AND FURTHER READING

Fields HL, Rowbotham M, Baron R. Postherpetic neuralgia: irritable nociceptors and deafferentation. *Neurobiol Dis* 1998; **5**: 206–27.

Levin MJ, Oxman MN, Zhang JH, *et al.* Varicella-zoster virus-specific immune responses in elderly recipients of a herpes zoster vaccine. *J Infect Dis* 2008; **197**: 825–35.

Oxman MN, Levin MJ, Johnson GR, *et al.* A vaccine to prevent herpes zoster and postherpetic neuralgia in older adults. *N Engl J Med* 2005; **352**: 2271–84.

Sanford M, Keating GM. Zoster vaccine (Zostavax): a review of its use in preventing herpes zoster and postherpetic neuralgia in older adults. *Drugs Aging* 2010; **27**: 159–76.

Schmader K. Herpes zoster and postherpetic neuralgia in older adults. *Clin Geriatr Med* 2007; **23**: 615–32.

Schmader K, Sloane R, Pieper C, *et al.* The impact of acute herpes zoster pain and discomfort on functional status and quality of life in older adults. *Clin J Pain* 2007; **23**: 490–6.

Volpi A, Gross G, Hercogova J, Johnson RW. Current management of herpes zoster: the European view. *Am J Clin Dermatol* 2005; **6**: 317–25.

50

Complex regional pain syndrome I (RSD) and II (causalgia)

Clinical presentation

Complex regional pain syndrome (CRPS) is the term used to describe a medical disorder with onset most often following an injury or trauma characterized by pain, vasomotor instability, reduced joint range of motion, swelling, trophic skin changes, and patchy bone demineralization. It may also follow a stroke or other vascular event such as a myocardial infarction. Often confusing is the fact that CRPS, a recently adopted term, has been preceded by numerous other previously used terms including reflex sympathetic dystrophy, causalgia, Sudeck's atrophy, shoulder–hand syndrome, and many others. In an attempt to reduce the number of terms used to describe these disorders, a consensus development panel suggested CRPS as the new term to be used. Unfortunately, the taxonomy can remain confusing at times.

There are two recognized forms of CRPS:
- CRPS type 1, previously referred to as reflex sympathetic dystrophy (RSD), is more common than type 2 and accounts for 90% of CRPS patients. No definitive nerve lesion as traditionally defined is present in CRPS type 1.
- CRPS type 2, previously referred to as causalgia, is associated with a definite nerve lesion.

The term *sympathetically maintained pain* (SMP) is *not* interchangeable with CRPS types I and II; it is used when it has been determined that the sympathetic nervous system is partially or completely contributing to the mechanism of the pain. SMP may or may not be present in patients with CRPS type 1 or 2, as well as in additional disorders such as post-herpetic neuralgia and others. The exact pathophysiology of CRPS is uncertain; however, most hypotheses suggest both peripheral and CNS factors that initiate and maintain this syndrome. Recent studies suggest that genetic factors may play a role in the development of CRPS.

CRPS presents initially as a localized/regional pain and sensory disorder associated with autonomic changes most often following an injury or traumatic event. Included among the reported initiating events are fractures, soft tissue injury, myocardial infarction, stroke, arthroscopic procedures of the knee, routine phlebotomy, and placement of a hemodialysis arteriovenous graft. Notably, the symptoms and especially the pain are of severity greater than that expected following the inciting event. The pain is frequently experienced concurrent with changes in skin color, edema, temperature change, or abnormal sudomotor activity. Many reports have emphasized that significant stress is present at the time of onset, and many feel that this may play an import pathogenetic role in the development of CRPS.

Signs and symptoms

CRPS commonly affects the extremities; however, it is uncommon for an individual patient to have all four limbs affected simultaneously. "Spread" of the signs and symptoms of CRPS from one limb to another has been reported, and the mechanism(s) underlying this is under active investigation. Autonomic abnormalities are common, including skin discoloration, abnormal sweating and hair growth, changes in urinary function including urgency, frequency, retention, or incontinence, and skin temperature changes. These being noted, the exact role of the sympathetic nervous system in producing all of the pain-associated and varied manifestations of CRPS is uncertain. The presentation of CRPS is frequently associated with myofascial trigger points as well.

The course of CRPS is often divided into three clinical stages, although not all agree about categorizing CRPS in this manner. Nevertheless, when seeing a patient with CRPS, it may be helpful to consider this approach.

- During **stage 1**, pain develops in the affected area, most often a limb. Aching, burning, allodynia, temperature sensitivity, edema in the involved region, and changes in skin temperature and color may occur.
- During **stage 2**, more soft tissue edema may be accompanied by shiny skin and thickening of the skin and soft tissues around affected joints.
- During **stage 3**, increasingly severe clinical findings may include dramatic reductions in joint range of motion leading to joint contractures as well as radiographic findings suggesting notable bone demineralization and trophic skin changes.

Early recognition of the signs and symptoms of CRPS can be challenging, partly because many injuries, such as an ankle sprain, may be associated with edema, skin hypersensitivity, and other similar complaints acutely. In the setting of an acute injury, trauma, or other condition known to be associated with CRPS as described above, one must be aware of the potential for the development of CRPS and recognize such when evaluating patients, who may complain of non-specific burning and aching pain even in the absence of objective findings. Keep in mind that most evidence supports that CRPS is optimally treated when the diagnosis is made earlier in its course, and that CRPS is primarily a clinical diagnosis.

Laboratory tests and diagnostic investigations

While there are no definitive blood tests that can be ordered to make the diagnosis of CRPS, blood work to rule out various forms of inflammatory arthropathies, vasculitis, connective tissue diseases, and certain infections known to be associated with joint complaints should be strongly considered by the clinician evaluating the patient with suspected CRPS. Autonomic testing, including measuring skin temperature and sweat production, may be helpful not only to assist in making the diagnosis but also in predicting who is likely to respond to sympathetic blockade as a treatment.

Electrophysiological testing, in the form of electromyography (EMG) and nerve conduction studies (NCS), may be helpful in selected patients in whom, after a detailed history and physical examination has been completed, the possibility of a major nerve injury has been raised. Keep in mind that the NCS examination is an examination of large myelinated nerve fiber function, and that pain and temperature sensation are subserved by small or unmyelinated nerve fibers, and consequently a "normal" NCS does not in any way rule out CRPS type 1.

Growing use of the results of 3 mm skin biopsy analysis for CRPS diagnostic purposes may prove to be a generally helpful diagnostic approach. Many pain specialists advocate the use of regional or intravenous sympathetic blocks (stellate ganglion, lumbar sympathetic, Bier) for both diagnostic and therapeutic reasons. The clinician must keep in mind that not all pain associated with CRPS is likely to be sympathetically maintained, and thus it may not be completely responsive to sympathetically directed therapies.

Imaging studies

Bone scintigraphy used in the acute stage of CRPS may reveal increased uptake in the region of peripheral joints of the involved extremity. Compared with plain radiography, scintigraphy is more sensitive and specific in early CRPS. Multiple studies support the use of triple-phase bone scan to help make the diagnosis of CRPS type 1.

Plain radiography may demonstrate osteopenia. Other less common x-ray findings include joint destruction, degenerative changes, and evidence of new bone formation. Plain radiographs of the involved extremities may show extensive demineralization, especially beyond the acute stage. MRI may be abnormal both acutely and in chronic settings of CRPS. Although CT scans may demonstrate osteoporotic changes in patients with CRPS, it is not clear if this is a more effective imaging tool than plain x-ray or scintigraphy for CRPS.

Differential diagnosis

Undoubtedly, early in the course of CRPS, there may be a number of other clinical disorders with overlapping and somewhat similar complaints to consider, including skin infection, peripheral vascular disease, deep venous thrombosis, cervical nerve root impingement, vasculitis, angioedema, progressive systemic sclerosis, rheumatoid arthritis, thoracic outlet syndrome disuse atrophy, Pancoast syndrome, various types of painful peripheral neuropathy, and conversion disorder.

However, a thorough history and detailed physical examination often helps to make an accurate diagnosis. For example, early in the course of CRPS patients may experience burning pain, various other abnormal sensations, and altered skin temperature, each of which may aid in making the diagnosis of CRPS.

Pharmacotherapy

CRPS appears to be most effectively managed when treated in a multimodal manner. Most would agree that the most effective approach to the management of CRPS is prevention. Measures that can be used in an attempt to accomplish this include early mobilization through passive and active strategies appropriate for the specific patient and use of vitamin C supplementation after fractures. Non-pharmacologic as well as interventional procedures may be utilized alongside pharmacologic therapies in order to achieve optimal patient outcomes.

Regrettably, very few medical therapies have been studied appropriately in patients with CRPS. There are a few medications that have been well studied, including various anticonvulsants such as gabapentin and pregabalin, nasal calcitonin, oral steroids, and the bisphosphonates. There are several published guidelines for the pharmacologic management of neuropathic pain in general, and these generally recommend tricyclic antidepressant (TCA) medications such as nortriptyline, doxepin, or amitriptyline as first-line therapy for neuropathic pain.

Consensus guidelines developed by a panel of providers/academicians with significant experience of treating CRPS suggest using non-steroidal anti-inflammatory drugs (NSAIDs) for some patients and opioid analgesics for those with severe pain. Please keep in mind that this is a consensus-based and not a clinical-trial-based set of recommendations.

Topical therapies, including topical lidocaine and capsaicin, may be of some help to certain patients. There are mixed data concerning the use of clonidine for CRPS.

Ketamine intravenous infusions are administered in certain centers and are being increasingly considered and studied as a potential treatment of CRPS for refractory patients. Intravenous immunoglobulin infusion (IVIG) is also being actively studied.

Non-pharmacologic approaches

Early referral to a physical and/or occupational therapist should be considered, not only to help with mobilization (as appropriate) of the affected areas but also for protective reasons. Not infrequently, the benefit of pharmacotherapy and/or interventional approaches can be enhanced through the implementation of an effective rehabilitation program. This can also include the use of mirror therapy. Experience suggests that such treatment is more helpful if initiated as soon as the diagnosis is established and hopefully before signs of chronic CRPS such as bony and skin changes are present.

Prompt and assertive early referral to an interventional pain specialist for appropriate pain management interventions such as nerve blocks may not only result in pain reduction but also allow CRPS patients to participate in an aggressive physical therapy program.

Experience also suggests that a patient with CRPS who understands more about the condition may be more willing to more vigorously participate in these therapies, as opposed to more passively receiving medical and interventional therapies.

At some point in the course of CRPS, many patients will benefit from – and some frankly require – evaluation and treatment by a behavioral health provider to address depression and anxiety, to learn stress management techniques, and to help optimize interpersonal relationships. Cognitive behavioral therapy (CBT) approaches may also be helpful, through guided imagery for example, in managing the pain associated with CRPS.

Tobacco use, specifically cigarette smoking, is a risk factor for the development of CRPS. This needs to be communicated to the patient with CRPS, and smoking cessation approaches should be implemented whenever possible.

Interventional procedures

The clinician should consider interventional approaches early in the course of CRPS, and especially if the patient is not responding to non-interventional therapies. Sympathetic ganglion block with local anesthetics, intravenous lidocaine, and/or phentolamine infusions may serve as diagnostic and/or therapeutic interventions for some patients with CRPS. Patients who respond to stellate ganglion blocks are said to have sympathetically maintained pain, and these tend to be more helpful earlier in the course of CRPS. Concurrent myofascial trigger points may be present, and these may be treated not only with physical rehabilitation but also with trigger-point injections.

Regional anesthetic procedures such as Bier blocks have not been shown to be of long-term benefit for most patients with CRPS. Epidural clonidine has been utilized as well.

Peripheral as well as spinal stimulation is increasingly utilized for the treatment of CRPS and might be considered when more conservative treatment measures have failed to help the patient.

Intrathecal use of baclofen (if increased muscle tone or dystonia is prominent), opioid and the non-opioid analgesic, or ziconotide may be considered for those patients with particularly severe pain.

Sympathectomy has been performed on many patients with CRPS, but there are no long-term data to highlight who is most likely to respond; nor have there been any high-quality controlled studies. Furthermore, the premise of performing this procedure is that the pain and other symptoms of CRPS are sympathetically maintained, and this is clearly not true for many patients with CRPS.

Follow-up

The treatment of CRPS is a very active and individualized process that will require regular follow-up by the healthcare provider coordinating and performing the treatment.

Prognosis

Few patients with CRPS are cured. Thus, relapse following treatment and the need for ongoing treatment monitoring is to be expected for many.

REFERENCES AND FURTHER READING

Allen G, Galer BS, Schwartz L. Epidemiology of complex regional pain syndrome: a retrospective chart review of 134 patients. *Pain* 1999; **80**: 539–44.

Kemler MA, Barendese GA, van Kleef M, *et al.* Spinal cord stimulation in patients with chronic reflex sympathetic dystrophy. *N Engl J Med* 2000; **343**: 618–24.

Moseley GL. Graded motor imagery for pathologic pain: a randomized controlled trial. *Neurology* 2006; **67**: 2129–34.

Stanton-Hicks M. Complex regional pain syndrome: manifestations and the role of neurostimulation in its management. *J Pain Symptom Manage* 2006; **31**: S20–4.

Stanton-Hicks MD, Burton AW, Bruehl SP, *et al.* An updated interdisciplinary clinical pathway for CRPS: report of an expert panel. *Pain Pract* 2002; **2**: 1–16.

51

Painful polyneuropathy

Clinical presentation

Polyneuropathy is a cause of significant pain and disability. Neuropathy refers to damage to a nerve or group of nerves resulting in loss of movement, sensation, or other function; the damage may be due to infection, disease, trauma, nutritional deficiency, or drugs. This review focuses on polyneuropathy (involvement of several nerve groups) syndromes that cause pain and/or paresthesia.

Polyneuropathy occurs symmetrically or asymmetrically, related to length (distal or proximal), and affects predominantly small-diameter or large-diameter sensory nerve fibers. Small sensory nerve fibers in the skin and viscera, such as C and A-delta fibers, transmit thermal and nociceptive stimuli, while large sensory nerves in muscles, joints, and tendons are responsible for proprioception. Both large- and small-diameter sensory nerve fibers may sustain damage that results in neuropathy, but since nociceptive function is generally controlled by the latter, many painful polyneuropathy syndromes are of the small-fiber type.

Neuropathic pain has many manifestations including paresthesia (a sensation of burning, "pins and needles" or prickling, itching, or tingling, with no apparent physical cause), hyperpathia (intense pain with repetitive stimuli), hyperalgesia (exacerbated pain produced by noxious stimulus), allodynia (non-noxious stimulus perceived as painful), phantom pain (pain in a part that has been surgically or traumatically removed or congenitally absent; it has been noted that congenital amputees have a very low rate of phantom limb pain as compared with traumatic amputees), or stimulus-evoked pain (pain elicited by stimulus after damage to sensory neurons). The experience of paresthesia may be illustrated by the common scenario of having one's foot "fall asleep," resulting in an irritating, tingling, or burning feeling that resolves spontaneously.

There are many potential causes for painful polyneuropathy, including: infections such as human immunodeficiency virus (HIV), Lyme disease (neuroborreliosis), or herpes zoster virus (shingles); disease states such as diabetes mellitus (DM) or amyloidosis; demyelinating diseases such as multiple sclerosis (MS) or chronic inflammatory demyelinating polyneuropathy; autoimmune disease such as Guillain–Barré syndrome; trauma such as due to spinal cord injury or amputation; nutritional deficiency such as B_{12} and thiamine deficiency seen in alcohol abuse; or drugs, such as chemotherapeutic agents, isoniazid, and others, or potential neurotoxins such as gold or arsenic. A partial list of medications that may be implicated in polyneuropathy is shown in Table 51.1.

The most common etiology of painful polyneuropathy is diabetes mellitus, which causes injury to both large- and small-diameter sensory nerves, referred to as painful diabetic peripheral neuropathy (PDPN). The sensory component generally manifests earlier than proprioceptive and motor dysfunction and may also remain more prominent. Typically, PDPN occurs as symmetric, distal pain/paresthesia in a stocking-and-glove distribution. The pain may be dull and aching, or lancinating, or burning. As the disease progresses, patients may complain of loss of balance or the inability to feel their feet, which can lead to serious sequelae such as occult fractures, diabetic ulcers, osteomyelitis, gangrene, and amputation. Other, non-painful manifestations of diabetic-induced neuropathy include the loss of sensation related to visceral structures, e.g., non-painful myocardial injury/infarction (silent ischemia) or motor function, e.g., loss of gastrointestinal motility (gastroparesis).

Demyelinating conditions such as multiple sclerosis, which are characterized by progressive loss of motor function, may or may not be accompanied by pain. A rare form of polyneuropathy is POEMS syndrome: the acronym stands for characteristic clinical changes of Polyneuropathy, Organomegaly, Endocrinopathy, M-protein gammopathy, and Skin changes. This peripheral neuropathy syndrome has motor dominance, however, and pain is not a primary concern.

Signs and symptoms

The onset of painful polyneuropathy that is caused by systemic disease states, medication use, or toxins is usually subtle and insidious. Patients may complain of loss of sensation (hypoesthesia or frank anesthesia), burning, tingling, or itching. Electric-shock-like symptoms may also occur: a characteristic finding in multiple sclerosis is Lhermitte's sign, described as a sudden, transient, electric-shock-like pain that is triggered by flexing the neck forward and races from the neck to the base of the spine.

Diabetic patients may report pulsating, sharp pains in the feet or hands as well as a sensation of tightness or burning. In addition to the aforementioned risks, the sensory manifestation of the inability to "feel one's feet" results in loss of balance, causing a tentative gait or frank ambulatory dysfunction. Observation of gait and careful routine inspection of the feet are important features of the clinical examination of all patients with known or suspected diabetes or other chronic progressive diseases.

Guillain–Barré syndrome, which typically follows a minor illness such as an upper respiratory infection, is a polyneuropathy of large-diameter nerve fibers

Table 51.1 Drugs with the potential to cause polyneuropathy

Cardic or blood pressure	Anti-infectives	Chemotherapeutic agents	Disease-modifying antirheumatic drugs	Antiretrovirals	Antiepileptics	Anti-alcohol	Toxins, others
Amiodarone	Cholorquine	Cisplatin	Etanercept	Didanosine	Phenytoin	Disulfiram	Arsenic
Hydralazine	Isoniazid	Docetaxel	Infliximab	Stavudine			Colchicine
Perhexilene	Metronidazole	Paclitaxel	Leflunomide	Zalcitabine			Gold
	Nitrofurantoin	Suramin					
	Thalidomide	Vincristine					

generally characterized by loss of motor function that can progress to paralysis; it may also be accompanied by pain and paresthesia. Spinal cord injury patients frequently report similar debilitating symptoms of lancinating, burning distal extremity pain below the sensory level of the injury.

Damage to small-diameter nerve fibers results in skin denervation causing characteristic changes such that simple visual inspection may offer clues to the underlying process. Signs of neuronal loss in distal polyneuropathy include thinning of skin, loss of hair, and muscle atrophy. Diabetic patients display subtle or obvious bony deformities of the foot (Charcot foot), callus formation, and ulcers. Patients may also exhibit autonomic nervous system signs such as unilateral increased sweating or tremors.

Loss of sensation to light touch, pinprick, and vibratory sensation are all signs of underlying neuropathy. The gold standard for clinical evaluation of sensory neuropathy is Semmes–Weinstein monofilament testing, defined as loss of sensation for 5.07/10 g monofilament. Superficial pain sensation may be tested by applying a sterile needle pinprick, first to a sensate region (such as the sternum) for reference and then in an irregular pattern to the sites being tested. Vibratory testing using the on–off method (onset and dampening of felt vibration) with a tuning fork is also useful for evaluation.

Laboratory tests and diagnostic investigations

There is no gold-standard laboratory test for evaluation or diagnosis of polyneuropathy. The American Academy of Neurology (AAN) has established practice parameters for diagnostic testing for distal symmetric polyneuropathy. The laboratory evaluation guidelines, which receive only a level C recommendation ("possibly effective, ineffective, or harmful in the specified population"), include measurement of blood glucose, serum B_{12} with metabolites (methylmalonic acid with or without homocysteine), and serum protein immunofixation electrophoresis.

It is well documented that assiduous glucose control may delay or slow the progression of disease in patients with diabetes mellitus. Thus, hemoglobin (Hb) A1c measurement with the goal of maintaining the lowest level possible is recommended. B_{12} and folate levels may indicate a nutritional source for distal polyneuropathy, perhaps related to medications (e.g., isoniazid) or alcohol abuse.

Electrodiagnostic studies (electromyography, EMG) can confirm the presence of large-fiber neuropathy but will not detect the presence of small-fiber neuropathy, as is the case in PDPN. Nerve biopsy confirms the presence of polyneuropathy but is to be avoided when the diagnosis can be made on clinical grounds.

An emerging technique for definitive diagnosis of painful diabetic polyneuropathy is a skin biopsy in which there is a clearly demonstrable decrease in the number of intraepidermal nerve fibers and decreased vascular structures, as well as trophic changes such as thinning of the epidermal layer. Pathologic specimens of epidermis in PDPN show unequivocal neuronal loss, changes that account for the clinical finding of pain/paresthesia.

Imaging studies

There are no specific imaging studies recommended for diagnosis of poly-neuropathy. Patients with suspicion for fracture, osteomyelitis, or other bony abnormalities should, however, be evaluated with routine radiographs, CT, or MRI as appropriate.

Differential diagnosis

The differential diagnosis of painful polyneuropathy includes compressive mono-neuropathies such as carpal, cubital, or tarsal tunnel syndrome, radiculopathy, lumbosacral plexopathy; inflammatory conditions such as plantar fasciitis; and vascular claudication, spinal stenosis, Raynaud's syndrome, or cervical spondylo-tic myelopathy.

Pharmacotherapy

The approach to painful polyneuropathy differs from that for most other painful conditions in that anti-inflammatory drugs have little or no efficacy for provid-ing analgesia; to date, there are no available treatments to restore normal nerve function. Anticonvulsants (carbamazepine, phenytoin, lamotrigine, topiramate), calcium channel ligands (gabapentin and pregabalin), secondary amine tricyclic (desipramine and norpramine) and serotonin–norepinephrine reuptake inhibitor (duloxetine, milnacipran) antidepressants, topical lidocaine, capsaicin, and other topical analgesics are considered first-line for treatment of polyneuropathy pain. Pregabalin and duloxetine are approved by the US Food and Drug Administration (FDA) for PDPN. Second-line agents include tramadol and other opioid analgesics.

A multicenter randomized controlled clinical trial of 159 subjects measured overall average daily pain intensity in patients with painful diabetic polyneuro-pathy treated with the opioid analgesic oxycodone. The treatment group received oxycodone CR doses of 10 mg every 12 hours titrated to a maximum dose of 60 mg every 12 hours (average dose 37 mg/day, range 10–99 mg). The treatment group demonstrated a significant reduction in pain score ($p = 0.002$); however, treated subjects had more adverse events than the placebo group, including constipation, itching, confusion, and sedation. In addition to these unpleasant side effects, the use of opioids for persistent pain is problematic because of the possibility of endocrinologic dysregulation and the potential long-term develop-ment of hyperalgesia.

A role for N-methyl-D-aspartate (NMDA) receptor antagonists (e.g., dextromethorphan, memantine, ketamine) in PDPN is emerging. Extensive preclinical research documents involvement of the NMDA receptor in central sensitization, neuropathic pain, and the development of analgesic tolerance. Clinical study results of single-entity NMDA receptor antagonists have suggested that on their own they are unlikely to act as analgesics. Potential side effects may also limit clinical utility, and currently there are no available NMDA receptor antagonists that are FDA-approved for use in painful polyneuropathy.

Non-pharmacologic approaches

The onset of PDPN has been touted by some authors as announcing the identification of an "at-risk" foot; hence, measures to prevent adverse outcomes such as diabetic foot ulcers, Charcot foot, and gangrene should be promptly instituted. This includes assiduous foot care, proper footwear with appropriate orthotics and pressure-leveling support, daily personal observation, and regular inspection by clinicians to identify areas of concern. It bears restating that several controlled trials have demonstrated the benefit of tight blood glucose control in diabetic patients for reducing or forestalling PDPN.

Acetyl-L-carnitine (ALCAR), a dietary substance found in plant and animal sources, is claimed to have antioxidant and neuroprotective qualities. Available as an over-the-counter supplement, this nutriceutical product may be useful for slowing the loss of neuronal tissue in polyneuropathy syndromes.

Self-management is the mainstay for care in all patients with pain, and this is certainly the case for painful polyneuropathy. Physical therapy to maintain range of motion, balance, and optimal ambulatory capacity, psychiatry to address symptoms of anxiety or depression, and psychological evaluation for cognitive behavioral therapy (CBT) are recommended for ongoing support and monitoring of these patients.

Interventional procedures

Transcutaneous electrical nerve stimulation (TENS) has been used with good results in patients with refractory polyneuropathy. Neuromodulation using spinal cord stimulation has been also been studied in refractory cases of polyneuropathy.

Follow-up

Patients with painful neuropathy suffer with a chronic, often progressive syndrome that may take a significant toll on quality of life and physical function. They require ongoing close monitoring for improvement, based on trials of medication and other treatment modalities. These patients must develop a therapeutic relationship based on trust and the willingness to attempt new interventions, as well as involving multiple disciplines, such as physical therapy and psychology, to forge a multimodal therapeutic plan.

Prognosis

The prognosis for painful polyneuropathy depends on the etiology of the painful condition. Those with an infectious cause such as shingles or neuroborreliosis may experience improvement and even complete resolution of the symptoms over time, whereas the outcome for patients with progressive, chronic disease such as diabetes or multiple sclerosis may not be so favorable.

REFERENCES AND FURTHER READING

Dworkin RH, O'Connor AB, Backonja M, *et al.* Pharmacologic management of neuro-pathic pain: evidence-based recommendations. *Pain* 2007; **132**: 237–51.

Gimbel JS, Richards P, Portenoy RK. Controlled-release oxycodone for pain in diabetic neuropathy: a randomized controlled trial. *Neurology* 2003; **60**: 927–34.

Pluijms WA, Slangen R, Joosten EA, *et al.* Electrical spinal cord stimulation in painful diabetic polyneuropathy: a systematic review on treatment efficacy and safety. *Eur J Pain* 2011; **15**: 783–8.

Sprice MC, Potter J, Coppini DV. The pathogenesis and management of painful diabetic neuropathy: a review. *Diabet Med* 2003; **20**: 88–98.

Wernicke JF, Pritchett YL, D'Souza DN, *et al.* A randomized controlled trial of duloxetine in diabetic peripheral neuropathy. *Neurology* 2006; **67**: 1411–20.

52

Pain in human immunodeficiency virus-related neuropathy

Clinical presentation

Although there have been significant advances made in the management of patients infected with human immunodeficiency virus (HIV), e.g., the highly active antiretroviral therapy (HAART), neurological sequelae of HIV have become increasing concerns, given the longer life span of afflicted individuals. Among these, peripheral neuropathies are especially common painful conditions encountered at every stage of disease progression. The peripheral neuropathies can be classified according to HIV stage and associated symptoms (Table 52.1).

Affecting as many as 30% of HIV-infected individuals, the most common manifestation of peripheral neuropathy is distal symmetric polyneuropathy (DSP). DSP is thought to be caused by cytotoxic immune processes arising from HIV infection, i.e., the activation of chemokines and cytokines within the dorsal root ganglion producing distal axonal degeneration of primary afferent fibers. It is similar to distal sensory neuropathies arising from other conditions (e.g., diabetes mellitus), and the characteristic pattern of that encountered with HIV is distal, symmetric, and predominantly sensory in nature, the longest axons being most vulnerable. Symptoms typically include spontaneous and evoked pain and numbness; motor effects are generally spared until very late in disease progression. Although DSP will be the primary focus of this chapter, distinctions between DSP and other HIV-related painful neuropathies will also be addressed.

It should be noted that DSP can also arise from exposure to antiretroviral agents, e.g., dideoxynucleoside reverse transcriptase inhibitors, and other agents commonly utilized in the management of HIV (Table 52.2). These agents are thought to precipitate pain via disruption of peripheral axonal mitochondrial activity, with symptoms that are indistinguishable from that associated with HIV-related DSP.

Patients presenting with weakness as a primary complaint, especially at sero-conversion and early stages of HIV infection, prompt concerns about demyelinating neuropathies, e.g., acute (AIDP) or chronic inflammatory demyelinating

Table 52.1 Neuropathies encountered in HIV

Class	Stage of illness	Features
Acute inflammatory demyelinating polyneuropathy (AIDP)	Early	Immune-mediated; usually acute Guillain–Barré syndrome with prominent weakness and possibly less prominent sensory symptoms
Chronic inflammatory demyelinating polyneuropathy (CIDP)	Early	Immune-mediated; chronic and relapsing motor weakness and possibly less prominent sensory symptoms; generally occurs later than AIDP
Plexopathies	Early	Can present with symptoms suggestive of brachial plexopathy
Herpes zoster (varicella) neuropathy	Transition	Neuropathic pain arising from varicella reactivation often occurring in the context of a dermatomal rash; although unusual, it is possible that *zoster sine herpete* (i.e., without commensurate rash) may occur
Mononeuritis multiplex (mild)	Transition	Immune-mediated; usually limited to a single or a few nerves, producing asymmetric sensorimotor neuropathy; usually resolves spontaneously
Autonomic neuropathy	Late	Symptoms depend on the extent to which the parasympathetic and sympathetic nervous systems are affected; patients can present with dizziness, syncope, tachycardia, diarrhea, or constipation
Progressive polyradiculopathy	Late	Cauda equina-like syndrome including numbness, weakness of the lower extremities, and sphincter dysfunction, which can progress to paraparesis often associated with cytomegalovirus (CMV) co-infection; other potential etiologies including lymphoma, syphilis, tuberculosis, and varicella
Mononeuritis multiplex (severe)	Late	Vasculitic or CMV co-infection; asymmetric motor and sensory symptoms ± cranial neuropathy, which can progress to become confluent; usually co-occurs with progressive polyradiculopathy or DSP
Distal sensory polyneuropathy (DSP)	Late	Immune-mediated; symmetric paresthesia, dysesthesia, and numbness; proceeding in a length-dependent manner with onset in the lower extremities and eventually extending in a stocking-and-glove manner

Table 52.1 (*cont.*)

Class	Stage of illness	Features
Mononeuropathies	Any stage	Cranial nerve neuropathies, e.g., facial palsy; and/or syndromes mimicking entrapment neuropathies; caused by tuberculosis, varicella virus (Ramsay Hunt syndrome); meningitis related to HIV
Toxic polyneuropathy	Any stage	Axonal mitochondrial dysfunction caused by medication/toxins; producing a symptom profile indistinguishable from DSP

Early stage, seroconversion and asymptomatic phase of illness T-lymphocytes (CD 4+) > 500/mm^3; Transition, CD 4+ > 200 and < 500/mm^3; Late stage, CD 4+ < 200/mm^3.
Adapted from Robinson-Papp & Simpson 2009, Pardo *et al.* 2001, Verma *et al.* 2005.

Table 52.2 Medications used in the management of HIV potentially contributing to toxic neuropathies

Class	Examples
Dideoxynucleoside antiretrovirals	Didanosine (ddI); stavudine (d4T); zalcitabine (ddC)
Pneumocystis pneumonia (PCP) prophylaxis	Dapsone
Antivirals	Foscarnet
Antibacterials	Metronidazole
Antimycobacterials	Isoniazid; rifampicin
Antineoplastics	Cisplatin; paclitaxel; vincristine; vinblastine

Adapted from Dalakas 2001.

polyneuropathy (CIDP). In these conditions, the motor weakness is most prominent, as compared with sensory symptoms. By contrast, asymmetric motor and sensory symptoms suggest progressive polyradiculopathy, mononeuritis multiplex, and focal radiculopathies, i.e., involving a single nerve root.

It should be pointed out that it is possible that more than one neuropathic condition can exist concurrently within the same individual. In later stages of HIV, as the CD4 counts decrease and immunodeficiency progresses, it is conceivable that neurologic insults can arise from co-infections (e.g., opportunistic infections) and other illnesses (e.g., diabetes mellitus), as well as from immune-mediated processes. The evaluation warrants an accurate patient history with attention to onset and course, location, quality, and intensity of pain symptoms as well as associated symptoms. Characterization of these features and diagnostic assessments will assist the clinician in determining the likely etiology, and the management approaches to be undertaken.

Signs and symptoms

Pain associated with polyneuropathy, and DSP in particular, is typically characterized as burning in the distal extremity, initially in the toes or the anterior surface of the foot, and which eventually extends proximally to the foot, ankle, and beyond. There may be associated paresthesias and numbness symmetrically. The symptoms evolve in a length-dependent manner, afflicting the most distal portions of long nerves. Eventually, there may be finger and hand involvement. The degree of pain can be variable, from burning to tingling to electric-like pain. In extreme forms, especially when accompanied by marked allodynia, patients may be unable to don socks or shoes, develop an antalgic gait, and experience sleep difficulties because of intolerability of pain associated with normally innocuous stimulation.

Neurologic examination typically reveals impairments in distal sensation, i.e., temperature and vibration. There may be associated decreased, or possibly hyperalgesic, response to pinprick stimulation, although proprioception is usually well preserved. The ankle reflexes may be depressed (or absent) as compared with reflex examination at proximal sites such as the patella.

HIV patients who present with complaints of weakness, by contrast, should prompt evaluation of other conditions including acute or chronic demyelinating polyneuropathy, polyradiculopathy, mononeuritis multiplex, and focal radiculopathies. Other physical findings may raise the index of suspicion that the neuropathy is attributable to other causative agents, e.g., co-infection. For example, the presence of a dermatomal rash may suggest varicella reactivation. Alternatively, evidence of cytomegalovirus (CMV) infection of other organs (e.g., pneumonia, retinitis, or gastroenteritis) should prompt diagnostic assessments intended to refute or confirm that the neuropathy might otherwise be related to CMV infection.

Laboratory tests and diagnostic investigations

Because DSP occurs at high rates among HIV-infected persons, patients who present with prototypic distal sensory abnormalities often do not require extensive laboratory assessments. However, informed by clinical history, it may be prudent to perform laboratory assessments to evaluate for other treatable causes of neuropathy, e.g., glycemic status and glucose tolerance, Vitamin B_{12} level, thyroid-stimulating hormone, rapid plasma reagin, and hepatitis serology.

Patients whose symptoms are at variance with those prototypically found in DSP may require more extensive laboratory investigations, e.g., to assess for opportunistic infections. For example, low CD4 counts and cerebrospinal fluid polymerase chain reaction (PCR) analysis may suggest CMV co-infection and would be essential to the work-up of CMV-related polyradiculopathy, whereas immunoassays (indirect fluorescent antibody test), serology (enzyme-linked immunosorbent assay, ELISA), viral culture, and PCR can be useful in clarifying whether the patient's symptoms are related to herpes zoster infection.

Although diagnostic assessments are rarely indicated for DSP, if there are atypical features such as motor weakness, or major asymmetries in symptoms or signs, consideration of supplemental diagnostic assessments can clarify diagnosis and specific treatment approaches (Table 52.3). In general, electromyographic (EMG) and nerve conduction studies (NCS) do not distinguish HIV-DSP from dideoxynucleoside-induced neuropathy, but can be useful in identifying polyradiculopathy and mononeuritis multiplex. For DSP, skin biopsy may unveil reduced intraepidermal nerve fiber density, the severity of which may correlate clinically with symptom severity and electrophysiological findings.

Imaging studies

Spinal imaging will not be helpful in suspected cases of DSP. Spinal MRI would be indicated in patients for whom there are concerns about the possibility of an underlying cervical or lumbar radiculopathy arising from spinal stenosis and/or disc herniation. For example, HIV patients presenting with abrupt onset of low back discomfort, with concurrent lower extremity sensory signs and motor weakness along with impairments of bowel or bladder function, may have MRI findings that reveal a mass or tumor suggesting lymphoma or tuberculosis, or meningeal enhancement and thickened spinal roots suggesting CMV-related polyradiculopathy. CT and radionucleotide bone scanning may detect vertebral fractures and spondylolisthesis, especially if there is a history of recent trauma.

Differential diagnosis

As indicated in the previous sections, the clinician must consider whether a patient's pain is associated with DSP or another HIV-related neuropathy (differentiated by HIV-associated distal painful sensory neuropathy's slower progression and emergence during a later stage of the disease). Because of the longer life span of HIV-afflicted patients, one must also consider other possible non-HIV-related medical causes of neuropathy. For example, based upon historical data, it may be prudent to consider neuropathies related to alcohol toxicity, vitamin B_{12} deficiency, and/or diabetes mellitus, among others. Toward this end, the clinician will need to consider the following differential diagnostic possibilities:
- alcoholic neuropathy
- diabetic neuropathy
- hepatitis C-related neuropathy
- human T-lymphotropic virus type 2 (HTLV-2)-related neuropathy

Table 52.3 Features of diagnostic assessments distinguishing distal symmetrical polyneuropathy (DSP) from polyradiculopathy and mononeuritis multiplex

Test	DSP	Polyradiculopathy	Mononeuritis multiplex
CSF analysis	Not applicable	Low glucose, elevated protein and polymorphonuclear pleocytosis; confirmed by CMV PCR	CMV PCR may confirm this as an etiology; although less common causes, e.g., herpes simplex, varicella virus, syphilis, may also require exploration
EMG	Possibly abnormal spontaneous motor unit changes reflecting distal degeneration and reinnervation	Reduced number of motor end unit action potentials; abnormal spontaneous motor unit changes in weakened muscles	Reduced number of motor end unit action potentials; may reveal denervation
NCS	Reduced amplitudes of sensory nerve action potentials, mildly symmetric reductions in conduction velocities, or mildly increased F-wave or H-reflex latencies	Reduced amplitudes or absent sensory nerve action potentials; prolonged or absent F-wave latencies	Asymmetric reductions in amplitudes of sensory nerve action potentials and compound muscle action potentials; H-reflex latencies may be prolonged or absent
MRI with contrast	Not applicable	Enhancement of meningeal cauda equina and thickened lumbosacral spine roots	Not applicable
Skin biopsy	Reduced epidermal small fiber density	Not applicable	Not applicable

CMV, cytomegalovirus; CSF, cerebrospinal fluid; EMG, electromyography; MRI, magnetic resonance imaging; NCS, nerve conduction studies; PCR, polymerase chain reaction. Adapted from Pardo *et al.* 2001, Verma *et al.* 2005.

- nutritional/metabolic neuropathy
- spinal stenosis/compression
- paraneoplastic neuropathy
- uremic neuropathy
- vasculitic neuropathy
- vitamin B_{12} deficiency-induced neuropathy

Pharmacotherapy

HIV patients with neuropathic pain may require trials of antidepressants, e.g., tricyclics (TCAs) or serotonin–norepinephrine reuptake inhibitors (SNRIs), and anticonvulsants, e.g., alpha-2-delta ligands such as gabapentin or pregabalin, among others, e.g., lamotrigine. Treatment approaches directed at mitigating pain associated with DSP have not been established on a solid foundation of empirical work; the proposed benefit of antidepressants and/or anticonvulsants is largely extrapolated from studies demonstrating efficacy in diabetic neuropathy and post-herpetic neuralgia. Additionally, there is a dearth of investigation comparing the efficacy of one approach versus another, or determining the efficacy of combined endeavors versus those administered in isolation. Caution would naturally be required with the use of any of these agents: for example, side effects may limit tolerability and resultant utility, and in some cases may be prohibitive – e.g., using TCAs with prominent anti-cholinergic side effects may be especially problematic in HIV patients with concurrent dementia.

Topical agents (e.g., lidocaine ointment gel or high-concentration capsaicin patch) have demonstrated promise in the mitigation of symptoms. These agents can be particularly helpful in patients who have difficulty tolerating orally administered medications.

Inadequate responses to the aforementioned agents may necessitate the addition of opioid analgesics (e.g., hydrocodone, transdermal fentanyl, and others), but the benefits always need to be balanced against potential adverse effects. Careful monitoring and risk stratification is warranted when considering opioid use in patients with substance abuse histories.

The management of toxic neuropathy, e.g., from antiretroviral use, can likewise benefit from the aforementioned pharmacologic approaches. However, these symptoms can sometimes be attenuated by dose reduction of the offending agent, or substitution of a non-neurotoxic alternative. Naturally, the latter options would have to be weighed against the potential risk of jeopardizing HIV virological control. Symptomatic improvement resulting from such measures may not be appreciated for several weeks after dose adjustment or medication discontinuation.

AIDP, CIDP, and severe cases of mononeuritis multiplex, especially of vasculitic origin, may benefit from corticosteroid treatment and administration of intravenous immunoglobin. In each of these, the clinician must carefully weigh the risks of further immunosuppression from the use of corticosteroids against potential benefits. CMV-related neuropathies, e.g., mononeuritis multiplex or progressive polyradiculopathy, may benefit from antiviral therapies including ganciclovir, foscarnet, or cidofovir. Notably, some of these (e.g., foscarnet) also have the potential of producing neuropathy. Aciclovir can be useful in expediting recovery in herpes zoster neuropathy.

Non-pharmacologic approaches

A number of psychological approaches (cognitive behavioral therapy [CBT], relaxation training, biofeedback) and physical approaches (transcutaneous electrical nerve stimulation [TENS], physical and occupational therapies) can be employed to assist with pain management strategies. However, the efficacy for many of these modalities has not yet been systematically investigated for use in HIV-related neuropathy.

Interventional procedures

Plasmapheresis may be useful in severe mononeuritis multiplex unresponsive to corticosteroids and intravenous immunoglobin. Severe refractory neuropathic symptoms, especially in patients with advanced disease requiring palliative care, may benefit from epidural analgesia. However, the effect of epidural analgesia is likely to be time-limited, and its utility in managing pain associated with HIV-related neuropathies has not been empirically established.

Follow-up

The frequency of patient follow-up is targeted toward monitoring of the efficacy of, and potential adverse side effects associated with, medication use and other treatments. Failure to achieve relief should prompt: (a) consideration of the accuracy of diagnosis; (b) assessment of alternative explanations for the persistent pain and/or coexisting conditions; (c) inquiry into patient adherence with medications; and (d) consideration of alternative treatment approaches to be undertaken. In refractory and disabling cases, continuous monitoring and employing several concomitant treatment approaches may be required to mitigate discomfort.

Prognosis

Neuropathy complicating the clinical course of HIV can be quite disabling, underscoring the need for early recognition of peripheral neuropathy and measures to address pain and functional capacity. Mild mononeuritis multiplex and AIDP generally have a good prognosis. Mild mononeuritis multiplex arising in the early stages of HIV is often self-limited, resolving spontaneously without treatment. CIDP, by contrast, has a progressive course, with patients displaying relapsing motor and sensory symptoms. Unfortunately, the presence of DSP with axonal degeneration is associated with a poor outcome; it is often relentless, but symptoms can be managed with analgesic agents. Severe forms of mononeuritis multiplex and CMV-related polyradiculopathies have a relentless progression and very poor prognosis.

REFERENCES AND FURTHER READING

Dalakas MC. Peripheral neuropathy and antiretroviral drugs. *J Peripher Nerv Syst* 2001; **6**: 14–20.

Evans SR, Ellis RJ, Chen H, *et al*. Peripheral neuropathy in HIV: prevalence and risk factors. *AIDS* 2011; **25**: 919–28.

Pardo CA, McArthur JC, Griffin JW. HIV neuropathy: Insights in the pathology of HIV peripheral nerve disease. *J Peripher Nerv Syst* 2001; **6**: 21–7.

Robinson-Papp J, Simpson DM. Neuromuscular diseases associated with HIV-1 infection. *Muscle Nerve* 2009; **40**: 1043–53.

Simpson DM, Kitch D, Evans SR, *et al*. HIV neuropathy natural history cohort study: assessment measures and risk factors. *Neurology* 2006; **66**: 1679–87.

Verma S, Estanislao L, Simpson D. HIV-associated neuropathic pain: epidemiology, pathophysiology and management. *CNS Drugs* 2005; **19**: 325–34.

53

Central pain and neurologic disorders

Clinical presentation, signs and symptoms

Central pain has been defined as pain that results from lesions of the central nervous system (CNS). Since central pain is associated with lesions of the CNS, it is considered a type of neuropathic pain.

Multiple distinct clinical conditions resulting in CNS lesions exist, and several of these will be discussed in more detail in this chapter. However, there are important general characteristics of central pain that should be noted:

(1) Central pain results from injury to somatosensory pathways in the CNS (spinal cord or brain).
(2) The injury may be massive or minimal; some individuals with central pain have no obvious sensory loss despite the severe pain.
(3) The onset of pain following the injury may be delayed.
(4) The pain is sometimes reversible.
(5) Three main components of central pain are: pain evoked by stimulation, steady and neuralgic-like pain, and spontaneous pain.
(6) The pathophysiology of central pain is not well understood.
(7) Treating central pain successfully can be very challenging.

The most common cause of central pain resulting from brain injury is that resulting from **stroke**. Brain-derived central pain may result from any type of lesion occurring at any level from the foramen magnum to the cerebral cortex. Seemingly paradoxically, the patient with central pain following a brain lesion may not have any clearly detectable sensory loss. Although it was previously thought to occur only as a result of thalamic lesions, it is now known that this type of pain can occur from any brain lesion affecting sensory processing areas. Of interest is that traumatic brain injury and craniotomy do not frequently result in central pain. The onset of brain central pain may be immediate, and most commonly it will occur within the first year following the injury; however, it may uncommonly have its onset more than 1 year after the injury. Brain central pain has been reported to be reversable following a stroke, or following the removal of a brain tumor.

Multiple sclerosis is a CNS demyelinating disorder that is frequently associated with pain. Painful conditions associated with multiple sclerosis include: acute transverse myelitis, spinal cord demyelination (myelopathy-related pain), spasticity, and trigeminal neuralgia (other secondary types of pain associated with multiple sclerosis, e.g. associated with osteoporosis, wheelchair positioning, are not included here).

Pain is very commonly experienced in patients with various movement disorders including **Parkinson's disease**. This progressive central condition, characterized most often by resting tremor, bradykinesia, and rigidity is often associated with cramping, complaints of muscular tightness, restless legs syndrome, and generally painful dysthesias in affected extremities.

Dystonia, a central condition associated with abnormal motor control of various muscle groups, can be quite painful and may be focal, multifocal, or generalized. Causes of dystonia include hereditary, post-traumatic, post-infectious, and idiopathic. Pain is a very commonly experienced symptom associated with dystonia.

Lesions of the spinal cord arising from a diverse group of medical conditions can result in central pain. The most common reported cause of spinal cord injury is **trauma**, with the cervical spinal region most commonly affected. The onset of spinal cord central pain is not infrequently delayed after the event that has caused it, and it has been reported in some instances to occur years post injury. In one series of spinal-cord-related central pain, 75% of patients reported pain that was burning, 44% evoked by normal or painful stimulation, 31% shooting, and 15% musculoskeletal-like. Patterns of sensory loss in this one series were quite variable, with 42% of patients experiencing complete sensory loss, 39% incomplete loss, 16% dissociated loss, and 3% no sensory loss. Central neuropathic pain is the most severe pain experienced after spinal cord injury, and it may be more intense at the transition areas from normal to abnormal sensation. When the spinal cord is injured at the level of the conus medullaris and above, the pain may be associated with painful muscle spasms and spasticity.

Syringomyelia refers to the development of a cystic cavitation (syrinx) within the central canal of the spinal cord. Causes of syringomyelia include congenital (in association with the Arnold–Chiari malformation), post-traumatic, associated with hematomyelia, post-infection, and in association with an intramedullary spinal cord tumor. The pain that may accompany syringomyelia is most often neuropathic, with patients experiencing burning, allodynia, and hyperalgesia at the same time that they experience numbness in the affected region. Facial pain may occur when the syrinx extends into the upper cervical spinal cord. If the syrinx affects the thoracic region, the patient may complain of abdominal pain or pain around the truncal region, and dissociated sensory loss and spasticity may be noted on examination.

Laboratory tests and diagnostic investigations

There are no general laboratory tests for this group of conditions. For patients with suspected multiple sclerosis, spinal fluid analysis and various electrophysiologic studies such as visual evoked responses may be necessary to make the diagnosis.

Imaging studies

Neuroimaging studies including MRI and in certain instances CT myelography are important diagnostic modalities to use when evaluating and treating a patient with central pain.

Differential diagnosis

Causes of central pain include trauma, vascular, infectious, inflammatory, demyelinating, hereditary, and neoplastic.

Pharmacotherapy

When medical therapies are considered for the management of central pain, one should keep in mind that although many treatments have been attempted, very few have been consistently helpful. Recently the US Food and Drug Administration (FDA) has approved pregabalin for the treatment of spinal cord injury pain.

Gabapentin, a medication with a similar mechanism of action as pregabalin, may be considered as well. One of the newer preparations of gabapentin, a gastroretentive form, has the advantages of being administered as a single dose at dinner time and much lower reported sedation and dizziness, the two most common adverse effects, when compared with traditional gabapentin.

Both pregabalin and traditional gabapentin are usually administered multiple times daily in order to be effective. In addition to pregabalin and gabapentin, other medications that may provide some benefit to patients with spinal cord injury pain include amitriptyline, desipramine, carbamazepine, lamotrigine, non-steroidal anti-inflammatory drugs (NSAIDs), clonazepam, oral baclofen, and tizanidine. Both baclofen and tizanidine are used to control spasticity, but each may have analgesic qualities as well. Medications that have not been shown to be helpful for spinal-cord-related central pain include trazadone, valproic acid, and mexilitine. The same medications may be considered for central pain related to brain injury, and studies have suggested that naloxone or propofol may be helpful as well.

For both spinal-cord-related central pain and brain-injury-related central pain, there are inconsistent results with the use of opioids for treating the chronic pain associated with these conditions.

Non-pharmacologic approaches

There are no known preventive strategies to consider for any type of central pain. Non-pharmacologic approaches must be considered, and these, depending upon the associated neurological impairment of the patient, may include urologic care, pulmonary care, wound care, optimizing wheelchair/general seating and positioning, treatment of spasticity and muscle spasms (which may be painful as well), proper nutrition, and physical and occupational therapy.

Interventional procedures

Interventional therapies for central pain have also been utilized, again with mixed and too often disappointing results. For patients with pain from spinal cord injury, peripheral nerve blocks may offer temporary but not sustained pain relief. Intravenous lidocaine infusions may also result in temporary pain relief, and some patients have experienced prolonged benefit with repeated infusions. These should only be completed in a monitored environment supervised by an experienced practitioner.

The use of botulinum toxin injection should be considered when painful spasticity and/or painful muscle spasms associated with the central pain are present. For some patients with more generalized spasticity, intrathecal baclofen via an implanted pump may be more appropriate than botulinum toxin injections, given the widespread involvement in that setting. Many patients with severe and widespread painful spasticity due to brain or spinal cord injury may benefit from thoughtfully combining both of these modalities.

In this instance, intrathecal baclofen would be helpful in reducing the more generalized spasticity, and botulinum toxin would be targeted in a more localized manner to address those areas that may be more resistant to treatment with intrathecal baclofen. These treatments combined or used singly certainly need to be individualized in a patient-centered manner to address the specific needs of specific patients. Other intrathecal treatment approaches for central pain include the use of intrathecalmorphine, clonidine, or ziconotide.

The above treatments are highly specialized and should only be offered by those practitioners with sufficient training and experience to do so. Particularly with respect to the use of intrathecal therapies, monitoring and ongoing care is not only vital to the success of the treatment but is imperative from a patient safety perspective. In order for these modalities to be used properly, it must be clear that the patient can and will be followed as closely as required by a properly trained and experienced practitioner for all aspects of intraspinal pump/medication management, including but not restricted to dose adjustment, pump refills, and all aspects of pump troubleshooting.

Spinal cord stimulation, which can be successful in the treatment of post-laminectomy pain, as well as for various other types of neuropathic pain, has not been shown to be consistently effective for central pain associated with spinal cord injury. Neurosurgical procedures such as deep brain stimulation, while not generally helpful for patients with central pain related to spinal cord injury, has been used with varying degrees of success (0–80%) for patients with central post-stroke pain.

Additional surgical treatments for central pain due to spinal cord injury include percutaneous radiofrequency rhizotomy, in which radiofrequency lesioning is directed towards specific nerve roots in an attempt to relieve allodynia and pain in the distribution of a particular nerve root. Cordectomy involves the transection of the spinal cord above the level of the area responsible for the pain. This is not typically an acceptable approach, as it is not always successful, and additionally cord transection would prevent any chance of restoration of spinal cord function in the future.

The dorsal root entry zone procedure (DREZ lesion) involves making a lesion in the pain fibers as they enter the dorsal horn of the spinal cord. It is not without its risks of injury as well. For each of the above procedures there is a very wide range of reported benefit or lack of benefit. Thus one must fully appreciate this spectrum of potential responses when considering these procedures for a patient.

Follow-up

There are no specific recommendations regarding follow-up for patients with central pain. If a patient is being managed with intraspinal medications via an implanted pump, or if a patient is being treated with botulinum toxin, those patients will require careful regular follow-up consistent with the modality (no less frequently than every 6 months – often more frequently for patients with pumps, and generally every 12 weeks for patients receiving botulinum toxin injections). If a patient is being treated medically, periodic follow-up is certainly recommended.

Prognosis

Central pain, a group of pain conditions arising from diverse causes, remains extremely challenging to treat effectively on a long-term basis. Prognosis in general is therefore guarded.

REFERENCES AND FURTHER READING

Finnerup NB, Baastrup C. Spinal cord injury pain: mechanisms and management. *Curr Pain Headache Rep* 2012; **16**: 207–16.

Hadjimichael O, Kerns RD, Rizzo M, *et al.* Persistent pain and uncomfortable sensations in persons with multiple sclerosis. *Pain* 2007; **127**: 35–41.

Hansen AP, Marcussen NS, Klit H, *et al.* Pain following stroke: a prospective study. *Eur J Pain* 2012; **16**: 1128–36.

Kim JS, Bashford G, Murphy TK, *et al.* Safety and efficacy of pregabalin in patients with central post-stroke pain. *Pain* 2011; **152**: 1018–23.

Klit H, Finnerup NB, Jensen TS. Central post-stroke pain: clinical characteristics, pathophysiology, and management. *Lancet Neurol* 2009; **8**: 857–68.

54

Phantom limb pain

Clinical presentation

Phantom limb pain represents a type of neuropathic pain that arises following amputation of a body part. Among the causes of amputation are included accidents, peripheral vascular disease, and less commonly osteomyelitis and neoplasms. Landmine explosions and subsequent injuries account for traumatic amputations as well.

Phantom pain can be viewed as a complex of several different experiences, all of which may occur in the same patient: (1) stump pain or residual limb pain occuring in the stump itself; (2) phantom limb sensation, which refers to non-painful sensations perceived in the missing limb; and (3) phantom limb pain, which refers to pain perceived in the missing limb.

There is general agreement from several studies that phantom pain is experienced by 60–80% of amputees. Phantom pain does not appear to depend upon the reason for the amputation, the patient's gender, the level, or the side of the amputation. Phantom pain most often begins the first week after the amputation, and often within 24 hours. Other reports have suggested that the onset of phantom pain can be delayed for years after the amputation.

Phantom pain is uncommon in congenital amputees, and in children who lose a limb under the age of 6. There is some evidence to support that theory that pain experienced in the limb before the amputation predisposes the patient to phantom pain.

Signs and symptoms

Almost always, phantom pain is not constant but intermittent. The pain may occur on a daily basis or episodically, occurring every few days or weeks. Pain duration can be seconds, minutes, hours, or less commonly longer. The pain is described as burning, shooting, stabbing, pricking, boring, squeezing, or throbbing, with boring, pricking, and shooting pain most commonly noted. The clinician might want to document exactly the way in which the patient with phantom pain describes it, since not uncommonly the description used is quite colorful.

The pain tends to be more common in the distal parts of the body such as the feet and toes or hands and fingers compared to more proximal areas such as the knees or elbows.

Apart from phantom pain, phantom limb sensations that may be experienced include kinesthetic sensations or sensations that involve the perception of desired limb movement, volume, limb length, and position of limb. The perception of limb distortion or limb shortening is fairly common. These sensations are more common soon after the amputation than later.

Laboratory tests and diagnostic investigations

No specific laboratory tests are required to make the diagnosis of phantom pain.

Imaging studies

No specific imaging studies are suggested when evaluating and treating the patient with phantom pain.

Differential diagnosis

As mentioned earlier, three main types of phantom sensations may occur in the same patient: stump pain, phantom limb sensation, and phantom limb pain.

Stump pain, or residual limb pain, is considered a peripheral neuropathic pain syndrome, while phantom limb pain is considered to more clearly involve CNS mechanisms. Patients with stump pain experience the pain localized to the stump.

Pharmacotherapy

Very few high-quality studies have been completed evaluating various pharmacologic therapies for patients with phantom limb pain. Medications such as topical capsaicin, tricyclic antidepressants, various anticonvulsants including pregabalin and gabapentin, and sodium channel blockers, which have been extensively studied in a number of other neuropathic pain states, have either not been adequately studied in phantom limb pain or are considered ineffective.

For some patients, reports have suggested that chronic opioid therapy may provide benefit, and other small studies or reports have suggested the potential benefit for some patients of intrathecal agents.

A small crossover study in 21 patients comparing intravenous calcitonin to placebo suggested not only a reduction in pain during the intravenous calcitonin infusion but continued benefit at 1-year follow-up.

In yet another small study involving 11 patients with phantom pain, intravenous ketamine notably reduced thresholds to mechanical stimulation as well as pain. Memantine, an oral N-methyl-D-aspartate (NMDA) receptor antagonist, was not successful compared to placebo in treating phantom pain.

Non-pharmacologic approaches

When a patient presents with phantom pain in a non-acute setting, the clinician should evaluate the patient for any treatable conditions that could be contributing to the ongoing pain. These include unrecognized and untreated depression as well as the presence of a stump neuroma that may be contributing to the pain.

Physical therapy and/or the use of a prosthesis have not been associated with pain reduction in patients with phantom pain. However, since the overall treatment goals include functional restoration, these treatments should be appropriately considered for patients with phantom pain as part of their overall treatment program.

Although the use of transcutaneous electrical nerve stimulation (TENS) has not been frequently associated with significant benefit, many would suggest a trial of such for patients with phantom pain, given its safety and possible benefit. TENS may provide short-term rather than long-term benefit. Other physical modalities such as ultrasound and acupuncture may also provide temporary relief in stump and phantom limb pain.

Mirror box therapy involves using a box with two mirrors in the center (one facing each way), to help alleviate phantom limb pain. In a mirror box the patient places the good limb into one side, and the stump into the other. The patient then looks into the mirror on the side with the good limb and makes "mirror symmetric" movements. If the patient views the reflected image of the good limb moving, it appears as if the phantom limb is also moving. Through the use of this it becomes possible for the patient to "move" the phantom limb, and to potentially release it from painful positions. The quality of evidence in formal studies to support this is low, but this modality is often used by the military following traumatic amputations.

Recently, graded motor imagery, combining mirror therapy with sensory discrimination training, has emerged as a possible therapy for phantom limb pain.

Interventional procedures

The concept that phantom pain can be prevented has been extensively evaluated, and there is evidence from a small study that a 72-hour preoperative epidural infusion of a local anesthetic with or without an opioid may be helpful in diminishing postoperative phantom pain for those patients who experienced preoperative pain in the affected limb.

Postoperative sciatic nerve blockade did not prevent phantom limb pain despite decreased opioid consumption. Several other studies have demonstrated the absence of benefit following postoperative perineural analgesia with respect to the development of phantom pain compared to those who were not treated. Timing of regional anesthesia may determine the pre-emptive effect on phantom limb pain.

Nerve blocks, and in particular sympathetic nerve blocks, have not been shown to be generally associated with long-term benefit in patients with phantom pain. The exception to this is the use of local anesthetic injection into the stump for patients with stump-related pain. Since there are reports that occasionally patients do experience long-term benefit from sympathetic blocks, the clinician might consider a trial of such in patients with intractable phantom pain.

Significant benefit from non-sympathetic blocks is even less common, and occasionally reports of increased pain following such treatment have been noted. Neurolytic (nerve-destructive) therapies including surgical procedures such as dorsal root entry zone (DREZ) lesions as well as chemical approaches to neurolysis have not been shown to benefit patients with phantom pain.

Mixed results have been documented in studies of deep brain stimulation and spinal cord stimulation for the management of phantom pain. Many other interventional treatments have been attempted for patients with phantom pain including neurectomy, stump revision, cordotomy, sympathectomy, and rhizotomy, without any consistent documented benefit.

Follow-up and prognosis

The natural history of phantom limb pain is uncertain. While many individuals will experience less pain and fewer symptoms over time, others will continue to experience high levels of pain despite multiple attempts at treatment. Treatment should be individualized to optimize outcome.

REFERENCES AND FURTHER READING

Kern U, Busch V, Müller R, Kohl M, Birklein F. Phantom limb pain in daily practice: still a lot of work to do! *Pain Med* 2012; **13**: 1611–26.

Moura VL, Faurot KR, Gaylord SA, *et al.* Mind-body interventions for treatment of phantom limb pain in persons with amputation. *Am J Phys Med Rehabil* 2012; **91**: 701–14.

Nikolajsen L, Jensen TS. Phantom limb pain. *Curr Rev Pain* 2000; **4**: 166–70.

55

Burn pain

Clinical presentation

There are an estimated 1 million burn injuries each year in the United States, with approximately 5% requiring acute hospitalization. The majority of burn victims are men in their thirties. Flame and scald burns are the most common types. Most burn injuries involve less than 10% of total body surface area. Smoke inhalation and blast injuries are frequently associated with burn injuries.

The early resuscitation and hemodynamic shifts over the first 48 hours may determine the prognosis after burn and concurrent injuries. Bacterial infection, sepsis, and organ failure after burn injuries are immediate concerns. Modern treatment of burn injuries comprises invasive and rehabilitative procedures that continue on a daily basis. Each of these interventions may cause further repeated pain, on top of that due to the original burn.

Signs and symptoms

Burns can be assessed by extent and depth, with concomitant injury and underlying disease further complicating the picture. The "rule of nines" is used to determine the extent of a burn, dividing the body surface area into 11 zones of 9% each: whole head and neck, anterior and posterior of upper trunk, anterior and posterior of lower trunk, each arm, and anterior and posterior of each leg. The genital area represents the final 1%.

The total burn surface area is estimated for second- and third-degree burns only. The extent of burn injuries should be evaluated on initial and subsequent examinations to launch the precise treatment strategy and to plan for transfer to a burn center, if indicated. First-degree burns (e.g., sunburn) demonstrate excellent capillary refill and no blister initially. There may be hyperalgesia and mild to moderate pain. Second-degree burns display blister formation due to partial-thickness injury to the dermis. Superficial second-degree burns involve only the upper, papillary dermis and are more likely to heal; deep second-degree burns involve the deeper, collagen-dense reticular dermis and are more likely to require surgical intervention. Thus, second-degree burns result in noticeable hyperalgesia and moderate to severe pain. Third-degree burns involve complete destruction of dermis including sensory and vascular structures. The extent of the loss of adnexal structures depends on the depth (degree) of the burn. Although the extent of acute pain due to third-degree burns is variable, it is usually present over transition zones between burned and intact skin.

The prognostic Burn Index calculates mortality rate from the sum of patient's age and percentage of burn in full thickness or deep partial thickness. Inhalation injuries may add 20% extra mortality. Recent advances in treatments, such as early excision of devitalized tissue and use of skin substitutes for early coverage, have reduced mortality rates after burn injuries.

Smoke inhalation comes hand in hand with burns, and may compromise airway sooner rather than later. The generalized edema following fluid resuscitation may involve soft tissues of the upper and lower respiratory tract. Early intubation to secure and maintain an airway should be considered for at least 2–3 days. Adult respiratory distress syndrome (ARDS) may develop 24–48 hours after severe inhalation injury.

Burn injuries covering over 20% of total body surface may result in widespread capillary leak and need judicious fluid replacement. The Parkland formula provides guidelines for fluid resuscitation with lactated Ringer's solution. The fluid requirement in the first 24 hours is estimated as 4 mL per kilogram of body weight per percent of burn over body surface area. Half of the calculated fluid requirement is administered in the first 8-hour period from the time of burn injury. The second half of the fluid is then divided equally into two 8-hour periods. The requirement of fluid replacement may escalate in deep burns and inhalation injury. Vital signs and monitoring of central venous pressure may determine adequacy of fluid resuscitation.

In the context of burn injuries, it is worth reviewing the commonly used pain terms established by the International Association for the Study of Pain (IASP):

- pain – an unpleasant sensory and emotional experience associated with actual or potential tissue damage, or described in terms of such damage
- allodynia – pain due to a stimulus that does not normally provoke pain
- hyperalgesia – an increased response to a stimulus that is normally painful
- hyperpathia – a painful syndrome characterized by an abnormal painful reaction to a stimulus, especially a repetitive stimulus, as well as an increased threshold
- dysesthesia – an unpleasant abnormal sensation, whether spontaneous or evoked

Physical examination of a burn injury patient usually reveals pain. The extent to which allodynia, hyperalgesia, and dysesthesia may occur varies, depending on the stage of burn injury and extent of wound care.

Laboratory tests and diagnostic investigations

The initial burn injury is only the emergent event that leads to local and systemic reactions of inflammation and probable multiple organ failure. Appropriate laboratory tests should be ordered at each phase of care. The sufficiency of fluid resuscitation may be gauged by urinary output and specific gravity.

Imaging studies

Plain radiography, CT, and MRI may be contemplated for comprehensive appraisal of any related injury in any victim with burn injuries.

Differential diagnosis

Burn pain may be categorized into several types. Acute pain is caused by the initial burn injuries. Procedural pain can be very intense as a result of wound debridement, limb and joint mobility exercises, therapeutic skin stretching, etc. Resting pain is constant in nature but less intense and not associated with activity. Breakthrough pain may occur whenever resting pain is under inadequate control. Postoperative pain is common after surgical interventions, especially in more severe burn injuries.

Second- and third-degree burn injuries involving dermis may result in imminent peripheral and central sensitization. Experimental models of these cellular alterations in burn injuries may provide a pathophysiologic concept to explore the mechanism of hyperalgesia, acute and chronic pain states.

Although acute and chronic pain often accompanies burn injuries, the differential diagnosis of intractable pain should always be guarded. Abdominal compartment syndrome with compromised respiratory function could be evolving in a case of severe burn injury. Early detection and abdominal decompression may be life-saving. All full-thickness burn and constricting eschar over the extremities, neck, and trunk may cause life-threatening ischemic injuries. Urgent escharotomy in the emergency department or operating room may save life and limb. High-voltage electrical burns may cause compartment syndromes of extremities due to extensive deep tissue necrosis and profound tissue swelling. Early diagnosis and intervention such as fasciotomy may salvage the limb in compartment syndrome caused by electrical burns and crush injury. Rhabdomyolysis and acute kidney injury should always be closely monitored for, especially in electrical burns and crush injury.

Pharmacotherapy

Non-opioid analgesics such as acetaminophen, non-steroidal anti-inflammatory drugs (NSAIDs), and cyclooxygenase-2 (COX-2) inhibitors may only work for mild burn pain, because of a ceiling effect on the dose–response relation of analgesia. Various anticonvulsants, tricyclic antidepressants (TCAs), serotonin–norepinephrine reuptake inhibitors (SNRIs), sodium channel blocking agents, and alpha-2 agonists have all been proposed for neuromodulation of burn pain that is not responding to conventional anti-nociceptive treatments.

Oral gabapentin as adjunctive treatment was studied in burn patients under standard pain therapy. There was reduced opioid consumption and lowered pain scores compared with the control group. The effect was attributed to neuro-modulation of hyperalgesia that extended beyond the pharmacologic action of gabapentin.

Opioids are the most regularly used analgesics in the treatment of burn pain. The pharmacokinetics of morphine could be altered in burn patients due to decreased volume of distribution and clearance, and increased elimination half-life. Long-acting oral opioids or sustained-release opioids may also provide continuous control of background pain. Short-acting or immediate-release opioids prior to any expected procedure are mandatory.

Gastrointestinal dysfunction and constipation may be common problems in burn injury. The majority of burn patients need opioids for pain management, which inhibit gastrointestinal motility and lead to adverse outcomes. Methylnal-trexone (MNTX) is a peripheral opioid antagonist approved for the treatment of opioid-induced constipation in advanced illness and palliative care when response to common laxative therapy is insufficient.

Anxiolytics are commonly prescribed as premedication for sedation and pain management prior to daily wound care and during surgical debridement. Patients with burn injuries and high state anxiety around the time of the procedure, or a high baseline score of burn pain, may benefit from low-dose benzodiazepines.

Non-pharmacologic approaches

Psychological counseling and coping skills to deal with decreased control are mandatory for burn injury patients and their loved ones.

Deep breathing and progressive muscle relaxation are important training modalities for burn patients in wound care and pain management. Behavioral interventions such as operant (reinforcement) conditioning are practical techniques in the management of burn pain. Cognitive restructuring techniques may include thought stopping and cognitive reappraisal. The healthcare team should encourage burn patients to participate in coordinating their schedules of medication and wound care. Regular schedules of pain medications may minimize the factors that exacerbate pain levels when medications are administered on an as-needed basis. In the management of anxiety and pain related to burn injuries, it is crucial to provide preparatory information about any impending procedures and the timeline of care.

Avoidance coping styles may involve distraction, imagery, music, hypnosis, and virtual reality.

Hypnosis has been documented in the effective management of pain and complications due to burn injuries. Anecdotal data support the timely incorporation of hypnosis as a means of augmenting pain control and wound healing in burn injuries.

Immersive virtual reality (VR) is a cognitive distraction technique that is interactive through the provision of multiple sensory inputs. Immersive VR may facilitate hypnotic induction and suggestion. The VR achieves analgesia by diversion of conscious attention away from concurrent nociception and attenuation of subjective pain experience. Functional brain imaging studies have validated pain modulations that are parallel and synergistic to opioid analgesia.

Interventional procedures

Patient-controlled analgesia (PCA) is a programmable drug delivery system that is activated via a push button by the patient. PCA may optimize pain medication delivery and improve satisfaction by engaging the patient in achieving the therapeutic level of the medication. Intravenous PCA with opioids may offer effective analgesia for background (basal) and procedural (on-demand) analgesia. PCA provides patients with a measure of control over the medical care of burns. However, parenteral opioids may cause sedation and impairment of a patient's capacity to initiate the on-demand process of intravenous PCA.

Inhaled nitrous oxide may provide effective and relatively safe analgesia without loss of consciousness. An awake, cooperative, and spontaneously breathing patient can self-administer a mixture of 50% nitrous oxide and oxygen.

Intravenous, intramuscular, or oral ketamine has been used for deep sedation in children undergoing extensive wound care procedures. Ketamine is a central-acting anesthetic and analgesic. It is a non-competitive N-methyl-D-aspartate (NMDA) receptor antagonist and interacts with opioid, muscarinic cholinergic, serotoninergic, and norepinephrine receptors. Ketamine may provide profound analgesia and amnesia while still maintaining spontaneous respiration. Ketamine is approved by the US Food and Drug Administration (FDA) as an adjunct for general anesthesia and procedural sedation such as in burn injury and dressing changes. Ketamine may offer an opioid-sparing benefit via the potentiation of opioid-induced analgesia, in addition to antagonism of NMDA receptors.

However, ketamine is a dose-dependent dissociative anesthetic that can produce unpredictable deep sedation, general anesthesia, and emergence delirium. An appropriate level of monitoring and expertise in airway management are mandatory in the use of ketamine for burn pain and wound care.

The anesthesiology service may extend into the burns unit outside of the operating room. There are new intravenous anesthetics (propofol), opioids (remifentanil), and inhalation agents (sevoflurane and desflurane) that provide rapid onset and short duration of action, fast awakening and recovery, and fewer side effects. Propofol is a gamma-aminobutyric acid (GABA) receptor agonist that can induce hypnosis and amnesia at lower doses than induction of general anesthesia. Other sedatives should be considered for use in the longer term, because of the various complications associated with prolonged use of propofol. Propofol should be discarded after 6 hours and tubing changed every 12 hours to avoid contamination due to its preparation with a lipid emulsion carrier that may support bacterial growth.

Postoperative pain management can be challenging, particularly when donor sites are harvested. The increased requirement for analgesics should be limited to less than 4 days. There are anecdotal reports of epidural anesthesia and analgesia used in patients with lower extremity burns. Epidural abscess may occur at indwelling catheters close to burn wound sites that are densely colonized with infectious organisms. Regional anesthesia of the lower extremity has been proposed for pain associated with donor site preparation in burn injuries. Topical local anesthetic use or intravenous lidocaine bolus and continuous infusion have been reported in pain management of acute burn injuries.

Follow-up

A requirement for fluid replacement of more than 150% of estimated volumes could be attributed to undetected injury or comorbidities that warrant intensive care. Any systemic infection or septic episode demands culture and selection of suitable antibiotic therapy. Various non-pharmacologic approaches offer adjunctive analgesia in burn pain, and can minimize the potential adverse effects related to any pharmacotherapy.

Prognosis

Electrical burn injuries may be under-recognized, and may lead to overwhelming events such as amputation due to compartment syndrome. The judicious detection and decompression of an extremity or abdominal compartment can be life-saving in burn injuries. Interdisciplinary and multimodal treatment of burn pain may facilitate recovery and functional rehabilitation.

More patients with huge burns are surviving, and these patients pose distinctive challenges in terms of physical and psychological rehabilitation, encompassing such issues as scarring, contractures, amputations, adjustment disorder, and intractable pain. We need to overcome the under-treatment of pain after burn injury and during burn care, to minimize adverse psychological and physical outcomes in this patient population, especially in children.

REFERENCES AND FURTHER READING

Bayat A, Ramaiah R, Bhananker SM. Analgesia and sedation for children undergoing burn wound care. *Expert Rev Neurother* 2010; **10**: 1747–59.

Browne AL, Andrews R, Schug SA, Wood F. Persistent pain outcomes and patient satisfaction with pain management after burn injury. *Clin J Pain* 2011; **27**: 136–45.

Cuignet O, Pirson J, Soudon O, Zizi M. Effects of gabapentin on morphine consumption and pain in severely burned patients. *Burns* 2007; **33**: 81–6.

Maani CV, DeSocio PA, Jansen RK, *et al.* Use of ultrarapid opioid detoxification in the treatment of US military burn casualties. *J Trauma* 2011; **71** (1 Suppl): S114–19.

Maani CV, Hoffman HG, Morrow M, *et al.* Virtual reality pain control during burn wound debridement of combat-related burn injuries using robot-like arm mounted VR goggles. *J Trauma* 2011; **71** (1 Suppl): S125–30.

McGuinness SK, Wasiak J, Cleland H, *et al.* A systematic review of ketamine as an analgesic agent in adult burn injuries. *Pain Med* 2011; **12**: 1551–8.

Parlak Gürol A, Polat S, Akçay MN. Itching, pain, and anxiety levels are reduced with massage therapy in burned adolescents. *J Burn Care Res* 2010; **31**: 429–32.

56

Acute postoperative pain management

Clinical presentation

The stress and metabolic response due to acute postoperative pain may present as tachycardia, hypotension, fever, hypercoagulability, ileus, and/or suppression of immune function. The adverse pathophysiology of acute pain may contribute to perioperative morbidity, especially in patients with underlying medical conditions.

Signs and symptoms

The activation of the sympathetic nervous system due to postoperative pain may contribute to cardiovascular events such as myocardial ischemia or infarction, dysrhythmia, and congestive heart failure. Postoperative hypercoagulability may cause deep venous thrombosis and subsequent pulmonary embolization; arterial thrombotic events may lead to myocardial ischemia and occlusion of any vascular graft.

Acute postoperative pulmonary dysfunction such as hypoxemia and pneumonia is very common after thoracic and upper abdominal surgery. Acute postoperative pain may contribute to rapid and shallow breathing and exacerbate respiratory efforts, worsening the decrease in functional residual capacity and the imbalance in the ventilation/perfusion (V/Q) ratio, thus resulting in atelectasis.

Acute pain and the stress response may contribute to the severity and duration of postoperative ileus and delay enteral feeding.

Physical examinations in patients with acute postoperative pain usually reveal allodynia, hyperalgesia, and dysesthesia, which may extend beyond the surgical wound site.

Laboratory tests and diagnostic investigations

The selection of laboratory tests is based on any particular need to differentiate etiology, guide ongoing treatment, and monitor progress in the management of acute postoperative pain.

Imaging studies

Appropriate imaging studies are indicated according to the individual case in the acute care of postoperative pain. The addition of contrast to standard CT and the use of MRI (with or without contrast) may help to rule out any suspicion of infection or neoplasm.

Differential diagnosis

It is prudent to rule out any adverse events related to surgery when a patient complains of severe pain despite appropriate pain management. Potential nerve irritation and neuropathic pain following surgery needs cautious assessment.

Acute flare-up of pain in opioid-tolerant patients can be challenging to manage. Patients may report more severe pain or hypersensitivity to any stimuli despite vigilant up-titration of opioids. *Opioid-induced hyperalgesia* describes a paradoxical response to opioid agonists resulting in an augmented perception of pain rather than an anti-nociceptive effect. The escalation of opioid doses may not reverse the state of opioid-induced hyperalgesia.

Pharmacotherapy

It is unlikely that any single drug or intervention will be sufficient to relieve moderate or severe acute pain. The best approach to the management of acute postoperative pain is to use multiple modalities (e.g., pharmacotherapy, non-pharmacologic methods, and/or regional anesthesia and analgesia). Although opioids are usually the foundation of acute pain management, as the dose increases so does the incidence of adverse events. Non-opioid and adjuvant analgesia minimize the escalation of opioid doses and attenuate the likelihood of opioid-induced hyperalgesia.

A number of pharmacologic, nutritional, and physical mediations are proposed to attenuate surgical stress and catabolic illness. Pre-emptive analgesia relies on the concept that analgesia started prior to a noxious event may prevent or reduce the magnitude and duration of post-injury pain and/or the development of chronic pain. Studies of pre-emptive analgesia have focused on non-steroidal anti-inflammatory drugs (NSAIDs), gabapentin, pregabalin, dextromethorphan, local anesthetics, and ketamine.

Absorption of acetaminophen may be decreased by postoperative stress and concomitant opioid use. The intravenous formulation of acetaminophen as a repeated dose over 24 hours (1 gram every 6 hours) is a safe and effective first-line analgesic agent for the treatment of mild to moderate acute pain in the perioperative setting of orthopedic and abdominal surgery. Intravenous acetaminophen is also indicated as an adjuvant for its opioid-sparing effect in moderate and severe acute postoperative pain.

NSAIDs and cyclooxygenase-2 (COX-2) inhibitors could provide an opioid-sparing effect to reduce postoperative nausea and vomiting, sedation, and respiratory depression. Single-dose intravenous ketorolac (Toradol) 30 mg is as effective as intravenous meperidine 50 mg for the relief of acute renal and biliary colic. However, NSAIDs have been linked to adverse events such as allergy and hypersensitivity, and gastrointestinal, hematologic, cardiovascular, renal, and hepatic dysfunction. The use of NSAIDs in acute postoperative pain needs attentive follow-up.

Opioids are prescribed as effective analgesia for moderate to severe acute postoperative pain. Patient-controlled analgesia (PCA) is a programmable drug delivery system that is activated via a push button. PCA improves satisfaction by engaging the patient to achieve the therapeutic level and optimize pain medication delivery. The cut-off age for children being able to apprehend and follow instructions on the use of PCA is 7 years or older. However, parenteral opioids may cause sedation and impairment of a patient's capacity to initiate the on-demand process of intravenous PCA.

Clonidine is an alpha-2-adrenergic receptor agonist with analgesic properties, but its systemic use has frequently been limited by side effects. Basic and clinical studies have shown that clonidine not only modifies the adrenergic component of pain perception but also has an important modifying effect on the neural and humoral response to tissue injury. Clonidine potentially offers a mechanism of modulating the transition from acute to chronic pain.

Ketamine is a non-competitive N-methyl-D-aspartate (NMDA) receptor antagonist. It may work as a central-acting anesthetic and analgesic. Ketamine may offer an opioid-sparing benefit via the potentiation of opioid-induced analgesia in addition to antagonism of NMDA receptors.

Anxiolytics are commonly prescribed as premedication for sedation and pain management in major wound care. Postoperative patients with high state anxiety and a severe baseline score of acute pain may benefit from low-dose benzodiazepines for a short duration.

Non-pharmacologic approaches

Psychological counseling, nutritional support, and physical and mental reactivation have all been proposed to facilitate recovery and rehabilitation in acute pain due to surgery or trauma or flare-up of chronic pain. Physical agents such as cold, heat, ultrasound, and electrical stimulation may provide adjunctive analgesia in the multimodal therapy of acute postoperative pain.

Interventional procedures

Regional anesthesia and analgesia, especially neuraxial blockade (epidural or spinal), have recently been implemented as part of comprehensive perioperative care, including acute pain management. There are useful somatic nerve blocks in the management of acute postoperative pain. Post-craniotomy pain can be relieved by occipital nerve and auriculotemporal nerve blocks. Cervical plexus block may help carotid and neck surgery. Brachial plexus block can be used for shoulder and upper extremity surgery. Intercostal nerve block can help rib fracture, chest tube, and chest wall pain. Median, radial, and ulnar nerve block can be considered in upper extremity and hand surgery. Ilioinguinal, iliohypogastric, and genitofemoral nerve block can help inguinal hernia repair and groin pain. Lumbar plexus and sciatic nerve block can help with pain from lower extremity surgery. Ankle block is commonly used in foot and ankle surgery.

The original indications for continuous nerve blocks were for perioperative care in orthopedic procedures, in either the inpatient or the ambulatory setting. Continuous nerve blocks may help acute pain management for upper and lower extremities, thoracic, abdominal, urologic, gynecologic, plastic, and trauma surgeries. The choice of infusion regimens of local anesthetics and supplements depends on the condition of the patient, the intensity of the surgical stress, and the need for immediate functional recovery. Continuous nerve blocks are effective in reducing opioid demand and related adverse events, accelerating recovery, and shortening the extent of hospital stay. Continuous nerve blocks provide a safer alternative to epidural analgesia in anticoagulated patients, particularly with low-molecular-weight heparin.

Epidural analgesia is a regional anesthesia technique that acts directly on the origin of the nerve supply and the pain impulses, and thus small doses of opioids combined with local anesthetics can achieve pain modulation. Local anesthetics can potentiate the analgesic properties of opioids and may even offer an anti-inflammatory effect. Afferent neural blockade by epidural anesthesia and analgesia may attenuate the neuroendocrine stress response. Epidural analgesia may be more suitable than intravenous analgesia in order to maintain the immunological homeostasis that may be altered by surgical stress, tumor growth, and pain.

Epidural analgesia with local anesthetic and opioid may improve the quality of analgesia compared with intravenous opioid PCA after major thoracic or abdominal surgery. However, patients need to be consented cautiously regarding the risks and benefits of regional analgesia versus alternative modalities for acute postoperative pain management.

Follow-up

Discharge planning should commence at an early stage to minimize the duration of polypharmacy and further opioid requirements. The specific coverage of prescription drugs and modalities of pain management all need to be considered on an individual basis. Multimodal analgesia and an integrated functional rehabilitation program may improve outcome and satisfaction in acute pain management.

Prognosis

The transition of acute postoperative pain to chronic post-surgical pain (CPSP) is a complex and poorly understood process. Common risk factors that lead to the development of CPSP may include pre-existing pain prior to surgery, psychological and environmental factors, and genetic susceptibility. Minimally invasive surgery with prevention of nerve damage and comprehensive multimodal analgesia before, during, and after surgery could help to reduce the incidence of CPSP.

REFERENCES AND FURTHER READING

Ali M, Winter DC, Hanly AM, *et al.* Prospective, randomized, controlled trial of thoracic epidural or patient-controlled opiate analgesia on perioperative quality of life. *Br J Anaesth* 2010; **104**: 292–7.

Chan AK, Cheung CW, Chong YK. Alpha-2 agonists in acute pain management. *Expert Opin Pharmacother* 2010; **11**: 2849–68.

Chandrakantan A, Glass PS. Multimodal therapies for postoperative nausea and vomiting, and pain. *Br J Anaesth* 2011; **107** (Suppl 1): 127–40.

Chelly JE, Ghisi D, Fanelli A. Continuous peripheral nerve blocks in acute pain management. *Br J Anaesth* 2010; **105** (Suppl 1): i86–96.

Neil MJ. Clonidine: clinical pharmacology and therapeutic use in pain management. *Curr Clin Pharmacol* 2011; **6**: 280–7.

Ramasubbu C, Gupta A. Pharmacological treatment of opioid-induced hyperalgesia: a review of the evidence. *J Pain Palliat Care Pharmacother* 2011; **25**: 219–30.

Schnabel A, Poepping DM, Gerss J, *et al.* Sex-related differences of patient-controlled epidural analgesia for postoperative pain. *Pain* 2012; **153**: 238–44.

Sinatra RS, Jahr JS, Reynolds L, *et al.* Intravenous acetaminophen for pain after major orthopedic surgery: an expanded analysis. *Pain Pract* 2012; **12**: 357–65.

57

Pain during pregnancy, childbirth, and lactation

Clinical presentation

Almost half of pregnant women report some type of back pain from the twelfth week of gestation until childbirth. The majority of back pain occurs in the lumbar and sacral regions; it is less likely in the cervical and thoracic areas, with sciatica the least likely complaint during pregnancy. Pain and disability from low back pain (LBP) and pelvic girdle pain (PGP) are quite common even with an uncomplicated pregnancy. Pain and disability can be determined as mild to moderate in most cases, and as severe in about 20% at 20–30 weeks during pregnancy.

Contributing factors associated with a higher risk may differ between LBP and PGP. A history of LBP, related or unrelated to previous pregnancy or partum, LBP surgery, and anxiety are the factors more strongly associated with pregnancy-related LBP. When these variables are taken into account, obstetric data from current or previous pregnancies and other variables do not show a significant association with LBP. The stage of pregnancy and depression have been linked with PGP. The incidence of radicular pain during pregnancy in women who have had microsurgical discectomy for lumbar disc herniation has been estimated at around 18%. Pregnancy does not substantially aggravate disease activity or severity in patients diagnosed with ankylosing spondylitis.

There are more options and evidence-based medicine for interventional procedures during labor and childbirth. Conservative approaches are usually recommended during pregnancy and lactation.

Signs and symptoms

Pregnancy-related LBP refers to pain in the lumbar region. PGP describes pain around the symphysis pubis, sacroiliac joints, iliac crest, gluteal region, and posterior thighs. The risk factors for LBP include strenuous work, and previous

LBP prior to pregnancy or during a previous pregnancy. The etiology of PGP may involve mechanical, traumatic, hormonal, metabolic, and degenerative changes during pregnancy. PGP usually begins in the second trimester and may resolve within several weeks to months after delivery.

Laboratory tests and diagnostic investigations

Laboratory evaluations of painful conditions are frequently non-specific during pregnancy. Appropriate tests may be ordered, based on any specific indications and clinical work-up.

Electromyography (EMG) and nerve conduction studies serve as safe and reasonably sensitive screening options in pregnant patients suffering from radicular pain that is associated with numbness and weakness of an extremity. LBP and PGP without radicular symptoms and signs do not need electrodiagnostic studies.

Imaging studies

Gestational age and fetal dose of absorbed radiation determine the risk of radiation exposure to the fetus and the mother. Significant risk of fetal malformation is increased especially at doses above 150 mGy. Radiation exposure should be avoided prior to the 15th week of gestation, since a dose as low as 50 mGy could still be detrimental to the fetus. MRI may be indicated during pregnancy if other non-ionizing imaging studies, such as ultrasonography, are unsatisfactory. There was no harmful effect related to MRI when it was ordered as an alternative to other ionizing radiation tests during pregnancy. Fluoroscopy for diagnostic or treatment purposes may deliver 10–50 mGy per minute of exposure time, and therefore should be avoided during pregnancy.

Differential diagnosis

It is crucial to distinguish LBP from posterior PGP during pregnancy by history, physical examination, and imaging studies. The posterior pelvic pain provocation test as described by Ostgaard *et al.* (1994) may help to delineate the source of posterior pelvic pain during pregnancy. The test is performed with the patient in the supine position with 90 degrees of flexion in the hip and knee on the side being tested. The examiner stabilizes the contralateral side of the pelvis over the anterior superior iliac spine and applies a light manual pressure to the patient's flexed knee along the longitudinal axis of the femur. The test is positive for PGP if the patient feels a familiar well-localized deep gluteal pain on the provoked side.

The appropriate physical therapy, exercise program, and functional restoration based on the etiology of the back and pelvic pain may help improve the outcome of each individual case.

Vigilant work-up is indicated for any new onset of severe headache, especially in the case of migraine-like symptoms and signs. A woman who has previously suffered from migraine may find that her symptoms are improved, or even in remission, during pregnancy.

Pharmacotherapy

The physiologic changes of pregnancy may have important clinical implications for the pharmacokinetics of drugs. Pregnant women may have an increased volume of distribution, decreased plasma protein concentration and altered drug binding, altered hepatic microsomal activity, and increased renal blood flow and glomerular filtration, all of which may affect drug metabolism and clearance.

The US Food and Drug Administration (FDA) introduced a five-category risk classification for medications taken during pregnancy in 1979:

- Category A – there is no increased risk of fetal abnormalities in well-controlled studies in pregnant women. There is no drug in this category.
- Category B – animal studies have not indicated a fetal risk, or animal studies have indicated a teratogenic risk but well-controlled human studies have failed to demonstrate a risk. Examples are acetaminophen, butorphanol, nalbuphine, caffeine, fentanyl, hydrocodone, methadone, meperidine, morphine, oxycodone, oxymorphone, prednisone, ibuprofen, naproxen, and indomethacin.
- Category C – studies have indicated teratogenic or embryocidal risk in animals, but no controlled studies have been done in women; or there have been no controlled studies in animals or humans. Examples are aspirin, ketorolac, codeine, gabapentin, pregabalin, lidocaine, mexiletine, nifedipine, propranolol, sumatriptan, sertraline, fluoxetine, and bupropion.
- Category D – there has been positive evidence of fetal risk, but in certain cases the benefits of the drug may outweigh the risks involved. Examples are amitriptyline, imipramine, paroxetine, diazepam, carbamazepine, phenobarbital, phenytoin, and valproic acid. All opioid analgesics are FDA risk category D over prolonged periods or in large doses near term.
- Category X – there has been positive evidence of significant fetal risk, and the risk clearly outweighs any possible benefit. An example is ergotamine.

In 2008 the FDA proposed discontinuing the use of these categories, relying instead on more detailed drug labeling, to include a risk summary, clinical considerations to support patient-care decisions and counseling, and a data section with more detailed information on the use of the drug in women who are pregnant, breastfeeding, or of child-bearing age. The proposed Pregnancy and Lactation Labeling Rule is not yet published.

The American Academy of Pediatrics outlined risk categories regarding transfer of drugs into human milk in 2001:

- Category 1 – strong evidence exists that serious adverse effects on the infant are likely with maternal ingestion of these medications during lactation. Examples are ergotamine and aspirin.
- Category 2 – the effects on human infants are unknown, but caution is urged. Examples are tricyclic antidepressants, fluoxetine, and benzodiazepines.
- Category 3 – these medications are compatible with breastfeeding. Examples are acetaminophen, non-steroidal anti-inflammatory drugs (NSAIDs), steroids, opioid agonists (except meperidine), opioid agonists–antagonists, local anesthetics, anticonvulsants, beta-blockers, sumatriptan, sertraline, and paroxetine.

Acetaminophen may be the medication of choice for mild back and pelvic pain during pregnancy and lactation. The short-term use of NSAIDs could be considered during the first and second trimesters. However, severe intractable pain may demand judicious prescription of opioids during pregnancy.

Non-pharmacologic approaches

Acupuncture is often recommended as a complementary and alternative medicine (CAM) modality for obstetric and gynecologic conditions. Twenty-four systematic reviews, covering a wide range of gynecologic conditions, were analyzed by Ernst *et al.* (2011). Even though nine of these reviews had clearly positive conclusions, there were still many contradictions and caveats. Evidence for acupuncture as a treatment modality for many obstetric and gynecologic conditions, including pain management, thus remains limited.

There is only limited evidence that transcutaneous electrical nerve stimulation (TENS) reduces pain in labor, and it does not seem to have any impact (either positive or negative) on other outcomes for mothers or babies. The use of TENS at home in early labor has not been evaluated. TENS is widely available in hospital settings, and women should have the choice of using it in labor.

Patient education, a pelvic belt, and cautious physical therapy may be beneficial for PGP in pregnancy.

Interventional procedures

Neurohumoral changes may modify the individual response to pain, with a possible higher pain threshold during pregnancy and in labor. However, pregnant patients may be more susceptible to anesthetics and analgesics.

There is enhanced neural blockade during pregnancy, due to changes in anatomy and physiology, with an estimated 25% reduction in segmental dose requirements to achieve epidural and spinal anesthesia.

Neuraxial techniques in pregnant patients with pre-existing back impairment or prior spine interventions could be challenging in labor and delivery suites.

A careful pre-procedure and preoperative examination remains mandatory, and patients should be sufficiently informed about technical aspects and possible relapses or progression of their disease. When necessary, patients should have additional technical and clinical evaluations as close as possible to any procedure or cesarean section delivery, to establish the baseline status. Most patients will benefit more from spinal (intrathecal) techniques than from less consistent epidural routes. High concentrations and volumes of local anesthetics should be avoided in neuraxial techniques at all times, especially in patients with nerve compression, large disc herniation, or spinal stenosis. Epidural steroid injection may be cautiously considered in cases of acute radicular pain correlated with irritation of a lumbar nerve root that fail to respond to other treatments.

The pain of childbirth in labor and delivery is arguably the most severe pain that women are likely to endure in their lifetimes. The pain from the early first stage of labor may ascend from dilatation of the lower uterine segment and cervix. The pain from the late first stage and second stage of labor is due to the descent of the fetus in the birth canal and the distension and ripping of tissues in the vagina and perineum. Non-pharmacologic modalities have been commonly used, but the effectiveness of these techniques generally lacks rigorous scientific study.

An assortment of non-pharmacologic techniques, systemic opioid analgesics, and neuraxial or other nerve blocks is presently used for labor analgesia. Patient-controlled analgesia (PCA) is a programmable drug delivery system that is activated via a push button by the patient. PCA may optimize pain medication delivery and improve satisfaction by engaging the patient in achieving the therapeutic level of medications. PCA offers patients some degree of control over their own medical care via a safe and efficient modality to achieve flexible analgesia. However, parenteral opioids cause sedation and impairment of a patient's capacity to initiate the on-demand process of intravenous PCA.

Neuraxial labor analgesia, such as epidural or combined spinal and epidural, may be the most effective modality of pain relief without maternal or fetal sedation during childbirth. The neuraxial analgesia commonly combines a low dose of local anesthetics with a lipid-soluble opioid (e.g., fentanyl or sufentanil). Neuraxial analgesia usually does not increase the rate of cesarean delivery as compared to traditional analgesia via systemic opioids.

A total of 1054 nulliparous women were randomized to traditional high-dose epidural, combined spinal epidural, or low-dose infusion. The women were followed up at 12 months postpartum by postal questionnaire to assess the incidence of long-term consequences. There were promising benefits of low-dose mobile (walking) epidural without any long-term disadvantages as compared to the high-dose epidural analgesia.

Epidural opioids may reveal similar side effects (respiratory depression, pruritus, nausea and vomiting) as systemic opioids. The lipophilic opioids (fentanyl, sufentanil) may have a faster onset but shorter duration, whereas hydrophilic opioids (morphine, hydromorphone) exhibit a slower onset but longer duration.

Delayed respiratory depression may occur in neuraxial (epidural, intrathecal) delivery of hydrophilic opioids.

Follow-up

Evaluation and treatment of back pain during pregnancy are restricted because of the relative contraindication of some imaging studies and the potential for adverse events associated with most pharmacotherapeutic and other interventions.

Prognosis

No significant differences were found in long-term backache after combined spinal epidural or low-dose infusion relative to high-dose epidural for labor pain and delivery. Clinical trial evidence showed no long-term disadvantages and possible benefits of low-dose mobile labor relative to high-dose epidural analgesia.

Further education of clinicians and patients may improve the outcome of pain management and quality of life during and after pregnancy and childbirth.

REFERENCES AND FURTHER READING

Dowswell T, Bedwell C, Lavender T, Neilson JP. Transcutaneous electrical nerve stimulation (TENS) for pain relief in labor. *Cochrane Database Syst Rev* 2009; (2): CD007214.

Ernst E, Lee MS, Choi TY. Acupuncture in obstetrics and gynecology: an overview of systematic reviews. *Am J Chin Med* 2011; **39**: 423–31.

Law R, Bozzo P, Koren G, Einarson A. FDA pregnancy risk categories and the CPS: do they help or are they a hindrance? *Can Fam Physician* 2010; **56**: 239–41.

Mens JM, Huis in't Veld YH, Pool-Goudzwaard A. Severity of signs and symptoms in lumbopelvic pain during pregnancy. *Man Ther* 2012; **17**: 175–9.

Ostgaard HC, Zetherström G, Roos-Hansson E. The posterior pelvic pain provocation test in pregnant women. *Eur Spine J* 1994; **3**: 258–60.

Vercauteren M, Waets P, Pitkänen M, Förster J. Neuraxial techniques in patients with pre-existing back impairment or prior spine interventions: a topical review with special reference to obstetrics. *Acta Anaesthesiol Scand* 2011; **55**: 910–17.

Wilson MJ, Moore PA, Shennan A, Lancashire RJ, MacArthur C. Long-term effects of epidural analgesia in labor: a randomized controlled trial comparing high dose with two mobile techniques. *Birth* 2011; **38**: 105–10.

Winder AD, Johnson S, Murphy J, Ehsanipoor RM. Epidural analgesia for treatment of a sickle cell crisis during pregnancy. *Obstet Gynecol* 2011; **118**: 495–7.

Wong CA. Advances in labor analgesia. *Int J Womens Health* 2010; **1**: 139–54.

58

Sickle cell disease

Clinical presentation

Sickle cell disease (SCD) or sickle cell anemia is an autosomal recessive disorder with abnormal hemoglobin (HbS). It arises from a single DNA base change that leads to an amino acid substitution of valine for glutamine in the sixth position on the beta-globin chain on chromosome 11.

A person without SCD has a genotype of HbAA. SCD refers to the homozygous genotype (HbSS). Sickle cell trait (SCT) is a heterozygous genotype (HbAS). The hemoglobin S gene is carried by 8% of African-Americans. It has been estimated that one in 400 African-American children may develop sickle cell anemia. The rate of sickling is usually proportional to the concentration of HbS and other hemoglobin. Red cell dehydration and formation of deoxyhemoglobin S due to acidosis and hypoxemia may all increase the prevalence of sickling. Patients with high fetal hemoglobin (HbF) levels may have a benign clinical course of SCD. The presence of HbF may reduce the incidence of sickling.

Signs and symptoms

SCD always presents with recurrent hemolytic anemia, clinical consequences, and painful episodes. The onset of SCD may be in the first year of life when the level of HbF falls. There may be a history of infection or folate deficiency prior to the onset of hemolytic or aplastic crises and severe anemia in SCD. Chronic hemolytic anemia may be associated with jaundice, pigment gallstones, splenomegaly, and non-healing leg ulcers.

Acute and chronic pain syndromes may occur in SCD. Acute pain is mostly related to vaso-occlusion. Acute vaso-occlusive crisis (VOC) due to clusters of sickle cells may result in acute painful episodes that involve the back, long bones, and chest. There is a possibility of thrombosis, strokes, and priapism during acute vaso-occlusive episodes lasting for hours to days. Ischemic necrosis of bone is vulnerable to staphylococcal osteomyelitis in SCD. The vital signs and laboratory tests are usually normal in acute VOC.

The pulmonary manifestations of SCD may include acute chest syndrome (ACS). Patients present with pleuritic chest pain, fever, acute dyspnea, and new pulmonary infiltration on chest radiography. The risk factors for the development of ACS may include high hemoglobin and white blood cell (WBC) count, acute anemic events, severe pain state, fever, cold weather, and pregnancy.

ACS may go on to develop into progressive hypoxemia, respiratory failure, and acute respiratory distress syndrome (ARDS), and death if exchange transfusion is not initiated in time. Chronic restrictive lung disease associated with SCD may result in pulmonary hypertension, dyspnea, and hypoxemia.

The hand–foot syndrome (dactylitis) presents with acute painful swelling of one or more extremities in infants and young children between 6 months and 2 years of age. The episode of dactylitis may resolve within 1 week and recur frequently. Priapism happens when sickle cells congest the corpora and prevent emptying of blood from the penis. Priapism may require surgical intervention if it does not respond to a conservative approach or exchange transfusion.

Chronic pain syndromes may be related to complications of SCD, such as non-healing leg ulcers, chronic osteomyelitis, avascular necrosis of humerus and femur, arthropathies, and collapse of vertebral body. All of these may result in chronic intractable pain.

Common neuropathic pain syndromes in SCD may include spinal cord infarction, ischemic optic neuropathy, and mental nerve neuropathy.

Laboratory tests and diagnostic investigations

The hematocrit is typically 20–30% in SCD, because of chronic hemolytic anemia. There are 5–50% of red blood cells (RBCs) with irreversibly sickled shapes, 10–25% are reticulocytes, and the remainder are accounted for by nucleated RBCs, RBCs with Howell–Jolly bodies, and target cells. There is an elevated WBC count (12 000– 15 000/μL) and high indirect bilirubin. Hemoglobin electrophoresis may reveal that HbS comprises 75–96% of hemoglobin in SCD. There is no HbA present in homozygous HbSS disease.

Patients with SCT have normal red blood cells on peripheral blood smear, without anemia. An SCT patient presents with 60% HbA and 40% HbS on electrophoresis.

Imaging studies

Radiography or CT may be indicated in chest pain associated with ACS. Small lung volume and diffuse interstitial infiltrates are usually seen in chest radiography in chronic restrictive lung disease in SCD. CT, MRI, or MRA may be considered in the work-up of headache or cerebrovascular accident. Bone scan may be used for bone pain, osteoarthritis, and aseptic bone necrosis in SCD. Ultrasonography may be the first step in the evaluation of abdominal pain, followed by CT or MRI if indicated.

Differential diagnosis

The questions most frequently asked by healthcare providers tend to center on differentiating acute VOC from acute pain crisis in patients with SCD.

Acute chest syndrome (ACS) has clinical symptoms similar to pneumonia, and thus acute infection is always on the list of differential diagnoses.

The differential diagnosis of acute abdominal pain in SCD could be challenging. The left upper quadrant syndrome may involve splenic sequestration that leads to functional asplenia and autosplenectomy. The right upper quadrant syndrome may comprise cholecystitis, hepatic sequestration or crisis, and intra-hepatic cholestasis. Other causes of acute abdominal episodes in SCD are bowel infarction or pseudo-acute surgical abdomen.

Acute multi-organ failure (AMF) presents with fever, rapid decrease in hemoglobin level and platelet count, non-focal encephalopathy, and rhabdomyolysis. AMF may even happen or relapse in SCD patients with only mild disease without chronic organ damage. The treatment of AMF may require aggressive blood transfusion or exchange transfusion for speedy recovery of organ failure.

Pharmacotherapy

Supplemental folic acid and pneumococcal vaccination are commonly recommended. Cytotoxic drugs increase HbF levels by stimulating erythropoiesis in more primitive erythroid precursors. Hydroxyurea at a dosage of 500–750 mg per day may reduce the frequency of acute pain crises in SCD. Prompt prophylactic broad-spectrum antibiotic whenever indicated may be crucial in SCD because of splenic dysfunction and immune deficiency.

In a study of children with SCD who complained of moderate to severe acute vaso-occlusive pain in the emergency department, first-line therapy with intravenous ketorolac and intravenous fluids resulted in adequate resolution of pain in an average of 53% of episodes. The assumed predictors of a likelihood to need additional intravenous analgesics are patients that report four or more painful sites and an initial pain score > 70 over a 0–100 verbal or visual pain scale (Visual Analog Scale, VAS).

The non-steroidal anti-inflammatory drugs (NSAIDs) or cyclooxygenase-2 (COX-2) inhibitors are commonly prescribed in acute and chronic pain. All NSAIDs have been linked to potential adverse events that may involve allergy and hypersensitivity, and gastrointestinal, hematologic, cardiovascular, renal, hepatic, bone healing, and CNS dysfunction. Acetaminophen can be used as an alternative in acute pain management of VOC and SCD, while systemic NSAIDs are prohibited because of side effects.

The intravenous formulation of acetaminophen as a repeated dose over 24 hours (1 gram every 6 hours) is a safe and effective first-line analgesic agent for the treatment of mild to moderate acute pain in the perioperative setting, or as an adjuvant for its opioid-sparing effect in moderate and severe pain. Intravenous acetaminophen is thus indicated when oral agents may be impractical, or when rapid onset with predictable therapeutic level is required in moderate to severe acute pain.

Adjuvant analgesics such as anticonvulsants, sodium channel blockers, tricyclic antidepressants (TCAs), and serotonin–norepinephrine reuptake inhibitors (SNRIs) are prescribed as off-label adjuvants for modulation of chronic pain syndromes in SCD. Benzodiazepines are commonly used as hypnotics and anticonvulsants. Anxiolytics may be prescribed as for anxiolysis or insomnia during acute pain in SCD.

The parenteral route of meperidine should be used with caution because of the risk of accumulation of its metabolite normeperidine, and the risk of seizure in acute crises of SCD. After the preliminary intravenous opioid titration has helped pain control, intravenous patient-controlled anesthesia (PCA) can be the next step. Oral opioids should always be considered whenever severe acute pain is under control by the intravenous route. Although opioids are commonly prescribed in acute flare-up of moderate to severe pain, their efficacy in the long-term management of chronic pain in SCD has not been well supported by evidence-based studies.

Non-pharmacologic approaches

It is crucial to continue intravenous hydration and adequate oxygenation in SCD by means of supplemental oxygen, and simple or exchange transfusion therapy as indicated in the case of hemolytic or aplastic crises with sickle cell production. An exchange transfusion may also be considered for the treatment of intractable pain crises, priapism, and stroke.

Incentive spirometry and deep breathing exercises may also help to reduce ACS in SCD. Close observation and rest are crucial in the acute phase of SCD. Physical modalities (e.g., heat, cold, ultrasound, electrical stimulation, massage, and manual therapy), water therapy and low-impact exercise programs, and complementary and alternative medicine (e.g., acupuncture) may all be valuable in the subacute and chronic phases of SCD.

A non-pharmacologic approach provides symptomatic relief and psychosocial support to minimize the adverse events frequently related to pharmacotherapy. An interdisciplinary and multimodal pain management model appears to decrease pain hospitalizations among the pediatric population with SCD in clinical studies.

Interventional procedures

There is no consensus regarding the use of diagnostic or therapeutic neural blockade in acute vaso-occlusive crisis or chronic pain related to SCD. Sympathetic block alone may not contribute to either confirmation or management of pain syndromes associated with SCD.

In one study, epidural analgesia with local anesthetics administered alone or in combination with fentanyl effectively and safely treated the pain of nine pediatric patients with sickle cell acute VOC crisis unresponsive to conventional pain management. Furthermore, early treatment of acute painful crises with epidural analgesia may improve oxygenation, a critical factor in the evolution of further sickling.

More than 50% of obstetric patients with SCD will have a pain crisis during pregnancy, and the management of these cases can be challenging. In a case study of SCD at 29 4/7 weeks of gestation with severe, debilitating leg and back pain, a lumbar epidural infusion provided pain relief for several days and facilitated discharge after weaning off opioids. Epidural anesthesia and analgesia may be considered as a potentially effective treatment for a severe sickle cell crisis in obstetric patients.

Follow-up

Pain management in sickle cell disease needs interdisciplinary and multimodal approaches for acute and chronic pain syndromes. It is prudent to set up appropriate criteria for discharge and to avoid lengthy or recurrent hospitalizations due to SCD. Further joint efforts to develop best patient care and treatment protocols, including pain management guidelines, are required in SCD.

Prognosis

Long-term transfusion therapy may reduce the risk of recurrent stroke in children with SCD. Pulmonary hypertension, cerebral infarction, spleen infarction, liver cirrhosis, renal failure, sepsis, aseptic necrosis, and retinopathy could all lead to a poor prognosis. Although life expectancy in SCD patients has improved significantly, multi-organ failure remains challenging in its clinical course.

REFERENCES AND FURTHER READING

Brandow AM, Weisman SJ, Panepinto JA. The impact of a multidisciplinary pain management model on sickle cell disease pain hospitalizations. *Pediatr Blood Cancer* 2011; **56**: 789–93.

Feliu MH, Wellington C, Crawford RD, *et al*. Opioid management and dependency among adult patients with sickle cell disease. *Hemoglobin* 2011; **35**: 485–94.

Glassberg J. Evidence-based management of sickle cell disease in the emergency department. *Emerg Med Pract* 2011; **13**: 1–20.

Miller ST, Kim HY, Weiner D, *et al*. Inpatient management of sickle cell pain: a 'snapshot' of current practice. *Am J Hematol* 2012; **87**: 333–6.

Niscola P, Sorrentino F, Scaramucci L, de Fabritiis P, Cianciulli P. Pain syndromes in sickle cell disease: an update. *Pain Med* 2009; **10**: 470–80.

Smith WR, Jordan LB, Hassell KL. Frequently asked questions by hospitalists managing pain in adults with sickle cell disease. *J Hosp Med* 2011; **6**: 297–303.

Yaster M, Tobin JR, Billett C, Casella JF, Dover G. Epidural analgesia in the management of severe vaso-occlusive sickle cell crisis. *Pediatrics* 1994; **93**: 310–15.

59

Pain in critical care

Clinical presentation

Pain in critical care is omnipresent and can be very challenging in evaluation and treatment. The sources of pain include surgery, invasive procedures, and monitoring devices on top of underlying injury, inflammation, and immobility. Pain, anxiety, and delirium can set up a vicious cycle leading to intensive care unit (ICU) psychosis.

Signs and symptoms

The stress and metabolic response due to trauma, surgery, medical illness and pain may manifest as fever, tachycardia, hypotension, hypercoagulability, and suppression of immune function. The adverse events of acute pain lead to activation of the sympathetic nervous system and hypercoagulability. Acute pain may contribute to cardiovascular events such as myocardial ischemia and infarction, dysrhythmia, and congestive heart failure. Hypercoagulability may cause deep venous thrombosis, pulmonary embolization, and occlusion of vascular grafts.

Pulmonary dysfunction such as hypoxemia and pneumonia is very common after trauma or thoracic and upper abdominal surgeries. Acute pain may cause rapid and shallow breathing with a decrease in functional residual capacity and an imbalance in ventilation/perfusion (V/Q) ratio, resulting in atelectasis.

A patient in ICU may not able to communicate the severity of pain experienced or the response to treatment. A simple approach for a communicative patient is to quantify pain intensity with a numeric rating scale such as from 0 to 10. For ICU patients unable to communicate verbally, the Critical-Care Pain Observation Tool (CPOT) is a behavioral scale recommended by experts for pain assessment. A pilot study in healthy subjects showed that the CPOT behavioral score was significantly correlated with self-report of pain intensity, and supported the clinical use of CPOT in ICU.

Laboratory tests and diagnostic investigations

The selection of appropriate laboratory tests depends on any particular requirement to differentiate etiology, guide treatment, and monitor progress in the management of acute pain in the critical care setting.

Imaging studies

Appropriate imaging studies will be indicated according to the individual case. The use of CT and MRI, with and without contrast, may help to rule out any suspicion of infection or neoplasm.

Differential diagnosis

Delirium is an acute reversible alteration of mental status that may contribute to worse long-term outcome. Dementia is a chronic illness with an advanced deterioration in memory and cognitive skills. The Confusion Assessment Method for the ICU (CAM-ICU) facilitates rapid and accurate assessment of delirium more effectively than Diagnostic and Statistical Manual of Mental Disorders (DSM-IV) criteria, and can evaluate inattention, altered level of consciousness, and disorganized thinking in a minimally sedated patient.

Pharmacotherapy

The specific physiological changes that ICU patients undergo will have direct impacts on the pharmacology of drugs, and on inter-patient differences in response. Objective assessment and vigilant titration of pain medications may lead to improvements in outcomes.

Non-steroidal anti-inflammatory drugs (NSAIDs) and cyclooxygenase-2 (COX-2) inhibitors could provide an opioid-sparing effect and reduce nausea and vomiting, sedation, and respiratory depression. NSAIDs have been linked to adverse events such as allergy and hypersensitivity, and gastrointestinal, hematologic, cardiovascular, renal, hepatic, and CNS dysfunction. NSAIDs should generally not be used in ICU, because of multiple systemic side effects.

Absorption of acetaminophen may be decreased by postoperative stress and concomitant opioid use. Intravenous acetaminophen is indicated when oral agents may be impractical or when rapid onset with predictable therapeutic dosing is required in moderate to severe acute pain. Earlier and greater cerebrospinal fluid (CSF) penetration occurs as a result of the earlier and higher plasma peak with intravenous administration of acetaminophen compared with oral or rectal routes. Clinical studies suggest that intravenous acetaminophen is a useful component in the multimodal analgesia model that reduces the use of opioids, extubation time, and opioid-related adverse effects after major surgery.

Opioids are prescribed as effective analgesia via the parenteral route for moderate and severe pain in ICU. Patient-controlled analgesia (PCA) is a programmable drug delivery system that is activated via a push button. PCA may optimize pain medication delivery and improve satisfaction by engagement of the patient to achieve the therapeutic level of medication. Intravenous opioid PCA has been commonly used and studied in acute pain management.

Pain, sedation, agitation, and delirium need always to be monitored in ICU, especially for patients on mechanical ventilation. Sedation regimens may cause or be correlated with depression and post-traumatic stress disorder throughout the ICU course. Potential withdrawal from sedation and analgesics may occur even after 1 week of extended medication use in ICU.

An understanding of commonly used medications is essential to formulate a sedation plan for the individual patient. The level of sedation should be measured and documented every 4 hours in ICU. The Ramsay sedation scale is commonly used as a guideline, with the following categories:
(1) patient is anxious and agitated, or restless, or both
(2) patient is cooperative, oriented, and tranquil
(3) patient responds to commands only
(4) patient exhibits brisk response to light glabellar tap or loud auditory stimulus
(5) patient exhibits a sluggish response to light glabellar tap or loud auditory stimulus
(6) patient exhibits no response
Benzodiazepines are commonly used as hypnotics and sedatives in ICU. Although midazolam offers rapid onset, the potentially prolonged sedative effect limits its application. Lorazepam has a slower onset of action and inactive metabolites. Diazepam is a rapid-onset but long-acting agent because of its active metabolite. The current trend is toward using a lighter level of sedation, with short-acting agents if possible.

Clonidine is an alpha-2-adrenergic receptor agonist with analgesic properties, but its systemic use was frequently limited by side effects. Dexmedetomidine (Precedex) is a selective alpha-2-adrenergic receptor agonist with affinity seven times greater than clonidine. It induces hypnosis that resembles a normal sleep pattern, with the patient being cooperative after easy arousal. The advantages of dexmedetomidine are sedation without respiratory depression and reduction of demand for opioid analgesia. Dexmedetomidine is indicated in the USA for the sedation of mechanically ventilated adult patients in ICU and non-intubated adult patients prior to and/or during surgical and other procedures.

Ketamine is a central-acting anesthetic and analgesic that is a non-competitive N-methyl-D-aspartate (NMDA) receptor antagonist. It may provide profound analgesia and amnesia while maintaining spontaneous respiration. However, ketamine is a dose-dependent dissociative anesthetic that can produce unpredictable deep sedation, general anesthesia, and emergence delirium.

Propofol is a gamma-aminobutyric acid (GABA) receptor agonist that can induce hypnosis, amnesia, and rapid arousal. Propofol at doses between 10 and 50 µg per kg per minute has been ordered only for short-term hypnosis in ICU. Propofol can only be administered efficiently and safely with comprehensive monitoring and well-trained staff such as in ICU.

Non-pharmacologic approaches

Cardiac surgery patients undergo extensive procedures and frequently have postoperative back and shoulder pain, anxiety, and tension while in recovery in ICU. Patients who received massage therapy had significantly decreased pain, anxiety, and tension after cardiac surgery. Patients were highly satisfied with the intervention, and no major barriers to implementing massage therapy were identified. Massage therapy was an important component of the healing experience after cardiac surgery.

There is a new protocol for acupuncture administration that was shown to be more effective than standard promotility medication in the treatment of delayed gastric emptying in mechanically ventilated neurosurgical patients. Acupoint stimulation at *Neiguan* (PC-6) may be a convenient and inexpensive option (with few side effects) for the prevention and treatment of malnutrition, and it may improve feeding balance in comparison with promotility drug treatment.

Delirium is characterized by fluctuating levels of arousal, and in the ICU setting this can be associated with sleep–wake cycle disruption, which in turn may be due in part to the reversal of day–night cycles. Proper lighting, noise reduction, relaxation, massage, and music therapy may all promote sleep in ICU. Appropriate control of pain and anxiety are crucial to avoid delirium. Overmedication with analgesics and sedatives may result in confusion and agitation, mandating intervention with haloperidol or a newer agent such as olanzapine.

Interventional procedures

Thoracic epidural, thoracic paravertebral, and intercostal blocks are among the top choices for patients with multiple rib fractures. These interventions present unique advantages and disadvantages, yet all provide similar efficacy in multiple rib fractures.

Regional anesthesia techniques and epidural infusions provide both somatic and sympathetic blockades. Appropriate management of acute pain and stress response with activation of the sympathetic nervous system may help to reduce the duration and severity of postoperative ileus. It may also facilitate timely continuation of enteral feeding in order to promote wound healing and decrease septic complications.

Follow-up

Critical care nurses provide thorough assessment in order to expedite the selection of proper treatment modalities including pharmacologic and non-pharmacologic modalities, and spiritual care intervention. The collaboration of an interdisciplinary team including pain specialists and palliative care may contribute to enhanced pain management and sedation in ICU.

Prognosis

Advances in non-invasive ventilation techniques and developments in the design of mechanical ventilators may result in ventilation that is more in tune with patient efforts and needs. These approaches may facilitate the adjustment of sedation strategies, thereby avoiding the protracted effects of drug accumulations and extreme immobilization and allowing physical therapy to be instituted earlier. The neuropsychiatric and neuromuscular benefits of minimizing opioid administration and facilitating earlier enteral nutrition could also be valuable.

REFERENCES AND FURTHER READING

Chlan LL, Weinert CR, Skaar DJ, Tracy MF. Patient-controlled sedation: a novel approach to sedation management for mechanically ventilated patients. *Chest* 2010; **138**: 1045–53.

Dolan EA, Paice JA, Wile S. Managing cancer-related pain in critical care settings. *AACN Adv Crit Care* 2011; **22**: 365–78.

Erstad BL, Puntillo K, Gilbert HC, *et al.* Pain management principles in the critically ill. *Chest* 2009; **135**: 1075–86.

Ho AM, Karmakar MK, Critchley LA. Acute pain management of patients with multiple fractured ribs: a focus on regional techniques. *Curr Opin Crit Care* 2011; **17**: 323–7.

Hoy SM, Keating GM. Dexmedetomidine: a review of its use for sedation in mechanically ventilated patients in an intensive care setting and for procedural sedation. *Drugs* 2011; **71**: 1481–501.

Memis D, Inal MT, Kavalci G, Sezer A, Sut N. Intravenous paracetamol reduced the use of opioids, extubation time, and opioid-related adverse effects after major surgery in intensive care unit. *J Crit Care* 2010; **25**: 458–62.

Patel SB, Kress JP. Sedation and analgesia in the mechanically ventilated patient. *Am J Respir Crit Care Med* 2012; **185**: 486–97.

Sawh SB, Selvaraj IP, Danga A, *et al.* Use of methylnaltrexone for the treatment of opioid-induced constipation in critical care patients. *Mayo Clin Proc* 2012; **87**: 255–9.

Skrobik Y, Ahern S, Leblanc M, *et al.* Protocolized intensive care unit management of analgesia, sedation, and delirium improves analgesia and subsyndromal delirium rates. *Anesth Analg* 2010; **111**: 451–63.

Tousignant-Laflamme Y, Bourgault P, Gélinas C, Marchand S. Assessing pain behaviors in healthy subjects using the Critical-Care Pain Observation Tool (CPOT): a pilot study. *J Pain* 2010; **11**: 983–7.

60

Pediatric pain

Clinical presentation

Previously believed to be inconsequential, pediatric pain, especially in neonates and young children, had long been dismissed as clinically irrelevant. Advances in developmental neurobiology, however, have revealed that pain transmission pathways are mature as early as 24 weeks gestational age. Increasingly, attention has been directed at explication of short-term (physiological alterations within the dorsal horn) and long-term sequelae (e.g., behavioral responses to subsequent painful stimulation) arising from untreated pain in children.

Acute pain conditions in children and adolescents are likely to be related to trauma/injury; illness such as otitis media, pharyngitis, meningitis, and pelvic inflammatory disease, among others; and medical procedures. Chronic and recurrent pain can be encountered in conditions such as rheumatoid arthritis, sickle cell anemia-related crises, complex regional pain syndrome, and terminal illnesses. The most common chronic and recurrent benign pain complaints in children and adolescents include headaches, abdominal pain, and musculoskeletal pain. The importance of anticipating painful experiences, recognizing the complexities involved in pain assessment, and implementing appropriate pain management strategies in pediatric patients is now well recognized.

Pain assessment

In order to effectively eliminate or assuage pain and suffering in children, clinicians need to use developmentally appropriate assessment tools and techniques (Table 60.1). A variety of pain assessment measures can be employed, depending on the age and the communication abilities of the child, e.g., self-report and observational indices. Pain assessment in infants requires observation of indicators of pain such as behavioral (e.g., facial activity, crying, and body movements) and physiological parameters (e.g., increased heart rate, respiratory

Table 60.1 Clinically useful pediatric pain assessment scales

Age group	Assessment scale	Description
Infants	CRIES [a]	Observational tool; relies on rating of pain behavior including crying, increased vital signs, facial expression, sleeplessness; useful for assessment of postoperative pain; ages 32 weeks of gestation – 6 months
	FLACC [b]	Observational tool; relies on rating of pain behavior including facial expression, leg movement, activity, cry, and consolability; useful for assessment of postoperative/post-procedural pain; age > 2 months
	COMFORT Scale [c]	Observational tool; requires unobtrusive observation for 2 minutes to rate alertness, calmness, respiratory response, physical movement, muscle tone, facial tension, blood pressure, and heart rate; useful for assessment of postoperative/post-procedural pain
Toddlers and preschoolers	FACES Scale [d]	Self-report scale; requires the child to select facial expressions along a visual scale that best describe the amount of pain experienced; useful for assessment of postoperative/post-procedural pain
	OUCHER Scale [e]	Self-report scale; 6 photos of children's faces indicating pain intensity; has corresponding 100-point vertical scale; useful for assessment of post-procedural pain; age ≥ 3 years
	Poker Chip [f]	Self-report scale; 4 poker chips represent "pieces of hurt"; the child is asked to provide how many pieces of hurt they experience; easy to administer; useful for assessment of post-procedural pain; ages 4–8 years
	CHEOPS [g]	Observational tool; relies on rating of pain behavior including cry, facial expression, child verbal, torso, touch, and legs; useful in assessment of postoperative/post-procedural pain; ages 1-7 years

Table 60.1 (*cont.*)

Age group	Assessment scale	Description
School age and adolescent	Coloured Analog Scale [h]	Self-report; modification of 10 cm horizontal VAS, gradations in color in 0.25 increments, with anchors of "no pain" and "most pain"; useful in the assessment of postoperative/ post-procedural and chronic pain; age $\geq$ 5 years
	FACES Scale	Self-report scale (described above); useful for assessment of postoperative/post-procedural and chronic pain
	VAS [i]	Self-report; one is asked to draw an "x" along a 10 cm horizontal line with anchors of "no pain" and "worst pain"; useful in the assessment of postoperative/post-procedural and chronic pain; age $\geq$ 5 years; the child must be able to comprehend proportions; intervals on numerical scales may not be equal from a child's perspective
	Pain Diary	Self-report; numerical ratings are repeated along with recording of other relevant information (e.g., time, activity, medication use); useful in older children and adolescents in determining patterns of pain and in teaching self-management strategies; requires commitment to make thoughtful and accurate entries
Non-communicative and cognitively impaired	Non-communicating children's pain checklist [j]	Observational tool; requires a 10-minute observation period to assess a compilation of behaviors reported by caregivers associated with potentially painful stimuli; useful in the assessment of postoperative/post-procedural, acute pain-related injury and chronic pain
	FLACC	Observational tool (described above); can be used in preverbal and cognitively impaired children $\leq$ 7 years

Table 60.1 (*cont.*)

Age group	Assessment scale	Description
	VAS	Self-report (described above); useful in the assessment of postoperative/ post-procedural pain in non-communicative children age $\geq$ 5 years

CRIES, crying, requires increased oxygen administration, increased vital signs, expression, sleeplessness; FLACC, faces, legs, activity, cry, consolability; CHEOPS, Children's Hospital of Eastern Ontario Pain Scale; VAS, Visual Analog Scale.
Sources:
[a] Krechel SW, Bildner J. CRIES: a new neonatal postoperative pain measurement score. Initial testing of validity and reliability. *Paediatr Anaesth* 1995; **5**: 53–61.
[b] Merkel SI, Voepel-Lewis T, Shayevitz JR, Malviya S. The FLACC: a behavioral scale for scoring postoperative pain in young children. *Pediatr Nurs* 1997; **23**: 293–7.
[c] Ambuel B, Hamlett KW, Marx CM, Blumer JL. Assessing distress in pediatric intensive care environments: the COMFORT scale. *J Pediatr Psychol* 1992; **17**: 95–109.
[d] Hicks CL, von Baeyer CL, Spafford PA, van Korlaar I, Goodenough B. The Faces Pain Scale-Revised: toward a common metric in pediatric pain measurement. *Pain* 2001; **93**: 173–83.
[e] Beyer JE, Denyes MJ, Villarruel AM. The creation, validation, and continuing development of the Oucher: a measure of pain intensity in children. *J Pediatr Nurs* 1992; **7**: 335–46.
[f] Hester NK. The preoperational child's reaction to immunization. *Nurs Res* 1979; **28**: 250–4.
[g] McGrath PA, Johnson G, Goodman J, *et al.* CHEOPS: a behavioral scale for rating postoperative pain in children. In Fields H, Dubner R, Cervero F, eds., *Advances in Pain Research and Therapy.* New York, NY: Raven Press; 1985; pp. 395–402.
[h] McGrath PA, Seifert CE, Speechley KN, *et al.* A new analogue scale for assessing children's pain: an initial validation study. *Pain* 1996; **64**: 435–43.
[i] Huskisson EC. Measurement of pain. *Lancet* 1974; **2** (7889): 1127–31.
[j] Breau LM, McGrath PJ, Camfield CS, Finley GA. Psychometric properties of the non-communicating children's pain checklist-revised. *Pain* 2002; **99**: 349–57.

rate, blood pressure, palmar sweating, decreased oxygen saturation). However, it should be recognized that such parameters may be more indicative of stress than pain.

In children and adolescents, self-reported assessments of pain are preferable; children as young as 3 years of age can be enlisted to report pain location, intensity, and quality. Assessment based upon observation of behavioral signs and physiologic parameters can be used adjunctively, but these may also be influenced by emotional distress – for example, incurred from being in unfamiliar settings or with unfamiliar people, anticipatory distress, etc. Stoic children, or those influenced by depression or fear, may not provide sufficient behavioral cues indicating the degree to which pain is experienced. Consequently, behavioral and physiological signs may be subject to misinterpretation, and should not be solely relied upon for pain assessment. Others who know the child well (e.g., caregivers or parents) can also be a resource upon which to rely to garner indicators of pain, but it is imperative to recognize that proxy assessments can potentially underestimate pain severity.

In contrast to acute pain, the assessment of chronic pain should also include an evaluation of psychosocial factors. Cognizant of the bidirectional influences of psychological states and social/environmental factors with medical disorders and their associated symptoms, including pain, a psychosocial inventory can potentially unveil, and otherwise explicate, the extent to which the patient's psychological makeup, the presence of psychological comorbidities, and the extent of social support and extenuating environmental circumstances contribute to, and are impacted by, the painful condition (Table 60.2). Provided by interview of the pain-afflicted patient as well as parents/caregivers, such efforts can inform, and thereby enrich, treatment endeavors. Though time-consuming, this phase of the examination can highlight those factors that ought to be addressed, which either potentially predispose, activate, and potentiate pain and disability, or which could otherwise undermine recovery and rehabilitation.

Pharmacotherapy

General principles underlying analgesic selection and the manner in which they are used are contingent upon several variables, including the anticipated levels and duration of pain, physiological development, and medical comorbidities. Medication should be dosed according to body weight. Intermittent and short-term pain may be managed adequately with an as-needed pain regimen. However, pain that is expected to persist warrants around-the-clock dosing at fixed intervals. Modifications in dosing and adjustments of administration intervals will need to be based on the assessments of the patient's response. Orally administered medications are preferable, but when immediate relief is required (e.g., during acute procedural pain) intravenous administration is indicated. Intramuscular administration of analgesics is generally avoided, as it is painful and because of concerns over variable absorption of the administered agent. Under certain circumstances, patient-controlled analgesia (PCA) may be a consideration in managing postoperative pain.

Non-opioid analgesics such as acetaminophen, non-steroidal anti-inflammatory drugs (NSAIDs), or cyclooxygenase-2 (COX-2) inhibitors are reasonable considerations to manage mild to moderate acute pain and chronic inflammatory pain in children and adolescents. Opioid analgesics are generally reserved for managing severe acute pain (e.g., postoperative), and for the management of moderate to severe chronic pain states (e.g., sickle cell crisis, cancer pain, and cystic fibrosis-related pain). Long-term opioid therapy for chronic non-malignant pain in children and adolescents remains controversial, as there are concerns regarding long-term sequelae, e.g., endocrine effects, as well as opioid tolerance,

Table 60.2 Psychosocial components of pain assessment for children and adolescents

Psychosocial factor	Examples	Possible intervention(s)
Psychological/ emotional states	Clarifying the relationship of pain to mood; identifying how beliefs and expectations impact pain experiences and perceived incapacitation; assess perceived controllability of pain and repertoire of self-soothing/coping strategies	Psychotherapy, e.g., CBT
Psychiatric comorbidities	Anxiety (including separation anxiety); depression; sleep disturbances	Child psychiatry consultation; psychotherapy; possible antidepressant or anxiolytic pharmacotherapy
Substance use	Drug/alcohol history	Family interventions to address access to/use of substances; coordinated treatment with substance abuse counselors
Adaptive functioning	Activities of daily living; impact on school attendance, academic achievement, participation in extracurricular activities; hobbies and leisure activities	Collaborative efforts with school counselors/teachers; parental education and family-based psychotherapies
Social roles	Interaction patterns between patient and others in the home; quality of peer relationships	Family-based psychotherapy; social skills training
Family-related issues	Impact of pain on other relationships within the home, e.g., between parents and between parents and other children; impact of pain on family functioning; financial impact	Family-based psychotherapy; marital therapy; educational approaches; community resources and social services

Adapted from Leo *et al.* 2011.

risks of misuse/dependence, etc. It should be noted that opioid clearance is reduced in infancy; the ability to metabolize opioids does not reach mature levels until approximately 6 months of life. Cytochrome P450 (CYP) metabolism is required to render certain opioids active (e.g., codeine), as well as to eliminate others (e.g., morphine). Immaturity of the CYP system may mean that a child is unable to obtain reasonable analgesic benefits from certain agents, and/or experiences significant adverse effects such as respiratory depression. Furthermore, toxicity and adverse effects may be apt to occur in children with renal or hepatic dysfunction – for example, morphine effects are protracted in patients with renal dysfunction. Selection of which opioid to use, therefore, would require careful consideration of the child's maturity and capacity to metabolize and/or eliminate the agent, along with medical comorbidities. In order to ensure that adequate pain management is uncompromised, anticipating and promptly addressing the adverse effects of opioid use (e.g., pruritis, nausea/vomiting, constipation, urinary retention, respiratory depression) is essential.

Anxiolytics or sedatives can be useful adjuncts to allay anxiety and distress prior to and during painful procedures. However, sole use of these agents is not advised, because anxiolytics and sedatives can potentially interfere with the child's ability to communicate pain severity.

Pharmacologic interventions for the management of chronic pain in children and adolescents have largely been extrapolated from research demonstrating efficacy in adult patients. There is limited evidence – e.g., case reports and open-label studies but relatively few controlled trials – to guide treatment recommendations. Co-analgesic agents, such as antidepressants, alpha-2-delta ligands, and other anticonvulsants, may be useful in the treatment of headache, neuropathic, and central pain states in children and adolescents. Although insufficient evidence exists to recommend the use of anticonvulsants for the treatment of neuropathy in children and adolescents, substantially more data support their utility in migraine prophylaxis. Similarly, the efficacy of antidepressants has not been systematically investigated, but the selection of these agents may be warranted, particularly in the context of psychological distress and comorbid psychiatric disorders, for example sleep and mood disorders.

Non-pharmacologic approaches

The utility of other treatment modalities in children, e.g., massage and transcutaneous electrical nerve stimulation (TENS), has not been extensively investigated. For example, massage may assist with alleviating burn pain encountered in children, but the generalizability of the usefulness of massage to other acute or chronic pain conditions in children or adolescents cannot be established. Similarly, there is, as yet, a lack of a solid foundation of empirical work upon which to base the utility of TENS in pediatric patients.

Behavioral and psychotherapeutic approach

Behavioral and psychotherapeutic strategies have a role in mitigating suffering and the potential morbidity associated with painful conditions. The modalities employed depend upon the child's stage of development and whether one is confronting acute or chronic pain.

For infants, measures to be undertaken can include holding and repositioning, swaddling, distraction with toys, use of a pacifier, sucrose administration, and breastfeeding. For younger children, the most widely used methods include those that emphasize modifying actions and behaviors surrounding, and thereby mastering, acute or chronic pain: for example, instruction on self-soothing measures such as imagery, relaxation, breathing techniques; distraction; and employing positive reinforcement to alleviate pain. Involving parents in such endeavors can enhance the likelihood that the techniques will be applied and maintained at home.

The bulk of investigations into the utility of psychotherapy in managing chronic and recurrent pain in older children and adolescents have focused on cognitive behavioral therapy (CBT). Through selected techniques – i.e., cognitive restructuring and coping skills training – patients are taught to become active participants in the management of their pain by identifying and restructuring maladaptive beliefs, and thereby minimizing the impact of distressing thoughts and feelings on how pain is experienced. Additionally, patients are taught to cultivate a repertoire of skills with which to more effectively manage distress. Although meta-analyses have revealed that CBT and relaxation training were effective in reducing pain intensity and frequency of headaches, recurrent abdominal pain, and fibromyalgia, there are noteworthy limitations in the extant literature regarding the efficacy of CBT. Outcome measures determining the impact on other domains, such as mood and/or psychiatric comorbidities, academic and functional restoration, were seldom examined. Additionally, studies examining the efficacy of CBT on other chronic pain conditions, for example recurrent musculoskeletal pain, are sparse – and thus the extent to which benefits generalize to such conditions cannot be affirmed with certainty.

Family interventions, maturational issues, and reintegration into the school setting

Chronic pain can produce significant life disruptions, for example by impeding activities and maturation, and interferes with family functioning. Educational and psychotherapeutic interventions involving the family are useful to provide information and support, and to instill consistent and reliable responses to the patient's pain. Such efforts allay parental distress and helplessness by providing a framework within which to better understand and address the child's pain. For example, patient- and family-directed educational approaches regarding implementation of sleep hygiene techniques can minimize pain-related sleep disturbances. Additionally, implementation of behavior modification and role playing may reduce behaviors that foster preoccupation with somatic concerns and the child's perceived incapacity – e.g. over-protectiveness and solicitousness – which could otherwise undermine rehabilitative efforts.

Children and adolescents with chronic pain may sustain particular social difficulties, such as reduced self-ratings of social competence and heightened victimization from peers, which impede maturational processes. Collaborative efforts with mental health providers may provide psychotherapy and skills training directed at fostering social competencies. Enlisting teachers and school counselors can be integral to facilitating the transition back into the school milieu, especially for children who have had protracted absences. In some cases, it may be necessary to coordinate accommodations to the school routine, gradually introduce extracurricular activities, and provide for supplemental instruction, e.g. tutoring and refinement of work habits and organizational skills, to enhance school attendance and academic success.

Interventional procedures

Regional analgesia can be utilized alone or in conjunction with general anesthesia to address intraoperative and postoperative acute pain management. Such measures, e.g., neuraxial (caudal, epidural, and spinal block) or peripheral nerve blockade, may improve patient comfort and possibly reduce total analgesic requirements, thereby minimizing potential medication-related adverse effects, including those from anesthetics and opioids. The decision to pursue interventional approaches should be based on the type of surgical procedure undertaken, the anticipated location of the pain, the absence of contraindications (i.e., systemic infection or coagulopathy), the patient's ability to cooperate with the procedure, and parental consent.

Follow-up and prognosis

Pediatric pain is best managed using multimodal and multisystem approaches. Although the range of needs can vary depending on the child's stage of development and on whether one is confronting acute or chronic pain, effective management can be enhanced by means of an interdisciplinary approach involving family members, pediatricians, child psychiatrists, and psychologists, along with other mental health practitioners, working collaboratively to treat pain and address psychosocial factors related to pain. Comprehensive pediatric care entails the judicious use of pharmacologic, behavioral and psychotherapeutic, interventional and rehabilitative approaches to ensure timely and competent management of pain and suffering.

REFERENCES AND FURTHER READING

American Academy of Pediatrics, Committee on Psychosocial Aspects of Child and Family Health. Task Force on Pain in Infants, Children, and Adolescents. The assessment and management of acute pain in infants, children, and adolescents. *Pediatrics* 2001; **108**: 793–7.

Goddard JM. Chronic pain in children and young people. *Curr Opin Support Palliat Care* 2011; **5**: 158–63.

Leo RJ, Srinivasan SP, Parekh S. The role of the mental health practitioner in the assessment and treatment of child and adolescent chronic pain. *Child Adolesc Ment Health* 2011; **16**: 2–8.

McGrath PJ, Walco GA, Turk DC, *et al.* Core outcome domains and measures for pediatric acute and chronic/recurrent pain clinical trials: PedIMMPACT recommendations. *J Pain* 2008, **9**: 771–83.

Murat I, Gall O, Tourniaire B. Procedural pain in children: Evidence-based best practices and guidelines. *Reg Anesth Pain Med* 2003; **28**: 561–72.

Yaster M. Multimodal analgesia in children. *Eur J Anaesthesiol* 2010, **27**: 851–7.

61

Geriatric pain

Clinical presentation

Aging increases the likelihood of developing one or more common painful conditions such as arthritis, low back pain, myofascial pain, cardiac or pulmonary disease, diabetes, stroke, and cancer. Geriatric pain (GP) refers to painful conditions that affect the elderly, defined as those aged 65 or older, with the "oldest old" being those over 85. The latter make up the fastest-growing cohort of the population in industrialized nations, and for this reason GP is an increasingly prevalent and important problem. Estimates of GP prevalence range from 40% to 80% of community-residing elders. According to studies, as many as 27% of institutionalized older persons do not receive any treatment for their pain. Acute pain, which may herald an underlying serious problem, warrants immediate attention; this review, however, focuses on the growing problem of persistent GP.

It is a geriatric fundamental to differentiate normal age-related change from disease; likewise, it is vital that clinicians recognize that pain is not a naturally occurring, expected part of aging. Rather, pain in older persons is likely due to an underlying disease or condition that will respond to treatment. Untreated painful medical conditions increase the risk for impaired physical and psychological functioning and reduce the quality of life of older persons.

Types of pain in the elderly

The existence of multiple coexisting etiologies for pain requires clinicians to determine whether the sources of pain are visceral, somatic, neuropathic, psychogenic, mixed, or unspecified. Multifactorial pain may require more than one intervention to address each component contributing to the pain.

Examples of nociceptive GP include coronary artery disease, back pain (myofascial, facet joint arthritis, and spondylosis), osteoarthritis, rheumatoid arthritis, osteoporosis, previous fractures, Paget's disease of bone, and polymyalgia rheumatica. Neuropathic pain may be due to central post-stroke pain, demyelinating disease, nutritional neuropathies, peripheral neuropathies, post-herpetic neuralgia, phantom limb, or trigeminal neuralgia. Examples of mixed pain include fibromyalgia and myofascial pain.

Degenerative joint disease is arguably the most common cause of pain in older persons, usually occurring in hips and knees but also in the cervical, thoracic, and lumbar spine and in the hands. Back pain may be due to spinal stenosis, osteoarthropathy, radiculopathy, compression fractures (osteoporosis), somatic dysfunctions, or myofascial syndromes. Pain caused by immobility and contractures, improper positioning, and pressure ulcers should not be overlooked. Peripheral vascular disease (claudication), headache, oral pathology, and chronic leg cramps are common concomitants of aging that may cause significant pain and disability.

Signs and symptoms

Comprehensive assessment is the foundation for accurate diagnosis and treatment of GP. Older patients should be asked about pain as part of routine evaluation, but there are barriers to assessment of pain in older individuals, including healthcare-provider, caregiver, patient, and institutional factors.

Healthcare providers may underestimate or ignore pain because of a perception that assessment is difficult and time-consuming, or they may be unfamiliar with appropriate assessment tools and treatment options available for GP. Caregivers may assume that pain is a normal part of aging which cannot be adequately managed. Patients may themselves believe that pain is to be expected with age. They may under-report pain because of fear about the meaning of pain (serious illness, death) or apprehension about undergoing invasive and potentially painful diagnostic tests. Patients with speech or cognitive deficits may have difficulty expressing what they are feeling; those with severe cognitive impairment or psychiatric illness may be unable to report and manifest behaviors such as agitation or combativeness as markers of pain. Institutional settings may lack systematic protocols for evaluation and treatment of pain.

The Joint Commission mandate to measure pain as the fifth vital sign has helped make pain scales available in all inpatient settings. Well-validated, easy-to-use pain scales include the numeric rating scale (NRS), the verbal descriptor scale (VDS), and the McGill Pain Questionnaire. The Visual Analog Scale, however, is not recommended for use in geriatrics as it is difficult for older persons to understand, especially those with cognitive difficulty, and has lower psychometric validity. Electronic health records may help document and trend pain scores, enabling both patient and clinician to track response to therapy and note improvement or deterioration. Keeping track of pain also allows patients to self-manage by modifying exacerbating conditions so as to minimize or avoid distress.

Patients with GP may present with physical limitations or decline in physical function, and they may tend to use non-specific terms to describe their pain, e.g., aching, boring, stiffness, or burning. Inadequately treated chronic GP can lead to social isolation, withdrawal, and depression; this may manifest as cognitive change ("pseudo-dementia"). Assessment of GP in patients with mild to moderate cognitive impairment requires direct questioning using terms synonymous with pain ("ache" or "discomfort"). Recognition of verbal and non-verbal pain-related behaviors, changes in usual activities or physical function, mood, and sleep are part of a complete geriatric pain assessment.

All older persons, especially those with moderate to severe cognitive decline who are unable to self-report, should be observed closely, and a thorough history of painful episodes and pain-related behaviors should be obtained. Pain should be monitored during movement and at rest. Facial expressions (grimacing, wincing), vocalization (crying, moaning, groaning, calling out), or postural changes (guarding, mobility change such as limping or resistance to moving) are all clear and convincing indicators of pain.

Physiologic changes affecting pain and therapeutics in the elderly

Observations of the effect of aging on pain have resulted in seemingly contradictory concepts: that pain perception with age is blunted (as noted in cases of silent ischemia during myocardial infarction) and that there is an age-related increase in development of neuropathic pain (as noted by the high incidence of post-herpetic neuralgia following herpes zoster infection). Discussion of these ideas is beyond the scope of this review, but the observations serve to assert the presence of GP as a unique biological construct. It is also clear that changes in pain perception with aging are heterogeneous and based on multiple physiologic and individual factors.

In addition to several sources for pain, the elderly have comorbid conditions that lead to polypharmacy, adverse drug interactions, and risk of iatrogenesis. Further, the aging body undergoes changes that directly impact the way older persons respond to medications: body composition change (increased fat-to-lean and fat-to-water ratios) alters drug absorption and distribution, and reduced hepatic and renal function alters metabolism and excretion. Irrespective of the effect of comorbidities, aging physiology itself requires selection and dosing adjustments of pharmacologic interventions for pain.

Table 61.1 summarizes major physiologic changes with aging that affect pharmacologic treatment.

Pharmacotherapy

Experts acknowledge that geriatric pharmacology is fraught with the potential for drug–drug interactions, adverse drug reactions, and iatrogenesis. Prescribing is

Table 61.1 Pharmacologic changes with aging

Pharmacologic concern	Change with normal aging	Common disease effects
Liver metabolism	Oxidation is variable and may decrease, resulting in prolonged drug half-life Conjugation is usually preserved First-pass effect usually unchanged Genetic enzyme polymorphisms may affect some CYP enzymes	Cirrhosis, hepatitis, tumors may disrupt oxidation but not usually conjugation
Renal excretion	Glomerular filtration rate (GFR) decreases with advancing age, resulting in decreased excretion	Chronic kidney disease may predispose further to renal toxicity
Transdermal absorption	Few changes in absorption based on age; may be related to patch technology used	Temperature and other specific patch characteristics may affect absorption
Gastrointestinal absorption or function	Slowing of GI transit time may prolong effects of continuous-release enteral drugs Enhanced opioid-related bowel dysmotility	Disorders that alter gastric pH and surgically altered anatomy may reduce absorption of some drugs
Active metabolites	Reduced renal clearance will prolong effects of metabolites	Renal disease Increase in half-life
Anticholinergic side effects	Increased confusion, constipation, incontinence, movement disorders	Enhanced by neurological disease processes
Distribution	Increased fat-to-lean body weight ratio may increase volume of distribution for fat-soluble drugs	Aging and obesity may result in longer effective drug half-life

Adapted from American Geriatrics Society Panel on Persistent Pain in Older Persons 2009.

further complicated by the fact that controlled clinical trials of analgesics have either completely overlooked geriatric patients, or have included only small numbers of this age group, leaving a dearth of evidence upon which to base recommendations. In general, clinicians treating GP are advised to avoid pre-scribing multiple-drug therapies with overlapping mechanisms of action or those that may have adverse pharmacokinetic interactions.

The American Geriatrics Society recently published the 2012 Beers Criteria Update for potentially inappropriate medication use in the elderly. The expert panel issued the following recommendations for analgesics to avoid or use with caution:

- Meperidine – not an effective oral analgesic in commonly used dosage and has the potential for neurotoxicity.
- Chronic use of non-COX-selective oral NSAIDs – potential to cause gastro-intestinal bleeding and peptic ulcer disease in high-risk groups, i.e., those over age 75 or taking oral or parenteral corticosteroids, antiplatelet medications, or anticoagulants.
- Oral NSAIDs – affect renal function and may cause acute or chronic renal failure, especially in older patients with concomitant hypertension, congestive heart failure or diabetes. Caution is advised even for short-term use. For short-term use or for patients having no other effective alternatives, NSAIDs with concomitant use of gastroprotective agents, e.g., proton pump inhibitor or misoprostol, may be considered.
- Tricyclic antidepressant medications and skeletal muscle relaxants – strong anticholinergic effects increase the risk for sedation, falls, and fractures.

Analgesic medications that may be useful for GP include the following:

- NSAID or other topical patches (e.g., lidocaine) may be applied directly to localized areas of pain; the risk for adverse drug reactions is mitigated by relatively low systemic absorption.
- Acetaminophen in doses lower than 3 g/day may be helpful for mild to moderate pain, alone or as a co-analgesic. However, caution should be used with higher doses in patients with hepatic insufficiency.
- Anticonvulsant, antidepressant, and membrane-stabilizing drugs have shown efficacy for treatment of neuropathic pain; sedation and the risk for falls may limit their use in older persons.

Opioids are known to have efficacy in a broad range of nociceptive and neuro-pathic painful conditions. The use of opioid analgesics for persistent, non-cancer pain remains controversial, but consensus groups note the relative safety of their use in carefully selected, closely monitored older patients. Issues of tolerance, side effects, and risk for misuse, abuse, and diversion must be considered as part of the evaluation of a patient with GP for chronic opioid therapy.

Because of individual variation in response, there is no one best opioid or "drug of choice," nor are there are guidelines specific to initiation, titration, and modi-fication of opioid analgesia in older persons. Therefore, the decision to use one drug over another must be based on clinician experience, patient health status and prior experience with analgesics or previous exposure to opioids, formulation availability, cost, and third-party coverage, as well as the attainment of therapeutic goals and predicted or observed harms. Recommendations for chronic opioid therapy in the elderly are limited by the lack of long-term studies supporting their safety and efficacy.

General recommendations for use of pharmacologic agents in older persons include knowing the actions, adverse effects, and toxicity profiles of all prescribed and over-the-counter medications, selecting therapies with a low risk of drug or nutrient interactions, and avoiding use of agents that may induce or inhibit cytochrome P450 (CYP) isoenzymes or prolong QTc interval.

All geriatric patients must be closely observed for signs of adverse drug reactions or drug–drug interactions during the first few weeks of any new therapy. Patients with persistent pain should be reassessed regularly for improvement, deterioration, or complications. In addition to the reduction of pain, focus should be placed on specific clinical endpoints such as functional capacity, behavior, mood, and sleep.

Non-pharmacologic approaches

Interventions that reduce or eliminate the need for analgesic medications are strongly recommended for older individuals, including physical therapy and rehabilitation modalities, manual medicine (osteopathic) techniques, and maintenance of ambulatory function through ongoing exercise (especially aquatherapy for those unable to tolerate weight-bearing activities). Complementary and alternative medicine (CAM) techniques such as balneotherapy and massage may prove to be of benefit. Patients who exhibit depression and poor coping skills will benefit from cognitive behavioral therapy (CBT) or psychiatric evaluation.

Interventional procedures

Please see various chapters on specific medical conditions.

Prognosis

The primary goal for adequate analgesia in the elderly is improved quality of life. An optimal approach emphasizes the best analgesic response that uses the fewest and lowest doses of medications for the shortest period of time, combined with multimodal therapies to maintain and enhance mood, sleep, and functional capacity.

REFERENCES AND FURTHER READING

American Geriatrics Society 2012 Beers Criteria Update Expert Panel. American Geriatrics Society updated Beers Criteria for potentially inappropriate medication use in older adults. *J Am Geriatr Soc* 2012; **60**: 616–31.

American Geriatrics Society Panel on Persistent Pain in Older Persons. Pharmacological management of persistent pain in older persons. *J Am Geriatr Soc* 2009; **57**: 1331–46.

Chou R, Fanciullo GJ, Fine PG, *et al.* Clinical guidelines for the use of chronic opioid therapy in chronic noncancer pain. *J Pain* 2009; **10**: 113–30.

Gagliese L. Pain and aging: the emergence of a new subfield of pain research. *J Pain* 2009; **10**: 343–53.

Herr K. Pain assessment strategies in older patients. *J Pain* 2011; **3**: S3–13

Reiser L. Pharmacological management of persistent pain in older persons. *J Pain* 2011; **12**: S21–9.

62

Cancer pain, palliative and end-of-life care

Clinical presentation

Morbidity and mortality rates from cancer continue to rise despite ongoing research to find a cure. At the same time, advances in detection and treatment allow cancer patients to live longer after diagnosis, some with active disease, some in remission, and some cured (cancer survivors). Metastases to bone or viscera are an obvious source of pain, but cancer survivors and patients in remission also experience acute and chronic pain as a consequence of surgical procedures, radiation, and chemotherapy. Since virtually every cancer patient will experience pain at some point during treatment or disease progression, the problem of cancer pain is an ongoing and growing healthcare concern.

Pain, the most common and feared result of cancer, may be nociceptive (visceral, somatic), neuropathic, or mixed (combination of painful etiologies). However, physical discomfort is not the only consequence of serious, life-limiting illness: psychological, existential, and social distresses are common in cancer as well as in many other terminal illnesses. Referred to as "total pain," this suffering necessitates thoughtful, well-coordinated care across multiple disciplines (medical, nursing, psychology, social service, pastoral care) to facilitate the best possible outcome for patients, families, and caregivers.

Studies suggest that cancer pain has mean prevalence estimates of 41% in the general adult cancer population (range 29–85%) and 75% in advanced cancer (range 53–100%); literature is sparse on cancer pain prevalence in cancer survivors. Neuropathic pain, estimated to cause 20% of discomfort in cancer patients and 40% when those with mixed pain are included, may result from treatments (chemotherapeutic agents, radiation) or it may be a result of comorbid disease.

Signs and symptoms

Sources of cancer pain include primary or metastatic tumor burden, diagnostic testing, postoperative pain, hormonal changes, chemotherapy, radiation, and infection. Nociceptive causes of cancer pain may be somatic (bone pain arising from pathologic fractures or bony metastases, chemotherapy-induced mucositis, radiation burns, surgical wounds, or diffuse musculoskeletal pain) or visceral (bowel or urinary obstruction, hepatic distension, ascites, pleuritis, or pericarditis). Neuropathic causes of cancer pain include spinal cord compression, painful polyneuropathy, cranial neuralgias, plexopathy, radiculopathy, leptomeningeal metastases, and paraneoplastic syndromes.

Many cancer patients have anemia, hypoxemia, and/or low left ventricular ejection fraction which result in profound fatigue. While not a painful state, fatigue is an extremely debilitating and distressing symptom. Cancer patients may have mixed nociceptive and neuropathic pain from several etiologies, as in cases of advanced carcinoma with metastases to bone, lungs, liver, and/or brain. Patients with complicated pain due to multiple etiologies may require rational polypharmacy and/or several therapeutic modalities for achievement of adequate analgesia.

Non-cancer terminal illnesses not immediately recognized as primary pain generators also cause pain. For example, end-stage cardiac disease causes angina, weakness, fatigue, and exercise intolerance, while advanced obstructive pulmonary disease is associated with chest wall pain, dyspnea, anxiety, and fatigue. Virtually all terminal disease states render patients progressively frail and immobile, predisposing them to the development of additional painful sequelae such as pressure ulcers, skin tears, upper and lower extremity contractures, fractures, deep venous thrombosis, cellulitis, osteomyelitis, pneumonia, and urinary tract infections.

Treating cancer and other serious or terminal illness involves comprehensive assessment of the patient's level of pain and all its potential sources. Using an appropriate rating scale, such discomfort should be evaluated for amount, location, frequency, duration, and type, as well as for precipitating, exacerbating, and alleviating factors. A review of the patient's current medical conditions, medications, and treatments should be combined with a thorough social and psychological evaluation, including attention to risk factors for depression, addiction, or non-adherence. Physical evaluation directed at establishing source(s) of pain must include a focused structural and neurological evaluation. Thorough assessment of previous treatments employed and identification of those that were successful is important for the development of a comprehensive palliative plan of care.

Diagnostic investigations and imaging studies

Imaging or other diagnostic studies may be useful in delineating the etiology of cancer pain, thus allowing specific interventional procedures or specialized pain regimens tailored to the cause to be implemented. Testing should be considered with the caveat that patients near the end of life may benefit more from withholding painful diagnostic tests than from any potential information that might be gained.

Clinical approach and goal of care

Involvement of the patient in advanced care planning and therapeutic plan of care is the cornerstone of palliative care, and should be part of the clinician–patient relationship for every patient with serious illness. Family and caregiver support is another vital part of the healthcare strategy. Optimal care-plan development to provide excellent analgesia involves participation of the patient, family, and caregivers with an interdisciplinary team of providers to (a) identify specific goals, (b) develop strategies for maximizing physical function, and (c) minimize psychosocial distress and unwanted symptoms.

Pain management goals of treatment for cancer pain and in palliative care are: (1) prevent discomfort when possible; (2) reduce baseline pain as much as possible through the use of long-acting analgesics, adjuvant medications, and/or therapeutic blocks; and (3) aggressively treat episodes of breakthrough pain, defined as acute transient and worsening. This discomfort may occur intermittently, associated with specific situations, e.g., turning or other movements (incident pain), or spontaneously without an apparent inciting event. Breakthrough pain requires immediate-release preparations, usually opioids, in addition to the patient's baseline, long-acting pain regimen.

Palliative care seeks to address patient needs both within and beyond the realm of physical pain. Palliative care is defined by the World Health Organization as the "active total care of patients whose disease is not responsive to curative treatment." Therefore, control of pain and other symptoms – e.g., psychological, social, and spiritual issues – is paramount. Palliative care is sometimes confused with hospice, a Medicare benefit established 30 years ago to provide formal care for individuals with terminal illness and limited life expectancy. According to the National Hospice and Palliative Care Organization (NHPCO), nearly 1.6 million Americans received hospice care in 2010. Palliative care, however, is not confined to patients facing the end of life and should be offered to all patients with pain, especially that due to chronic and/or serious illness. As reported by the Center to Advance Palliative Care (CAPC), 85% of US hospitals with 300 or more beds utilize palliative care teams to assist with symptom management and advance care planning.

Ideally, palliative care is provided in addition to potentially curative treatment options. When it is clear that cure is no longer possible, palliative care seeks to focus goals of care so as to maximize quality of life, which may include (but is not limited to) the election of the hospice benefit for end-of-life care. Thus, all hospice patients receive palliative care, but not all palliative care patients receive hospice care.

Pharmacotherapy

Table 62.1 lists important steps in the use of medications to treat pain classified as chronic, persistent, or end-of-life, regardless of etiology.

Table 62.1 Pharmacologic management of chronic, persistent, or end-of-life pain

---

(1) Select appropriate analgesic drug
(2) Prescribe appropriate dose of drug
(3) Administer drug by appropriate route
(4) Schedule appropriate dosing interval
(5) Prevent persistent pain and relieve breakthrough pain
(6) Titrate dose of drug aggressively
(7) Prevent, anticipate, and manage side effects of the drug
(8) Consider sequential trials of opioid analgesics
(9) Use appropriate co-analgesic drugs

Adapted from Levy & Samuel 2005.

Opioids are the drugs of choice for cancer pain, and also for moderate to severe non-cancer pain that impairs function or quality of life. Individual patients respond differently to medications, so there is no "best" opioid for pain. Clinicians must assess whether an alternative medication has a better risk–benefit profile and if not, determine whether the potential benefits of opioid analgesia outweigh risks for an individual patient.

Opioid dose titration is based on analgesic responsiveness; side effects (e.g., sedation, nausea, pruritus, myoclonus, constipation) must be closely monitored. While tolerance to sedation and nausea develop over time, constipation requires prophylaxis with stool softeners and motility agents as a routine part care for *every* patient receiving opioids. Intractable, distressing side effects such as myoclonus (more commonly seen in patients with renal or hepatic insufficiency), pruritis, or seizures necessitate a swift change to another opioid (opioid rotation) at an equivalent dose. An equianalgesic table (Table 62.2) is useful for calculating doses to be used in opioid rotation.

Commonly used co-analgesics include acetaminophen and non-steroidal anti-inflammatory drugs (NSAIDs). Acetaminophen, first-line therapy for mild to moderate pain, is often combined with short-acting opioids as a co-analgesic (e.g., oxycodone/acetaminophen). Note that the acetaminophen component of combination medications may limit titration to full analgesic effect because of its hepatotoxic dose range of 3 g per 24 hours. NSAIDs have insufficient evidence for their use as primary analgesics for cancer pain but are valuable co-analgesics and useful for bone pain (etiology for pain due to bone metastasis is prostaglandin release).

It is generally advisable to prescribe opioids that are not combined with co-analgesics such as acetaminophen or NSAIDs, so that the opioid can be up-titrated to full analgesic response without concern for liver, renal, or gastric toxicity.

Adjuvants are treatments given in addition to a primary or initial therapy. In this discussion, the term *adjuvant* refers to medications that facilitate the primary treatment through mitigation of side effects (e.g., laxatives to treat

Table 62.2 Equianalgesic doses of opioid analgesics

Oral (PO) dose (mg)	Analgesic	Intravenous (IV) dose (mg)
150	Meperidine [a]	50
100	Codeine [a,b]	60
15	Hydrocodone [a,c]	—
15	Morphine [d]	5
10	Oxycodone [e]	—
10	Methadone [f]	5
4	Hydromorphone [d]	1.5
2	Levorphanol	1
—	Fentanyl [g]	—

Adapted from Levy & Samuel 2005.

Equianalgesic doses listed were obtained from a variety of studies; this table is meant to be a practical guide for initial dosing, with the exact dose to be determined in each patient by individual titration.

Dose interval: every 4 hours except for: meperidine, every 2–3 hours; levorphanol, every 4–6 hours; methadone, every 6–12 hours; controlled-release morphine, every 8 or 12 hours depending on formulation; controlled-release oxycodone, every 12 hours; transdermal fentanyl, every 48–72 hours.

[a] Not recommended for severe pain.

[b] Acetaminophen + codeine combinations contain 325 mg of acetaminophen with either 15 mg, 30 mg, or 60 mg of codeine. Codeine doses above 1.5 mg/kg are not recommended because of increased toxicity.

[c] Acetaminophen + hydrocodone combinations contain 325 mg of acetaminophen with 2.5–10 mg of hydrocodone. Ibuprofen + hydrocodone combinations contain 200 mg of ibuprofen with 2.5–10 mg of hydrocodone.

[d] Rectal suppositories available. Per rectum (PR) dose is equal to PO dose.

[e] Acetaminophen + oxycodone combinations contain 325–650 mg of acetaminophen with 2.5–10 mg of oxycodone. Aspirin + oxycodone combinations contain 325 mg of aspirin with 2.5–10 mg of oxycodone.

[f] There is increased risk of toxicity from delayed accumulation of methadone. In opioid rotation, start methadone at 10–50% of equianalgesic dose calculated from table, depending on daily dose of morphine.

[g] Transdermal fentanyl dose should be calculated as follows: μg/h fentanyl every 3 days = mg of morphine PO every 12 hours. Oral transmucosal fentanyl citrate dosage must be determined by individual titration. Fentanyl units should be applied to the buccal mucosa over a 15-minute period for breakthrough pain. Dose may be repeated in 15 minutes if needed. Unit dose should be increased if patient needs more than 8 units per day.

opioid-induced constipation, antihistamines to treat pruritus, antiemetics to treat nausea/vomiting) and/or they may have efficacy for problems apart from the primary complaint of pain.

Adjuvant medications commonly used in palliative care include the following:

• Gabapentin is used for painful peripheral neuropathic pain and for cancer-related neuropathic pain.

- Antidepressants, which have limited evidence for cancer-related neuropathic pain, are useful to reduce postoperative neuropathic pain in breast cancer patients and have the synergistic effect of improving mood.
- Cannabinoids (e.g., dronabinol) have limited evidence for cancer pain but have been useful as antiemetic therapy (nabiximols is approved for cancer pain in Canada, United Kingdom, and parts of Spain).
- Corticosteroids, useful for reducing edema from brain metastasis, have limited evidence for their use as primary analgesics except for their anti-inflammatory effects in bone pain, and they may improve overall well-being.

Other treatments for bone pain include bisphosphonates, which may be effective for painful bone metastases; however, calcitonin is not clearly effective for bone metastasis pain. Denosumab (treatment for osteoporosis) has US Food and Drug Administration (FDA) approval for prevention of spine/axial skeletal events including pathologic bone fractures and bone pain requiring radiation (see below).

Non-pharmacologic approaches

Complementary and alternative measures include manual medicine techniques, massage, and aroma and music therapy. Psychological counseling and pastoral care are important modalities for patients suffering from cancer and chronic pain syndromes, and for those facing the end of life.

Radiation may be used both in an attempt to cure and for palliation: radioisotopes may provide pain relief in patients with metastatic bone pain. Radiofrequency ablation may be effective for pain relief of bony metastases. Single-fraction radiotherapy may be as effective as multiple fractions for relieving metastatic bone pain, but it is associated with higher re-treatment and pathological fracture rates.

Interventional procedures

When routine pharmacologic therapy fails to achieve adequate analgesia, interventional procedures may be helpful for selected patients with specific disease states. Intrathecal ziconotide, a toxin derived from a sea snail, has been shown to reduce pain in adults with cancer or AIDS and pain refractory to opioids. Celiac plexus block may reduce opioid use and constipation and slightly reduce pain in adults with pancreatic cancer, and chemical splanchnicectomy may reduce pain in patients with unresectable pancreatic cancer.

Patients with intractable bone pain from cancer-related vertebral fracture may be considered for vertebroplasty and kyphoplasty. The decision to refer for interventional procedures, with full informed consent by the patient, should be made as part of an ongoing dialog between the patient and the interdisciplinary team, keeping in mind the overall goals of care.

Follow-up and prognosis

Cancer prognoses are individual, based on the stage of illness and the overall medical condition of each patient. The goal of enhanced quality of life is paramount for these patients. When cure is not possible, the goals of palliative care are to provide support with difficult medical decision making, interdisciplinary expertise in care planning and coordination, excellent pain and symptom management, and psychological and spiritual support and comfort.

REFERENCES AND FURTHER READING

Bennet MI, Rayment C, Hjermstad M, *et al.* Prevalence and aetiology of neuropathic pain in cancer patients: a systematic review. *Pain* 2012; **153**: 359–65.

Burton AW, Fine PG, Passik SD. Transformation of acute cancer pain to chronic cancer pain syndromes. *J Support Oncol* 2012; **10**: 89–95.

Levy MH, Samuel TA. Management of cancer pain. *Semin Oncol* 2005; **32**: 179–93.

Portenoy RK, Lesage P. Management of cancer pain. *Lancet* 1999; **353**: 1695–700.

Svendsen KB, Andersen S, Arnason S, *et al.* Breakthrough pain in malignant and non-malignant diseases: a review of prevalence, characteristics and mechanisms. *Eur J Pain* 2005; **9**: 195–206.

63

Opioid tolerance, physical dependence, and addiction

Opioid medications have long been employed to produce analgesia in acute and cancer-related pain conditions. Increasingly, there has been a trend toward utilizing opioid therapy to address the severity of pain, improve quality of life, and enhance functional restoration of patients afflicted with chronic pain states refractory to other treatments. Physicians are confronted with the challenge of balancing the potential benefits of opioid therapy, especially if prescribed long-term or for patients with non-malignant chronic pain conditions, with the potential risks of opioid misuse, physical dependence, abuse, and addiction. Although the focus of this chapter will be to address concerns pertaining to opioid use, the principles apply equally to other medications within the pharmacologic arsenal which can likewise possess abuse potential, including certain muscle relaxants such as carisoprodol, benzodiazepines such as alprazolam or diazepam, and N-methyl-D-aspartate (NMDA) receptor antagonists such as ketamine, among others.

Definition of key terms

The presence of tolerance and/or physical dependence is a cardinal sign upon which the diagnosis of substance dependence, e.g., alcohol dependence, is based. However, tolerance and physical dependence are inevitable occurrences in the context of appropriate, regular, ongoing opioid therapy for patients with enduring pain, and therefore cannot be reasonably relied upon to delineate when opioid use has become problematic.

Tolerance

Tolerance is a pharmacodynamic phenomenon resulting in adaptation to an effect of a medication. It can be manifested as the perception of (a) a diminished effect with the same dose/frequency of a drug regimen, or (b) a need for a higher dose/frequency of a medication to maintain the same level of desired effect that had previously been appreciated with lower doses or less frequent dosing. Tolerance may develop to any effect of an opioid. In some cases, tolerance to, and therefore attenuation of, adverse effects of a prescribed agent would be desirable (e.g., the respiratory depressant effects of opioids), whereas tolerance to desired analgesic effects can be unfavorable.

Tolerance may be mediated by cellular processes, for example alterations in second-messenger systems such as the upregulation of the cyclic adenosine monophosphate (cAMP) pathway; downregulation of opioid receptors; and/or increases in and activation of NMDA and other receptor systems with effects that oppose the analgesia produced by opioids. (It has been suggested that use of NMDA antagonists such as ketamine can reverse tolerance.)

The rate at which tolerance develops, and the extent to which it develops, can vary considerably. Some patients can acquire sufficient analgesic benefits with a stable opioid regimen for prolonged periods, while others may require periodic dose escalations to sustain analgesic benefit. Tolerance, however, is but one of many factors that must be considered to account for a diminished perceived effectiveness of an opioid analgesic over time.

Physical dependence

Like tolerance, physical dependence is a pharmacologic process resulting in adaptation to regular use of the medication. It is characterized by overt physical and psychological withdrawal effects that arise from abrupt cessation, rapid dose reduction, or administration of an antagonist. In general, withdrawal symptoms are characterized by the over- or underactivity of physiological functions that are normally inhibited or stimulated, respectively, by the medication. Signs of opioid withdrawal can include yawning, rhinorrhea, lacrimation, piloerection, mydriasis, gooseflesh, nausea, vomiting, diarrhea, abdominal cramping, myoclonus, sweating, anxiety, and dysphoria. Unlike benzodiazepine withdrawal, for example from alprazolam, withdrawal from opioids does not produce life-threatening symptoms (i.e., delirium or seizures), but the symptoms are nonetheless very distressing.

Although the duration of administration required to produce physical dependence is not known, it may occur with regular use of an opioid for as brief a period as 2 weeks. Withdrawal can be avoided by gradual dose reductions in an attempted dose taper, and attenuated by administration of clonidine, an alpha-2 agonist (to reduce the elevations in blood pressure, diarrhea, and sweating that can accompany withdrawal).

Inappropriate use

Inappropriate medication use is denoted by the terms misuse, abuse, and addiction. Recent investigations suggest that there have been substantive increases in the rates of emergency room presentations of patients ascribable to opioid analgesic abuse and misuse. Naturally, safety concerns arise about potentially serious injury or death arising from unintentional overdose that can occur in the context of inappropriate opioid use. Abuse and addiction refer to maladaptive behavior patterns around medication/substance use which can lead to psychological, interpersonal, functional, and social impairments.

Misuse

Misuse refers to the utilization of a medication for an indication other than that for which it was intended – for example, a patient who makes use of an opioid for its sedative effects or to allay anxiety, independent of distress or sleep interference produced by pain. Misuse can occur sporadically, and it often arises from misunderstanding the intended purpose of the opioid. Patient education regarding the appropriate uses of prescription medication and the hazards of misuse may be sufficient to dissuade further occurrences. Habitual misuse, especially using a medication in a manner that is unintended, e.g., crushing to inject or insufflate an opioid that is intended for oral use, are likely to reflect abuse or addiction.

Abuse

Patients who abuse prescription opioids display a pattern of recurrent medication use, despite its deleterious effects on aspects of functioning. Although hazardous, the pattern of use does not reflect the degree of loss of control over use (or psychological dependence) that is encountered among persons with addiction. Some examples include using an opioid in situations that are physically hazardous, e.g., driving or operating heavy machinery and thereby incurring potential harm to self or others; recurrent legal problems related to substance use, such as charges for driving while under the influence of an opioid; recurrent use despite its adverse impact on one's functioning, impeding one's ability to fulfill role responsibilities and/or leading to social and interpersonal problems.

Addiction

Addiction is considered a psychiatric disorder characterized by features of compulsive use and/or loss of control over use of a medication or substance. Generally, the impairments incurred by addiction tend to be more severe and pernicious than those associated with abuse, implying more widespread dysfunction. Conceptually, loss of control can take a number of forms reflective of psychological dependence, including: (a) using a medication in ever-increasing amounts, despite deleterious effects; (b) repeated failed attempts to control one's use of the medication; (c) going to inordinate lengths to acquire, use, and recover from medication use; (d) giving up many aspects of one's self-care and social and recreational interests because of the use of the substance (instead of pain); and (e) persistent use despite having ongoing psychological and physical adverse effects produced by the use of the medication.

Risk management strategies

Except in cases of acute injury, cancer, or management of pain associated with surgical procedures which are likely to necessitate use of opioids to achieve pain relief, clinicians must be cognizant of measures that should be undertaken to address the risks of misuse, abuse, and addiction when contemplating opioid analgesics in chronic pain (Table 63.1). A comprehensive history, physical examination, and related diagnostic assessments are necessary to corroborate the patient's complaints and specify, if at all possible, the etiology of the pain and delineate appropriate courses of treatment. Long-term opioid therapy is likely to be best employed in patients with physical findings and definitive conditions that manifest with moderate to severe pain. Pain conditions with poorly defined etiologies, or for which there is evidence of strong psychosocial influence of the pain severity ratings, or possible somatoform disorders, may predict poor response to therapy, including long-term opioid treatment.

A detailed history and thorough review of medical records can unveil whether conventional and evidence-based approaches for the particular type of pain with which the patient presents have been previously undertaken. It is prudent, for past treatment failures, to ascertain whether previous medications (including multi-drug therapy regimes) were given a reasonable trial, e.g., dosed appropriately and of sufficient duration, before being deemed to have failed. Similarly, it is necessary to review whether non-pharmacologic interventions were previously attempted, including invasive approaches (e.g., injection therapies and neural blockade, implanted devices, surgical interventions), physical and occupational therapy, other rehabilitative approaches (e.g., work hardening program, TENS units, psychotherapeutic interventions), and the extent to which appreciable benefits or adverse effects were encountered. The aforementioned review will inform whether a trial of opioid treatment is reasonable or whether any untested treatment approaches, particularly those with favorable risk–benefit ratios, are warranted before initiation of, or concurrent with, opioid therapy.

One must consider whether a trial of opioid therapy carries with it undue risks that outweigh potential benefits. These can include risks of harm caused by pharmacologic effects of the opioids (e.g., toxicity in patients with hepatic and/or renal dysfunction), sleep apnea or other respiratory compromise, or concerns about potentially deleterious effects arising from co-administered medications such as sedatives or benzodiazepines. Lastly, consideration must be directed at determining whether there are concerns about the patient's ability to adhere to responsible and reliable medication use, e.g., risks of abuse or addiction. The factor that most predicts abuse or addiction appears to be a prior or current personal or familial history of substance abuse/dependence. Use of a screening assessment, such as the Opioid Risk Tool (ORT) or the Screener and Opioid Assessment for Patients with Pain (SOAPP), is essential and can assist in identifying those individuals for whom more intensive monitoring would be required during the course of therapy. Other potential risk factors suggested in the

Table 63.1 Strategies to mitigate risk when employing opioid therapy

Comprehensive assessment (history, physical examination, and related diagnostic
  assessments)
Review current and previously attempted treatment approaches employed
Know what medications are prescribed and by whom
Screen for the risk of opioid use disorder
Screen for psychiatric comorbidities and psychological distress
Provide informed consent
Use a mutually agreed treatment agreement/plan stipulating:
. Opioids are to be provided by a single clinician
. A single pharmacy is to be used
. The frequency of office follow-up visits
. How lost/stolen/misplaced prescriptions will be managed
. Risk management strategies, e.g., pill counts, random urine drug testing
Establish parameters for goals of therapy and define how treatment success will be
  determined, e.g., demonstrable improvements in activities of daily living (ADL),
  resumption of customary role responsibilities, etc.
Structure monitoring and concurrent treatment strategies according to level of risk for
  opioid misuse
Implement concurrent treatment strategies, e.g., concurrent therapies to improve function
  (physical therapy, occupational therapy, psychotherapy, substance-disorder-related
  treatment), multidisciplinary treatment
Apprise patients of potential hazards:
. Avoid combining opioids with sedative/hypnotics, benzodiazepines, or alcohol
. Reduce opioid dose during upper respiratory tract infections or asthmatic episodes
. Never take a prescription pain medication unless it is prescribed by the treating clinician
. Do not take more doses than prescribed without consulting with the treating clinician
. Avoid using prescription pain medication to facilitate sleep
. Secure prescription pain medications, e.g., to guard against accidental ingestion by
  children or pets and to prevent theft
. Avoid sharing pain medications with others
Follow-up:
. Monitor analgesic efficacy, adverse effects, impact on functioning and ADL, aberrant
  drug-taking behavior
. Assess whether modifications in treatment approaches are warranted
. Coordinate care with and manage medication prescribed by other providers

literature have included psychiatric comorbidities, younger age (< 45 years), male
gender, prior history of sexual abuse, prior history of sociopathy (i.e., illegal
behaviors), cigarette smoking, and poor social supports. Psychiatric or psychological assessment to screen patients for psychiatric comorbidities and
psychological distress that may otherwise impede treatment progress and contribute to the risk of abuse or addiction may be warranted. Patients with concurrent illicit-substance-related disorders are likely to require formal treatment
before initiation of long-term opioid therapy.

Based upon the above preliminary review, it may then be appropriate to pursue opioid therapy. Patients must be apprised of the potential risks of long-term opioid use (physical dependence, withdrawal, addiction, etc.) before treatment initiation as part of the full disclosure and informed consent process. Use of a mutually agreed treatment agreement can be helpful to establish the goals of treatment, specify how the opioids are to be prescribed and taken, delineate expectations regarding concomitant therapies, and establish the parameters for clinic monitoring and follow-up. The agreement should also delineate the indications for tapering or discontinuing opioid therapy, such as in circumstances where there is lack of progress in achieving therapeutic goals, intolerable adverse effects, or repeated or serious aberrant drug behaviors.

Regular follow-up of patients is necessary to evaluate tolerability of adverse effects, efficacy, and patterns of use. Monitoring must encompass an assessment of the adequacy of analgesia; adverse effects; response to treatment (i.e., demonstrable improvement in adaptive functions such as activities of daily living, and in quality of life, and resumption of functional capabilities); participation in and progress achieved through concomitant treatment approaches (e.g., physical and occupational therapy, psychotherapy, concurrent substance abuse treatment); changes in psychiatric comorbidities and mental status; and identification of aberrant drug-related behaviors suggestive of misuse, abuse, addiction, or diversion. Review of the patient's pain dairy can reveal the impact of treatment on day-to-day functioning and may show patterns of use that unveil whether dosing modifications are required, e.g., to address end-of-dose failures. Tracking of phone calls and requests for refills (especially for lost or stolen prescriptions), pill counts, and the results of periodic random urine toxicology screens are prudent to undertake and discuss with the patient during clinical visits. The clinician should recognize that some of these measures (e.g., pill counts) can be unreliable. Isolated reports of lost medication should not be ignored, and consideration should be given to possible cognitive impairments (idiopathic or iatrogenic, i.e., medication-induced). Repeated instances of lost prescriptions may be a concern and may require safeguards, for example having a reliable source dispense and monitor medication use.

Clinical considerations when confronted with aberrant drug-related behavior

There are several factors that must be considered when a patient's analgesic requirements increase (Table 63.2). Some behaviors – e.g., using medications more often than the prescriber intended, running out of medication prematurely and making requests for additional analgesics, supplementing what was provided by the prescriber with another's medications, among others – can be disconcerting and worrisome because these behaviors, on the surface, might suggest features of abuse or addiction. However, the emergence of such behaviors should not lead

Table 63.2 Differential of plausible factors underlying aberrant drug-related behaviors

---

Suboptimal analgesia (inadequate dosing or irregular use)

Progression of a pathologic process or emergence of another pain-producing condition

Breakthrough pain, either idiopathic or incident

End-of-dose failure

Opioid tolerance

Inadequate adherence to treatment, e.g., secondary to cognitive impairments and/or psychiatric disorders

Unrealistic expectations as to what the medication is expected to achieve

Co-administration of a drug that induces cytochrome metabolism (and diminished effectiveness) of the prescribed medication

Psychiatric comorbidity or psychological distress, which predispose to greater perceived incapacitation and pain rating augmentation

Genetic factors that render responsiveness to one analgesic less effective than to another

Diversion of prescription medication for profit

Misappropriation, e.g., theft of medication, perpetrated by others

Medication abuse or addiction

---

to summarily discharging the patient from treatment. Instead, these behaviors must be identified and acknowledged by the clinician and addressed with the patient directly so as to uncover the motives underlying the behavior. Failure to do so may impart a tacit acceptance of inappropriate medication use. Conversely, failure to clarify the motives underlying such behaviors can impede recognition of inadequately treated pain. In some cases, out of desperation arising from failure to obtain relief, a patient may resort to manipulation, demanding and entitled behaviors, exaggerated expressions of distress, etc., to enlist the clinician to provide solutions to his/her plight. This would be consistent with pseudoaddiction. The clinician must consider an extensive differential before necessarily concluding that abuse or addiction is present. On the other hand, one must recognize that pseudoaddiction and abuse or addiction can plausibly co-occur in the same individual.

Several strategies can be employed to address problems associated with suboptimal analgesia. Use of long-acting opioids may be preferred over long-term use of short-acting agents to avoid end-of-dose failure and potential risks of abuse. Inadequate analgesia may warrant dose adjustments, trials of opioid rotation, co-administration of co-analgesic agents (antidepressants and anticonvulsants) or weak analgesics (non-steroidal anti-inflammatory drugs and/or acetaminophen), and trials of non-pharmacologic therapies and complementary therapies. In each case, the treatment approaches invoked will need to be individualized and implemented in joint negotiation with the patient. Collaborative interdisciplinary approaches must always be considered in difficult-to-manage cases, and especially for patients with current or prior history of substance abuse. Participation in ongoing treatment from addiction specialists, substance abuse treatment, and concurrent psychiatric and/or psychotherapy may be particularly prudent in such cases, especially to enhance patient education, address psychiatric comorbidities, and cultivate a repertoire of skills to more effectively manage pain and related psychosocial stressors.

By contrast, behaviors that signal probable abuse or addiction include: (a) acquiring medication from "off-the-street" or illegal sources; (b) engaging in illegal behavior to acquire pain medication or money with which to purchase drugs from illegal sources, e.g., stealing, prostituting oneself or others; (c) misrepresenting oneself clinically, e.g., falsifying information or failing to disclose visits to emergency rooms or other clinicians from whom opioids have been acquired; (d) stealing drugs; (e) prescription forgery; and (f) selling prescription medications to acquire those of higher abuse potential or street value. In such cases, it may be important to take measures to safely taper and discontinue opioid therapy. Referral to formal substance disorder treatment under such circumstances is warranted.

REFERENCES AND FURTHER READING

Chou R, Fanciullo GJ, Fine PG, *et al*. Clinical guidelines for the use of chronic opioid therapy in chronic noncancer pain. *J Pain* 2009; **10**: 113–30.

Gourlay DL, Heit HA, Almahrezi A. Universal precautions in pain medicine: a rational approach to the treatment of chronic pain. *Pain Med* 2005; **6**: 107–12.

Højsted J, Sjøgren P. Addiction to opioids in chronic pain patients: a literature review. *Eur J Pain* 2007; **11**: 490–518.

Manchikanti L, Giordano J, Boswell MV, *et al*. Psychological factors as predictors of opioid abuse and illicit drug use in chronic pain patients. *J Opioid Manag* 2007; **3**: 89–100.

Passik SD, Kirsh KL, Donaghy KB, Portenoy RK. Pain and aberrant drug-related behaviors in medically ill patients with and without histories of substance abuse. *Clin J Pain* 2006; **22**: 173–81.

Index

abatacept 264
abdominal pain, functional. *See* irritable bowel
    syndrome
abduction and external rotation (AER) 64
abductor pollicis brevis 93
acetaminophen
    brachial plexopathy 61
    cancer pain 356
    cervical facet syndrome 52
    cervical radiculopathy 57
    compression fractures 182
    costosternal/costochondral/costovertebral
        syndromes 110
    critical care pain 332
    geriatric pain 351
    interstitial cystitis 158
    lumbar post-laminectomy pain syndrome 213
    lumbar spinal stenosis 198
    migraine 5
    osteoarthritis 262
    pediatric pain 341
    pelvic pain 164
    piriformis syndrome 194
    post-lumbar-puncture headache 25
    postoperative pain 316
    pregnancy pain 321–2
    sickle cell disease 328
    tension headache 15
    thoracic spinal pain 127
acetyl-ʟ carnitine 286
Achilles reflex 219, 234, 240
aciclovir
    herpes zoster 271
    HIV-related neuropathy 294
activities of daily living (ADLs) 97, 227
acupuncture
    irritable bowel syndrome 144
    lumbar spinal stenosis 198
    migraine 6
    osteoarthritis 265

    pregnancy pain 322
    thoracic spinal pain 128
acute chest syndrome 326–7
acute multi-organ failure 327
adalimumab 264
addiction 362
adrenocorticotropic hormone (ACTH),
        post-lumbar-puncture headache 25
Adson (scalene) maneuver 63
adult respiratory distress syndrome 308, 326
aerophagia 138
age-related pharmacologic changes 352
alcohol, abstinence from 135
allodynia 121, 148, 222, 291, 298, 308
almotriptan 5
amitriptyline
    central pain 299
    fibromyalgia pain syndrome 254
    temporomandibular joint pain 34
amyotrophic lateral sclerosis 282
anakinra 264
analgesic rebound headache. *See* medication-
    overuse headache
ankle arthritis 238–42
    clinical presentation 238–9
    differential diagnosis 240
    follow-up 242
    management 240–1
    physical examination 239–40
ankylosing spondylitis 108, 110, 126, 175, 186,
    208, 263
    bamboo spine 126
    differential diagnosis 127
anterior cruciate ligament injuries 233
anterior interosseus nerve 93–4
anticonvulsants
    burn pain 310
    cervical radiculopathy 48
    cervicobrachial pain 57
    complex regional pain syndrome 278

entrapment neuropathies 150
geriatric pain 351
lumbar radiculopathy 188
phantom limb pain 304
polyneuropathy 285
sickle cell disease 328
thoracic outlet syndrome 65
thoracic spinal pain 127
antidepressants
geriatric pain 351
intercostal neuralgia 117
irritable bowel syndrome 143
pediatric pain 343
See also tricyclic antidepressants, *and specific drugs*
antihistamines, in interstitial cystitis 158
antispasmodics 143
aquatherapy, in sacroiliac pain 209
arachnoiditis 186, 213
arcade of Frohse 92–4, 96
Arnold–Chiari malformation 298
arteriovenous fistula 39
arthritis
ankle, foot, and toe 238–42
elbow 83–7
hand and wrist 97–100
hip 217–21
knee 227–31
shoulder 67–71
arthroplasty
elbow 87
hip 221
knee 230
shoulder 71
thumb interposition 100
aspirin
back pain 176
compression fractures 182
migraine 5
pelvic pain 164
tension headache 15
assistive devices 230
aura, in migraine 1
avascular necrosis 217

back pain 167–78
clinical presentation 167–9
differential diagnosis 174–5
follow-up 178
imaging studies 174
laboratory tests 173
management 175–7

prognosis 178
red flags 170
signs and symptoms 169–73
yellow flags 170
baclofen
central pain 299–300
complex regional pain syndrome 279
trigeminal neuralgia 30
Baker's cyst 227
bamboo spine 126
benzodiazepines, in back pain 176
biceps reflex 42
biceps tendinitis 73
Bier blocks 279
biofeedback
cervicobrachial pain 57
post-thoracotomy pain syndrome 122
bisacodyl, irritable bowel syndrome 142
bisphosphonates
cancer pain 358
complex regional pain syndrome 278
compression fractures 182
side effects 182
bladder pain syndrome 156
bone mineral density 180
botulinum toxin
central pain 300
cervicobrachial pain 57
cluster headache 11
interstitial cystitis 159
migraine 6, 21
neck strain/sprain 44
piriformis syndrome 194
temporomandibular joint pain 35
Bouchard's nodes 97
brachial plexopathy 52, 59–62, 104
clinical presentation 59
differential diagnosis 60
follow-up 61
imaging studies 60
laboratory tests 60
management 61
prognosis 62
signs and symptoms 59
brachial plexus block 61, 65, 123, 317
breast milk, drugs in 321
Brown-Séquard syndrome 125
bruxism 32
bullous contact dermatitis 270
bullous pemphigoid 270
Burn Index 308
burn pain 307–13

burn pain (cont.)
  clinical presentation 307
  differential diagnosis 309
  follow-up 312
  imaging studies 309
  laboratory tests 309
  management 309–12
  prognosis 312
  rule of nines 307
  signs and symptoms 307–8
bursitis
  elbow 83–7
  hip 217–21
  knee 227–31
  shoulder 72–6
butalbital 5
butorphanol, pregnancy pain 321
butterbur
  migraine 6
  tension headache 17

caffeine
  analgesic combination 5, 15
  post-lumbar-puncture headache 25
  pregnancy pain 321
calcium pyrophosphate disease 229, 231
cancer pain 353–9
  clinical presentation 353
  follow-up and prognosis 359
  goals of care 354–5
  imaging studies 354
  management 355–8
  signs and symptoms 353–4
capsaicin
  complex regional pain syndrome 278
  herpes zoster 272
  intercostal neuralgia 117
  meralgia paresthetica 224
  phantom limb pain 304
  polyneuropathy 285
carbamazepine
  central pain 299
  entrapment neuropathies 150
  herpes zoster 271
  occipital neuralgia 39
  polyneuropathy 285
  side effects 29
  trigeminal neuralgia 29
cardiac surgery, post-surgical pain 120–3
carotid artery dissection, differential diagnosis 9
carotidynia 34
carpal pressure test 98, 103

carpal tunnel syndrome 64, 93–5, 102–6
  clinical presentation 102–3
  differential diagnosis 104
  follow-up 106
  imaging studies 104
  laboratory tests 104
  management 104–6
  prognosis 106
  risk factors 102
  signs and symptoms 103
cauda equina syndrome 197, 215
causalgia. *See* complex regional pain syndrome
celecoxib, back pain 176
celiac disease 134, 140
celiac plexus 131
celiac plexus block 135, 358
central neuropathic pain 298
central pain 297–302
  clinical presentation and signs 297–8
  differential diagnosis 299
  follow-up 301
  imaging studies 299
  laboratory tests 299
  management 299–301
  prognosis 301
cervical dystonia 55–8
cervical facet syndrome 51–4
  clinical presentation 51
  differential diagnosis 52
  follow-up 53
  imaging studies 52
  laboratory tests 52
  management 53
  prognosis 54
  signs and symptoms 51
cervical myelopathy 48
cervical nerve root compression 104
cervical plexus block 317
cervical radiculopathy 46–9
  clinical presentation 46
  differential diagnosis 47–8
  follow-up 49
  imaging studies 47
  laboratory tests 47
  management 48–9
  prognosis 49
  signs and symptoms 46
cervicobrachial pain 55–8
  clinical presentation 55
  differential diagnosis 56
  follow-up 58
  imaging studies 56

laboratory tests 56
management 57
prognosis 58
signs and symptoms 55
cervicobrachial syndrome 52
cervicogenic headache 39, 43
Charcot foot 239, 284
Charcot–Marie–Tooth disease 239
chemical neurolysis 123
CHEOPS scale 338
chest pain 107–13
chest wall pain 111
chickenpox 268–9
children, pain in. *See* pediatric pain
chondroitin sulfate, in osteoarthritis 262
chondromalacia patella 229
Chopart's joint 239–40
chronic daily headache 18–22
    clinical presentation 18
    differential diagnosis 19–20
    follow-up 22
    laboratory tests 19–20
    management 21
    prognosis 22
    signs and symptoms 18–19
chronic pelvic pain 157
cidofovir, in HIV-related neuropathy 294
cisapride, in irritable bowel syndrome 143
clonazepam, in central pain 299
clonidine
    complex regional pain syndrome 279
    critical care pain 333
    postoperative pain 316
club foot 239
cluster headache 4, 8–12
    chronic 19
    clinical presentation 8
    differential diagnosis 9
    episodic 19
    follow-up 12
    imaging studies 9
    laboratory tests 2
    management 10–11
    prognosis 12
    signs and symptoms 8–10
coccydynia 152–5
    clinical presentation 152
    differential diagnosis 153–4
    follow-up 155
    imaging studies 153
    laboratory tests 153
    management 154–5

prognosis 155
    signs and symptoms 152–3
coccygalgia. *See* coccydynia
coccygectomy 155
coccygeoplasty 155
codeine, in cancer pain 357
co-enzyme Q10, in migraine 6
cognitive behavioral therapy
    cervicobrachial pain 57
    coccydynia 154
    complex regional pain syndrome 279
    fibromyalgia pain syndrome 256
    herpes zoster 272
    interstitial cystitis 159
    irritable bowel syndrome 144
    lumbar post-laminectomy pain syndrome 214
    myofascial pain syndrome 247
    pediatric pain 344
    polyneuropathy 286
    post-thoracotomy pain syndrome 122
colonoscopy, in irritable bowel syndrome 140
Coloured Analog Scale 339
COMFORT Scale 338
complex regional pain syndrome (CRPS) 60, 123,
    275–80
    clinical presentation 275–6
    differential diagnosis 277
    follow-up 280
    imaging studies 277
    laboratory tests 277
    management 278–9
    prognosis 280
    signs and symptoms 276
compression (approximation) test 207
compression fractures 180–4
    clinical presentation 180–1
    differential diagnosis 182
    follow-up 183
    imaging studies 182
    laboratory tests 181
    management 182–3
    prognosis 183
    signs and symptoms 181
computed tomography. *See* CT
conjunctival injection 9
cordectomy 301
corticosteroids
    carpal tunnel syndrome 105
    chronic daily headache 21
    epidural injection
        cervical radiculopathy 49
        lumbar radiculopathy 189

corticosteroids (cont.)
    lumbar spinal stenosis 198
    neck strain/sprain 44
    thoracic spinal pain 128
  post-lumbar-puncture headache 25
  tennis/golfer's elbow 91
costosternal/costochondral/costovertebral
    syndromes 107–13
  clinical presentation 107–8
  differential diagnosis 110
  follow-up 113
  imaging studies 109
  laboratory tests 109
  management 110–12
  prognosis 113
  signs and symptoms 108–9
COX-2 inhibitors
  back pain 176
  brachial plexopathy 61
  burn pain 309
  cervical facet syndrome 52
  cervical radiculopathy 48
  cervicobrachial pain 57
  costosternal/costochondral/costovertebral
    syndromes 110
  critical care pain 332
  herpes zoster 271
  intercostal neuralgia 116
  interstitial cystitis 158
  lumbar facet syndrome 202
  lumbar radiculopathy 188
  osteoarthritis 262
  pediatric pain 341
  postoperative pain 316
  post-thoracotomy pain syndrome 122
  sickle cell disease 327
  thoracic spinal pain 127
CPOT. See Critical-Care Pain Observation Tool
C-reactive protein 261
CRIES pain scale 338
critical care pain 331–6
  clinical presentation 331
  differential diagnosis 332
  follow-up 335
  imaging studies 332
  laboratory tests 332
  management 332–4
  prognosis 335
  signs and symptoms 331
Critical-Care Pain Observation Tool (CPOT) 331
Crohn's disease 263
  See also inflammatory bowel disease

cryoanalgesia 123
cryoneurolysis, in occipital neuralgia 40
crystal arthropathies 238
CT
  brachial plexopathy 60
  burn pain 309
  central pain 299
  cervical radiculopathy 47
  cervicobrachial pain 56
  coccydynia 153
  irritable bowel syndrome 139
  lumbar post-laminectomy pain syndrome 212
  lumbar radiculopathy 186
  meralgia paresthetica 223
  pancreatitis 133
  pelvic pain 163
  thoracic spinal pain 126
cyclobenzaprine
  fibromyalgia pain syndrome 254
  temporomandibular joint pain 34
cyclooxygenase-2 inhibitors. See COX-2
    inhibitors
cyclosporine, in interstitial cystitis 158
cystitis. See interstitial cystisis

deep brain stimulation
  cluster headache 11
  phantom limb pain 306
degenerative joint disease
  ankle, foot and toe 238–42
  elbow 83–7
  hip 217–21
  knee 227–31
  pain 348
  shoulder 67–71
  spine 205
  wrist 97
denosumab
  cancer pain 358
  compression fractures 183
depakote, in migraine prevention 6
desipramine
  central pain 299
  fibromyalgia pain syndrome 254
  polyneuropathy 285
dexmedetomidine, in critical care pain 333
dextromethorphan, in polyneuropathy 286
diabetes mellitus 133
diabetic peripheral neuropathy 282
diabetic truncal neuropathy 112
diazepam, in critical care pain 333
dicyclomine, in irritable bowel syndrome 141

diffuse idiopathic skeletal hyperostosis (DISH) 126
dihydroergotamine 5
  cluster headache 11
diltiazem, in cluster headache 10
disc herniation 185
discography, in cervical radiculopathy 47
disease-modifying antirheumatic drugs (DMARDs) 264
DISH 126
distal interphalangeal joints 97
distraction (gapping) test 206
divlaproex sodium, in tension headache 16
DMARDs 264
dorsal root entry zone (DREZ) procedure 61, 301
dowager's hump 181
drug abuse 362
drug misuse 362, 365–7
Duchenne muscular dystrophy 239
duloxetine
  fibromyalgia pain syndrome 254–5
  herpes zoster 271
  polyneuropathy 285
dural puncture headache. See post-lumbar-puncture headache
dysesthesia 121, 308
dysmenorrhea 163
dyspareunia 153, 162
dyspepsia 138
dystonia 298

Eagle syndrome 34
elbow
  bursitis 83–7
  tennis/golfer's 88–91
elbow arthritis 83–7
  clinical presentation 83
  differential diagnosis 85
  follow-up and prognosis 87
  imaging studies 86
  laboratory tests 85
  management 86
  physical examination 84–5
  signs and symptoms 83–4
elbow nerve entrapment 92–6
  clinical presentation 92–3
  differential diagnosis 94–5
  follow-up 96
  laboratory tests and imaging studies 95
  management 95–6
  physical examination 93–4
elbow replacement 87

electrodiagnostic testing
  carpal tunnel syndrome 104
electromyography. See EMG
eletriptan 5
EMG
  brachial plexopathy 60
  cervical facet syndrome 52
  cervical radiculopathy 47
  cervicobrachial pain 56
  complex regional pain syndrome 277
  groin pain 149
  lumbar facet syndrome 201
  polyneuropathy 284
  pregnancy pain 320
  tennis/golfer's elbow 90
  thoracic outlet syndrome 64
  thoracic spinal pain 126
endometriosis 157, 161–6
  clinical presentation 161–2
  differential diagnosis 163
  imaging studies 163–4
  laboratory tests 163
  signs and symptoms 162–3
epicondylitis, lateral/medial. See tennis/golfer's elbow
epidural analgesia 317, 329
epidural blood patch 25
epigastric pain 138
epilepsy 1
ergotamine 5
erythema exudativum multiforme 270
erythrocyte sedimentation rate (ESR)
    osteoarthritis 261
    thoracic spinal pain 126
escharotomy 309
estrogens, and bone mineral density 182
etanercept 264
extensor carpi radialis longus muscle 88
extensor indicis proprius 89
eyelid swelling 9

FABER sign. See Patrick's test
FACES Scale 338
facet arthropathy 125
facial asymmetry 33
famciclovir, in herpes zoster 271
femoroacetabular impingement 217–18, 220
femorotibial joint 227
fentanyl 134
    cancer pain 357
    HIV-related neuropathy 294
    pregnancy pain 321

feverfew, in migraine 6
Fibromyalgia Impact Questionnaire 257
fibromyalgia pain syndrome 32, 52, 111, 245,
    248–57
  clinical presentation 249–50
  differential diagnosis 56, 253, 257
  follow-up 256
  imaging studies 252
  laboratory tests 252
  management 253–7
  prognosis 257
  signs and symptoms 250–2, 257
  tender point locations 257
FLACC pain scale 338–9
flexor carpi ulnaris 88, 92, 94
flexor digitorum profundus 85, 93
flexor digitorum superficialis 104
  weakness 103
flexor pollicis longus 93, 104
fluoxetine
  fibromyalgia pain syndrome 254
  tension headache 16
foot arthritis 238–42
  clinical presentation 238–9
  differential diagnosis 240
  follow-up 242
  imaging studies 240
  management 240–1
  physical examination 239–40
Fortin finger test 206
foscarnet, in HIV-related neuropathy 294
fractures
  compression 180–4
  ribs 111, 121
  sternum 111
  vertebral 125
frovatriptan 5
functional abdominal pain. *See* irritable bowel
    syndrome

gabapentin
  burn pain 310
  central pain 299
  complex regional pain syndrome 278
  entrapment neuropathies 150
  fibromyalgia pain syndrome 254
  herpes zoster 271
  HIV-related neuropathy 294
  intercostal neuralgia 117
  lumbar radiculopathy 188
  lumbar spinal stenosis 198
  meralgia paresthetica 224

migraine prevention 6
  occipital neuralgia 39
  phantom limb pain 304
  polyneuropathy 285
  post-lumbar-puncture headache 25
  trigeminal neuralgia 30
Gaenslen's test 186, 206
gallstones 133
gamma knife surgery in trigeminal neuralgia 31
ganciclovir, in HIV-related neuropathy 294
genitofemoral nerve 146
genitofemoral neuralgia 146
  clinical features 147
    Tinel's sign 148
  differential diagnosis 149–50
geriatric pain 347–52
  age-related pharmacologic changes 352
  assessment 348–9
  clinical presentation 347
  management 349–52
  physiologic changes affecting 349
  prognosis 352
  types of 347
Gillet test 206–7
globus pharyngis 138
glossopharyngeal neuralgia 34
glucosamine sulfate, in osteoarthritis 262
golfer's elbow. *See* tennis/golfer's elbow
gout 229, 231, 238, 263
grip, evaluation of 98
groin pain 146–51
  clinical presentation 146–8
  differential diagnosis 149–50
  follow-up 151
  imaging studies 149
  laboratory tests 148–9
  management 150
  prognosis 151
  signs and symptoms 148
Guillain–Barré syndrome 282

hallux rigidus 240
hallux valgus 240–1
hand and wrist arthritis 97–100
  clinical presentation 97–8
  differential diagnosis 99
  follow-up 100
  imaging studies 99
  laboratory tests 99
  management 99–100
  signs and symptoms 98
hand–foot syndrome 326

hands-up test 64
Hawkins test 78
headache
    cervicogenic 39, 43
    chronic daily 18–22
    cluster 4, 8–12
    medication overuse 5
    migraine 1–7
    migrainous 4
    post-lumbar-puncture 23–6
    tension 4, 13–17
Heberden's nodes 97
hematocrit 132
hemicrania continua 19
hemicrania, chronic paroxysmal 19
hemiparesis, in migraine 1
hemoglobin S 325
herpes simplex virus 270
herpes zoster 116, 122, 125, 268–74
    clinical presentation 268–9
    differential diagnosis 9, 270
    follow-up 273
    laboratory tests 270
    management 270–3
    prevention 272
    prognosis 273
    signs and symptoms 269–70
herpetic neuralgia. See herpes zoster
hiccups 138
highly active antiretroviral therapy (HAART)
    288
Hill–Sachs deformities 69
hip arthritis/bursitis
    clinical presentation 217–18
    differential diagnosis 219
    follow-up 221
    imaging studies 219
    management 219–21
    signs and symptoms 218–19
hip replacement 221
HIV-related neuropathy 288–96
    clinical presentation 288–91
    differential diagnosis 292, 296
    drugs causing 296
    follow-up 295
    imaging studies 292
    laboratory tests 291
    management 294–5
    prognosis 295
    signs and symptoms 291
    types of 296
Hoffmann's sign 42, 48

Horner's syndrome 9
H-reflex 186
human immunodeficiency virus. See HIV-related
    neuropathy
Hunner's ulcers 156
hyaluronans 265
hydrocodone 134
    cancer pain 357
    HIV-related neuropathy 294
    pregnancy pain 321
hydrogen breath test 139
hydromorphone, in cancer pain 357
hyoscyamine, in irritable bowel syndrome 141
hyperalgesia 115, 121, 298, 308
    opioid-induced 315
hyperpathia 121, 308
hypnic headache 19
hypnosis, for burn pain 311
hypoesthesia 223

ibandronate, prevention of compression
    fractures 182
ibuprofen
    back pain 176
    cluster headache 11
    pregnancy pain 321
    tension headache 15
idiopathic skeletal hyperostosis. See DISH
iliohypogastric nerve 146
iliohypogastric neuralgia 146
    clinical features 147–8
    differential diagnosis 149–50
ilioinguinal nerve 146
ilioinguinal neuralgia 146–51
    abdominal weakness 148
    clinical features 151
    differential diagnosis 149–50
iliotibial band syndrome 219
iliotibial band tendinitis 232, 234, 236
immersive virtual reality 311
indomethacin
    chronic daily headache 21
    hemicrania continua 19
    pregnancy pain 321
infectious arthritis 263
inflammatory bowel disease 134, 140
infliximab 264
intercostal muscle injury 111
intercostal nerve block 117, 123
intercostal nerves 114
intercostal neuralgia 112, 114–19
    clinical presentation 114–15

intercostal neuralgia (cont.)
　differential diagnosis 116
　follow-up 118
　imaging studies 116
　laboratory tests 116
　management 116–18
　prognosis 119
　signs and symptoms 115
interstitial cystitis 155–60
　clinical presentation 156
　differential diagnosis 157–8
　follow-up 159
　imaging studies 157
　laboratory tests 156
　management 158–9
　prognosis 160
　signs and symptoms 156
irritable bowel syndrome 137–45
　clinical presentation 137
　differential diagnosis 140, 145
　follow-up 144
　imaging studies 140
　laboratory tests 139
　management 140–5
　prognosis 145
　signs and symptoms 137–9

joint laxity 32
jump sign 244

ketamine
　burn pain 311
　complex regional pain syndrome 278
　critical care pain 333
　polyneuropathy 286
　postoperative pain 316
ketoprofen
　cluster headache 11
　tension headache 15
ketorolac
　cluster headache 11
　post-lumbar-puncture headache 25
　postoperative pain 316
knee arthritis/bursitis 227–31
　clinical presentation 227
　differential diagnosis 229
　follow-up 231
　imaging studies 229
　laboratory tests 229
　management 229–31
　physical examination 228–9
　signs and symptoms 232–4

knee replacement 230
knee sprain/tendinitis 232–7
　clinical presentation 232
　differential diagnosis 235
　follow-up 236
　imaging studies 235
　management 235–6
　physical examination 234–5
　prognosis 236
　signs and symptoms 232–4
kyphoplasty 183
kyphosis 171, 175

lacrimation 9
lactation. *See* pregnancy/lactation, pain in
lactose intolerance 139
lamotrigine
　central pain 299
　HIV-related neuropathy 294
　polyneuropathy 285
　trigeminal neuralgia 30
laser therapy, in temporomandibular joint pain
　35
lateral collateral ligament sprain 233
lateral femoral cutaneous nerve 222–3
levorphanol, in cancer pain 357
Lhermitte's sign 282
lidocaine
　cervical facet syndrome 53
　complex regional pain syndrome 278
　herpes zoster 272
　HIV-related neuropathy 294
　intercostal neuralgia 117
　meralgia paresthetica 224
　polyneuropathy 285
ligament of Struthers 92–4, 96, 104
limaprost, in lumbar spinal stenosis 198
lipase 132
Lisfranc joint 239
lithium carbonate
　chronic daily headache 21
　cluster headache 10
Lloyd's test 181
loperamide, in irritable bowel syndrome 141
lorazepam, in critical care pain 333
lordosis 32
low back pain 319
lubiprostone, in irritable bowel syndrome
　142
lumbar facet syndrome 200–3
　clinical presentation 200
　differential diagnosis 202

follow-up 203
imaging studies 201
laboratory tests 201
management 202–3
prognosis 203
signs and symptoms 200–1
lumbar post-laminectomy pain syndrome
211–16
clinical presentation 211–12
differential diagnosis 213
follow-up 215
imaging studies 212
laboratory tests 212
management 213–14
prognosis 215
signs and symptoms 212
lumbar puncture headache. *See* post-lumbar-
puncture headache
lumbar radiculopathy 185–91, 217
clinical presentation 185
differential diagnosis 186, 213
follow-up 190
imaging studies 186–7
laboratory tests 186
management 187–90
prognosis 190
lumbar spinal stenosis 196–9
clinical presentation 196
differential diagnosis 197
follow-up 198
imaging studies 197
laboratory tests 197
management 198
prognosis 199
signs and symptoms 196

macroamylasemia 132
magnesium, in migraine 6
magnetic resonance angiography. *See* MRA
magnetic resonance imaging. *See* MRI
malabsorption 133
mastectomy, post-surgical pain 120–3
McGill Pain Questionnaire 273, 348
McMurray's click test 235
medial antebrachial cutaneous nerve 95
medial collateral ligament 233
median nerve
compression. *See* carpal tunnel syndrome
decompression 96, 106
entrapment 92
neuropathy 95
medication-overuse headache 5, 15–16, 19

management 21
memantine
phantom limb pain 305
polyneuropathy 286
meniscus tears 235
meningioma 39
meperidine
cancer pain 357
geriatric pain 351
pregnancy pain 321
sickle cell disease 328
meralgia paresthetica 222–6
clinical presentation 222
differential diagnosis 224
follow-up 225
imaging studies 223
laboratory tests 223
management 224–5
prognosis 225
metacarpal phalangeal joints 84, 98
fusion 100
methadone
cancer pain 357
pregnancy pain 321
methotrexate, in interstitial cystitis 158
methylcobalamin, in lumbar spinal stenosis 198
methylnaltrexone, in burn pain 310
methylprednisolone, in cervical radiculopathy 48
migraine 1–7
aura 1
chronic 18, 21
clinical presentation 1–2
differential diagnosis 4
follow-up 6
imaging studies 4
incidence 1
laboratory tests 2
management 4–6
pain characteristics 2
phases of 1
premonitory phase 1
prognosis 7
prophylaxis 5
signs and symptoms 2
without aura 7
migrainous headache 4
military maneuver 63
milnacipran
fibromyalgia pain syndrome 254–5
polyneuropathy 285
miosis 9
mirror therapy

mirror therapy (cont.)
  complex regional pain syndrome 279
  phantom limb pain 305
mittelschmerz 162–4
molluscum contagiosum 270
morphine 134
  cancer pain 357
  pregnancy pain 321
MRA, in cervicobrachial pain 56
MRI
  back pain 174
  brachial plexopathy 60
  burn pain 309
  central pain 299
  cervical 43
  cervical radiculopathy 47
  cervicobrachial pain 56
  cluster headache 9
  coccydynia 153
  complex regional pain syndrome 277
  costosternal/costochondral/costovertebral
    syndromes 109
  elbow nerve entrapment 95
  hip arthritis/bursitis 219
  HIV-related neuropathy 292
  knee sprain/tendinitis 235
  lumbar post-laminectomy pain syndrome 212
  lumbar radiculopathy 187
  lumbar spinal stenosis 197
  meralgia paresthetica 223
  migraine 2
  occipital neuralgia 38
  pelvic pain 163
  pregnancy pain 320
  rheumatoid arthritis 262
  rotator cuff tear 79
  shoulder bursitis/tendinitis 75
  temporomandibular joint 33
  tennis/golfer's elbow 89
  tension headache 14
  thoracic spinal pain 126
  trigeminal neuralgia 28
multiple myeloma 39
multiple sclerosis 282, 298
muscle relaxants 194
  back pain 176
  brachial plexopathy 61
  cervicobrachial pain 57
  lumbar facet syndrome 202
  post-thoracotomy pain syndrome 122
  thoracic spinal pain 127
myalgia, infection-related 112

myelitis 39
myelography, in central pain 299
myofascial pain syndrome 52, 55, 122, 213,
    243–8
  clinical presentation 243
  differential diagnosis 245, 248
  follow-up 248
  imaging studies 245
  laboratory tests 244
  management 245–7
  prognosis 248
  signs and symptoms 243–4

nalbuphine, in pregnancy pain 321
naproxen 5
  back pain 176
  cluster headache 11
  pregnancy pain 321
  temporomandibular joint pain 34
  tension headache 15
naratriptan 5
nasojejunal tube feeding 134
nausea and vomiting 138
  in migraine 2
neck strain/sprain 41–5
  clinical presentation 41
  differential diagnosis 43
  follow-up 44
  imaging studies 43
  laboratory tests 43
  management 43–4
  prognosis 45
  signs and symptoms 41–3
Neer test 78
nerve blocks. See specific nerves
nerve conduction studies
  brachial plexopathy 60
  cervical facet syndrome 52
  cervical radiculopathy 47
  thoracic outlet syndrome 64
  thoracic spinal pain 126
nerve entrapment
  elbow 92–6
  median nerve 92
  radial nerve 92
  ulnar nerve 85, 92
nervus intermedius decompression 11
neuralgia
  glossopharyngeal 34
  ilioinguinal 146–51
  intercostal 112, 114–19
  occipital 37–40

post-herpetic 125
neuroablation
    cervical facet syndrome 53
    postsurgery pain 123
    thoracic spinal pain 128
neurofeedback, in cervicobrachial pain 57
neurogenic arthropathy 263
neuromodulation
    cervical radiculopathy 49
    occipital neuralgia 40
    post-thoracotomy pain syndrome 123
neuropathic pain 281, 353
    central 298
    See also polyneuropathy
neurotomy, in lumbar facet syndrome 203
new daily persistent headache 19, 21
nimodipine, in cluster headache 10
nitrous oxide 311
NMDA receptor antagonists
    burn pain 311
    critical care pain 333
    polyneuropathy 286
    postoperative pain 316
non-communicating children's pain checklist 339
non-steroidal anti-inflammatory drugs.
        See NSAIDs
norpramine, in polyneuropathy 285
nortriptyline, in fibromyalgia pain syndrome 254
NSAIDs
    back pain 175
    brachial plexopathy 61
    burn pain 309
    cancer pain 356
    carpal tunnel syndrome 105
    central pain 299
    cervical facet syndrome 52
    cervical radiculopathy 57
    cervicobrachial pain 57
    cluster headache 11
    coccydynia 154
    compression fractures 182
    costosternal/costochondral/costovertebral
        syndromes 110
    critical care pain 332
    elbow arthritis 86
    elbow nerve entrapment 95
    foot and ankle arthritis 241
    geriatric pain 351
    hand and wrist arthritis 99
    herpes zoster 271
    hip arthritis/bursitis 220
    intercostal neuralgia 116

interstitial cystitis 158
    knee arthritis/bursitis 230
    lumbar facet syndrome 202
    lumbar post-laminectomy pain syndrome 213
    lumbar radiculopathy 188
    lumbar spinal stenosis 198
    migraine 5
    neck strain/sprain 43
    osteoarthritis 262
    pediatric pain 341
    pelvic pain 164
    piriformis syndrome 194
    post-lumbar-puncture headache 25
    postoperative pain 316
    post-thoracotomy pain syndrome 122
    sacroiliac pain 208
    sickle cell disease 327
    temporomandibular joint pain 34
    tension headache 15
    thoracic spinal pain 127
numeric rating scale (NRS) 348
nutation 205

occipital nerve block 39
    cluster headache 11
occipital neuralgia 37–40
    clinical presentation 37
    differential diagnosis 38–9
    follow-up and prognosis 40
    imaging studies 38
    laboratory tests 38
    management 39–40
    signs and symptoms 37–8
occlusal appliances 35
older people, pain in. See geriatric pain
olecranon bursitis 83–6
Opioid Risk Tool (ORT) 363
opioids 360–7
    abuse 362
    addiction 362
    back pain 176
    burn pain 310
    cancer pain 356
    critical care pain 333
    geriatric pain 351
    migraine 5
    misuse 362, 365–7
    pediatric pain 341
    physical dependence 361
    postoperative pain 316
    risk management 362–5, 367
    tolerance 360

orofacial pain 32–6
osmophobia, in migraine 2
osteoarthritis 258–67
   clinical presentation 258–60
   differential diagnosis 262, 266
   distinguishing features 266
   follow-up 266
   hand 97
   imaging studies 262
   laboratory tests 261–2
   management 264–6
   prognosis 266
   signs and symptoms 259–61
osteopenia 277
OUCHER Scale 338
oxcarbazepine, in trigeminal neuralgia 30
oxycodone
   cancer pain 357
   pregnancy pain 321
oxygen therapy, in cluster headache 11
oxymorphone, in pregnancy pain 321

pain 308
pain diary 339
painful bladder syndrome 156
palliative care 355
   See also cancer pain
pancreatectomy 135
pancreatic duct stenting 135
pancreatic fibrosis 133
pancreatitis 131–6
   acute necrotizing 134
   causes 136
   clinical presentation 131
   differential diagnosis 133
   follow-up 135
   imaging studies 133
   laboratory tests 132–3
   management 134–5
   prognosis 136
   signs and symptoms 131
pancreatojejunostomy 135
paraffin bath 100
Parkinson's disease 298
paroxetine
   fibromyalgia pain syndrome 254
   irritable bowel syndrome 141, 143
pars interarticularis 168
Parsonage–Turner syndrome 59
patella reflex 219, 229, 234
patella tendinitis 234
patellofemoral joint 227

patient-controlled analgesia 311, 316
Patrick's test 169, 172, 186, 206–7
pectoral muscle strain 111
pediatric pain 337–46
   assessment 337–41, 345
   clinical presentation 337
   follow-up and prognosis 345
   management 341–5
pelvic pain 161–6
   clinical presentation 161–2
   differential diagnosis 163
   follow-up 165
   imaging studies 163–4
   laboratory tests 163
   management 164–5
   prognosis 166
   signs and symptoms 162–3
persistent idiopathic facial pain 32
pes anserine bursitis 227–8, 230–1
PET
   brachial plexopathy 60
   compression fractures 182
Phalen's test 103
phantom breast syndrome 121
phantom limb pain 303–6
   clinical presentation 303
   differential diagnosis 304
   follow-up and prognosis 306
   management 304–6
   signs and symptoms 303
phenytoin
   herpes zoster 271
   polyneuropathy 285
   trigeminal neuralgia 30
phonophobia
   migraine 2
   tension headache 14
photophobia 43
   migraine 2
   tension headache 14
physical dependence 361
physical therapy
   costosternal/costochondral/costovertebral
      syndromes 112
   elbow arthritis 86
   elbow nerve entrapment 96
piriformis sign 193
piriformis syndrome 192–5
   clinical presentation 192
   differential diagnosis 193
   follow-up 195
   imaging studies 193

management 194–5
prognosis 195
signs and symptoms 192–3
plasmapheresis, in HIV-related neuropathy 295
platelet-rich plasma (PRP) 91
pneumothorax 118
POEMS syndrome 282
Poker Chip scale 338
polymyalgia rheumatica 263
polyneuropathy 281–7
    clinical presentation 281–2
    differential diagnosis 285
    follow-up 286
    imaging studies 285
    laboratory tests 284
    management 285–6
    prognosis 287
    signs and symptoms 282–4
polysulfate sodium, in interstitial cystitis 158
positron emission tomography. See PET
posterior cruciate ligament injuries 233
posterior interosseus nerve compression 89
post-herpetic neuralgia 125, 268
    differential diagnosis 9
post-lumbar-puncture headache 23–6
    clinical presentation 23–4
    differential diagnosis 24
    follow-up and prognosis 26
    imaging studies 24
    laboratory tests 24
    management 25
    signs and symptoms 24
postoperative pain 314–18
    clinical presentation 314
    differential diagnosis 315
    follow-up 318
    imaging studies 315
    laboratory tests 315
    management 315–17
    prognosis 318
    signs and symptoms 314
post-thoracotomy pain syndrome 120–3
    clinical presentation 120
    differential diagnosis 121
    follow-up 123
    imaging studies 121
    laboratory tests 121
    management 122–3
    prognosis 123
    signs and symptoms 120
pramipexole, in fibromyalgia pain syndrome 254
precordial catch syndrome 112

prednisone
    cluster headache 10
    pregnancy pain 321
pregabalin
    central pain 299
    complex regional pain syndrome 278
    entrapment neuropathies 150
    fibromyalgia pain syndrome 254–5
    herpes zoster 271
    HIV-related neuropathy 294
    intercostal neuralgia 117
    lumbar radiculopathy 188
    meralgia paresthetica 224
    phantom limb pain 304
    polyneuropathy 285
pregnancy/lactation, pain in 319–24
    clinical presentation 319
    differential diagnosis 320
    follow-up 324
    imaging studies 320
    laboratory tests 320
    management 321–4
    prognosis 324
    signs and symptoms 319
    teratogens 321
prepatellar bursitis 227–8, 230–1
primary stabbing headache 19
proctalgia fugax 153
prolotherapy, in piriformis syndrome 194
pronator quadratus 104
propantheline, in irritable bowel syndrome 141
propofol, in critical care pain 334
propranolol, in migraine prevention 6
prostate-specific antigen (PSA) 181
proton pump inhibitors (PPIs) 180
proximal interphalangeal joints 97
proximal median nerve compression 104
pseudo-dementia 349
pseudogout 263
psoriatic arthritis 263
ptosis 9

Q angle 192

radial nerve
    compression 93–5
    decompression 96
    entrapment 92
radial tunnel syndrome 90
radiculopathies 73
radiofrequency ablation
    cancer pain 358

radiofrequency ablation (cont.)
  occipital neuralgia 40
  sacroiliac pain 209
radiofrequency neuroablation. *See* neuroablation
radiofrequency rhizotomy 301
radiography
  burn pain 309
  carpal tunnel syndrome 104
  complex regional pain syndrome 277
  costosternal/costochondral/costovertebral
    syndromes 109
  elbow arthritis 86
  groin pain 149
  hand and wrist arthritis 99
  intercostal neuralgia 116
  knee arthritis/bursitis 229
  lumbar post-laminectomy pain syndrome 212
  osteoarthritis 262
  pancreatitis 133
  post-thoracotomy pain syndrome 121
  shoulder bursitis/tendinitis 74
  thoracic spinal pain 126
radionuclide bone scanning. *See* scintigraphy
Ramsay Hunt syndrome 269
Ramsay sedation scale 333
range of motion
  hip 218
  knee 229
reactive arthritis 263
reflex sympathetic dystrophy 65
Reiter syndrome 108, 110
relaxation therapy, in cervicobrachial pain 57
rheumatism. *See* osteoarthritis, rheumatoid
    arthritis
rheumatoid arthritis 127, 258–9
  diagnostic criteria 266
  differential diagnosis 262, 266
  distinguishing features 266
  elbow 84
  follow-up 266
  imaging studies 262
  laboratory tests 261–2
  management 262–6
  prognosis 266
  signs and symptoms 259
rheumatoid factor 261
rhinorrhea 9
rhizotomy
  lumbar facet syndrome 203
  occipital neuralgia 40
rhomboid weakness 74
riboflavin, in migraine 6

ribs 107
  fracture 111, 121
  slipping 111
rifaximin, in irritable bowel syndrome 142
rituximab 264
rizatriptan 5
Roos stress test 64
rotator cuff 67, 69
  focal testing 74
rotator cuff tear 77–81
  clinical presentation 77
  differential diagnosis 78
  follow-up 80
  imaging studies 79
  laboratory tests 78
  management 79–80
  prognosis 81
  signs and symptoms 77–8
rotator cuff tendinitis 73
rumination 138

sacral nerve stimulation, in interstitial cystitis
    159
sacroiliac joints 204
sacroiliac pain 204–6
  differential diagnosis 208
  follow-up 209
  imaging studies 207
  laboratory tests 207
  management 208–9
  prognosis 210
  red flags 208
  signs and symptoms 206–7
salmon calcitonin, in compression fractures 182
schwannoma 39
sciatic nerve blockade 306
sciatica 192–5
  clinical presentation 192
  differential diagnosis 193
  follow-up 195
  imaging studies 193
  management 194–5
  prognosis 195
  signs and symptoms 192–3
scintigraphy
  complex regional pain syndrome 277
  costosternal/costochondral/costovertebral
    syndromes 109
  intercostal neuralgia 116
  post-thoracotomy pain syndrome 121
  thoracic spinal pain 126
scleroderma 263

scoliosis 32, 171, 175
Screener and Opioid Assessment for Patients
    with Pain (SOAPP) 363
selective estrogen receptor modulators.
    See SERMs
selective serotonin–norepinephrine reuptake
    inhibitors. See SNRIs
Semmes–Weinstein monofilament testing 284
septic arthritis 99
sergeant's patch 78
SERMs, in prevention of compression fractures
    182
serum amylase 132
shoulder arthritis 67–71
    clinical presentation 67
    follow-up and prognosis 71
    imaging studies 69
    laboratory tests 69
    management 70–1
    mimics 70
    physical examination 68–9
    signs and symptoms 68
shoulder bursitis/tendinitis 72–6
    clinical presentation 72
    differential diagnosis 74
    imaging studies 74
    laboratory tests 74
    management 75
    physical examination 73–4
    signs and symptoms 72–3
shoulder–hand syndrome. See complex regional
    pain syndrome
shoulder impingement 78
shoulder replacement 71
sickle cell disease 325–9
    clinical presentation 325
    differential diagnosis 327
    follow-up 329
    imaging studies 326
    laboratory tests 326
    management 327–9
    prognosis 329
    signs and symptoms 325–6
sickle cell trait 326
sigmoidoscopy, in irritable bowel syndrome
    139
single photon emission computed tomography.
    See SPECT
Sjögren's syndrome 263
smoke inhalation 308
SNRIs
    burn pain 310

cervical radiculopathy 48
fibromyalgia pain syndrome 255
herpes zoster 271
neck strain/sprain 43
polyneuropathy 285
post-thoracotomy pain syndrome 122
sickle cell disease 328
thoracic outlet syndrome 65
thoracic spinal pain 127
somatosensory evoked potentials
    brachial plexopathy 60
    thoracic outlet syndrome 64
spasmodic torticollis 55
spastic torticollis 55
SPECT, in compression fractures 182
spinal column 168
    anatomic landmarks 169
spinal cord injury 298
spinal cord stimulation 214, 300
    interstitial cystitis 159
spinal manipulation 177
spinal pain, thoracic. See thoracic spinal pain
splanchnicectomy 135
spondylolisthesis 52, 169, 213
spondylosis 52, 56, 169
sprains
    knee 232–7
    neck 41–5
Spurling's sign 43, 46, 64, 89, 103
steatorrhea 134, 140
stellate ganglion block 66, 123
sternalis syndrome 111
sternum fracture 111
straight leg raising test 193
stroke 297
    differential diagnosis 1
strontium ranelate, prevention of compression
    fractures 182
subacromial bursitis 72
subarachnoid hemorrhage
    differential diagnosis 9
subcostal nerve 114
subdeltoid bursitis 72
Sudeck's atrophy. See complex regional pain
    syndrome
sumatriptan
    cluster headache 11
    migraine 5
SUNCT syndrome 18–19
    management 21
superior labral anterior to posterior (SLAP)
    lesions 78

sympathetically maintained pain 275
syringomyelia 298
systemic lupus erythematosus 258, 263

tarsal bones 239
TART mnemonic 172
tegaserod, in irritable bowel syndrome 143
temporal (giant cell) arteritis 9
temporomandibular joint pain 32–6
    clinical presentation 32
    differential diagnosis 34
    follow-up 36
    imaging studies 33
    laboratory tests 33
    management 34–6
    prognosis 36
    signs and symptoms 32–3
tendinitis 52
    knee 232–7
    shoulder 72–6
tenesmus 153
tennis/golfer's elbow 88–91
    clinical presentation 88
    differential diagnosis 89
    laboratory tests and imaging studies 90
    management 90–1
    signs and symptoms 88–9
tenosynovitis 102
TENS
    brachial plexopathy 61
    cervical radiculopathy 48
    herpes zoster 272
    interstitial cystitis 159
    lumbar radiculopathy 189
    pediatric pain 343
    phantom limb pain 305
    polyneuropathy 286
    post-thoracotomy pain syndrome 122
    pregnancy pain 322
tension headache 4, 13–17
    chronic 18, 21
    clinical presentation 13
    differential diagnosis 14–15
    follow-up 17
    imaging studies 14
    laboratory tests 14
    management 15–17
    prognosis 17
    signs and symptoms 14
theophylline, post-lumbar-puncture headache
    25
thigh thrust test (posterior shear test) 207

thoracic nerve root block 117
thoracic outlet syndrome 52, 63–6, 104
    clinical presentation 63
    differential diagnosis 65
    follow-up 66
    imaging studies 64
    laboratory tests 64
    management 65
    prognosis 66
    signs and symptoms 63–4
thoracic radiculopathy 125
thoracic spinal nerves 114
thoracic spinal pain 125–9
    clinical presentation 331
    differential diagnosis 127
    follow-up 128
    imaging studies 126
    laboratory tests 126
    management 127–8
    prognosis 128
    signs and symptoms 125–6
thoracotomy, post-surgical pain 120–3
tic douloureux. See trigeminal neuralgia
Tietze's syndrome 108
timolol, in migraine prevention 6
Tinel's sign 98, 103, 148, 223
tizanidine
    central pain 299
    fibromyalgia pain syndrome 254
    myofascial pain syndrome 245
tolerance 360
topiramate
    chronic daily headache 21
    migraine prevention 6
    polyneuropathy 285
total pain 353
tramadol
    compression fractures 182
    costosternal/costochondral/costovertebral
        syndromes 110
    fibromyalgia pain syndrome 254
    intercostal neuralgia 116
    myofascial pain syndrome 245
    osteoarthritis 262
transcutaneous electrical nerve stimulation.
        See TENS
transverse carpal ligament 102
trapezius weakness 74
Trendelenburg gait 218–19
triceps weakness 103
tricyclic antidepressants
    burn pain 310

cervical radiculopathy 48
geriatric pain 351
herpes zoster 271
interstitial cystitis 158
irritable bowel syndrome 141, 143
lumbar radiculopathy 188
migraine prevention 6
occipital neuralgia 39
phantom limb pain 304
post-thoracotomy pain syndrome
        122
sickle cell disease 328
temporomandibular joint pain 34
tension headache 16
thoracic outlet syndrome 65
thoracic spinal pain 127
trigeminal neuralgia 27–32, 34
    clinical presentation 27–8
    differential diagnosis 9, 29
    follow-up and prognosis 31
    imaging studies 28–9
    laboratory tests 28
    management 29–31
    signs and symptoms 28
triptans 5
    post-lumbar-puncture headache 25
    See also individual drugs
trochanteric bursitis. See hip arthritis/bursitis

ulcerative colitis 263
    See also inflammatory bowel disease
ulnar entrapment neuropathy 64
ulnar nerve
    compression 92, 98
    entrapment 85, 92
    neuropathy 89, 93, 95
    palsy 84
ultrasound
    pancreatitis 133
    shoulder bursitis/tendinitis 75
urethral syndrome 157

valaciclovir, in herpes zoster 271
valgus deformity 228
valproic acid

cluster headache 10
    herpes zoster 271
varicella zoster virus. See herpes zoster
varus deformity 228
vaso-occlusive crisis 325, 327
venlafaxine
    fibromyalgia pain syndrome 254
    herpes zoster 271
ventilation/perfusion (V/Q) scanning 109
verapamil
    chronic daily headache 21
    cluster headache 10
    migraine prevention 6
verbal descriptor scale (VDS) 348
vertebrae
    compression fractures 180–4
    fractures 125
vertebral bodies 168
vertebral fractures 126
Visual Analog Scale (VAS) 339, 348
vitamin B_2, in tension headache 17

wallet neuritis 192
whiplash-associated disorders (WAD)
        41, 64
    See also neck strain/sprain
Williams flexion exercises 177
Wright (shoulder brace) position 63
wrist arthritis. See hand and wrist arthritis
wrist bracing 100

xiphisternal syndrome 111
x-rays. See radiography

Yeoman's test 186

ziconotide
    in cancer pain 358
    in complex regional pain syndrome 279
Zollinger–Ellison syndrome 134, 140
zolmitriptan 5
zoster sine exanthema 269–70
zoster sine herpete 269
zygapophyseal joint syndrome. See cervical facet
        syndrome